Helicobacter pioneers

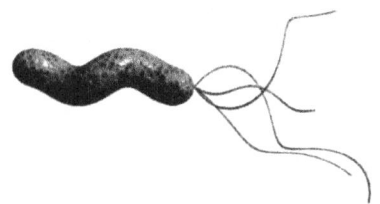

Helicobacter pioneers

Firsthand accounts from the scientists who discovered helicobacters, 1892–1982

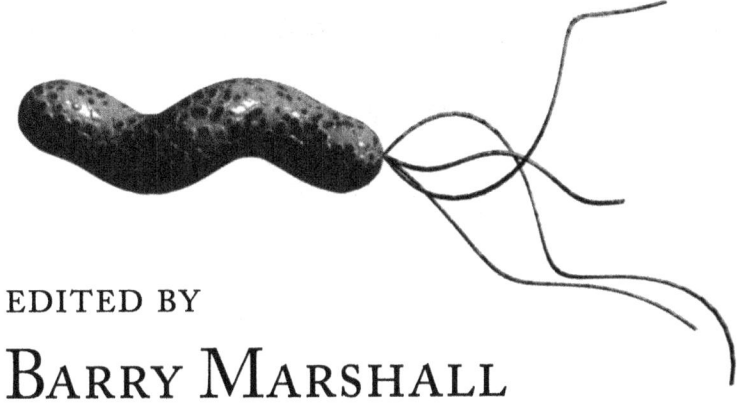

EDITED BY

BARRY MARSHALL

Professor of Microbiology
University of Western Australia

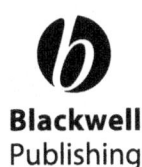

Blackwell
Publishing

© 2002 Blackwell Science Asia Pty Ltd

Published by Blackwell Science Asia Pty Ltd

First printed 2002

Editorial Offices
550 Swanston Street
Carlton South
Victoria 3053, Australia

Osney Mead,
Oxford OX2 0EL, UK

25 John Street,
London WC 1N 2BL, UK

23 Ainslie Place
Edinburgh EH3 6AJ, UK

350 Main Street, Malden
MA 02148-5018, USA

10, rue Casimir Delavigne
Paris 75006, France

Other Editorial Offices
Blackwell Publishing Wissenschafts-Verlag
GmbH, Kurfürstendamm 57
Berlin 10707, Germany

Iowa State University Press
A Blackwell Publishing Company
2121 S. State Avenue
Ames, Iowa 50014-8309, USA

Blackwell Publishing KK
MG-Kodenmacho Building, 3F
7–10 Kodenmacho, Nihombashi
Chuo-ku, Tokyo 103-0001, Japan

Designed and typeset by Lauren Statham, Alice Graphics

DISTRIBUTORS
Blackwell Publishing Asia Pty Ltd
550 University Street
Carlton South
Victoria 3053, Australia
Orders
Tel: +61 3 9347 0300
Fax: +61 3 9347 5001
info@blacksci-asia.com.au
www.blacksci-asia.com.au

North America
Blackwell Publishing
Commerce Place
350 Main Street, Malden
MA 02148-5018, USA
Orders
Tel: +1 617388 8250
        +1 800759 6102
Fax: +1 617388 8255

Canada
Copp Clark Professional
200 Adelaide Street West
3rd Floor,
Toronto, Ontario M5H 1W7
Orders
Tel: +1 416597 1616
        +1 800815 9417
Fax: +1 416597 1616

United Kingdom
Marston Book Services Ltd
PO Box 87
Oxford, OX2, 0DT, UK
Orders
Tel: +44 1865 791155
Fax: +44 1856 791927
Telex: 837515

Cover

Helicobacter pylori attached to a mucus-secreting epithelial cell taken from a biopsy of Susumu Ito's stomach. (First published in Heidel US, Code CF (eds). *Handbook of Physiology*. Section 6: *Alimentary Canal*, Vol. 2: *Secretion*. Washington DC: American Physiological Society, 1967.)

Cataloguing-in-Publication Data

Marshall, Barry J.

Helicobacter pioneers: firsthand accounts from the scientists who discovered helicobacters, 1892–1982.

Bibliography.

Includes index.

ISBN 0 86793 035 7.

1. Helicobacter. 2. Bacteriology—History. 3. Bacteriologists. I. Title.

579.32

Contents

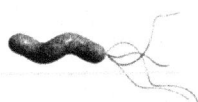

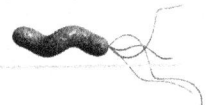

Foreword

'*Helicobacter* Pioneers' is the crowning achievement of a lifetime's work by Barry Marshall. The fascinating tale of Marshall and Warren's identification and elucidation of *Helicobacter pylori* and its role in the pathogenesis of peptic ulcer disease runs the gamut of Greek tragedy to Moliere farce and Hollywood drama. The protagonist is the shadowy and often sinister helicobacter organism, flagellating against the undulating backdrop (an outline of the stomach and duodenum) to the proscenium (iconic medical opinion). Against the swirling mists of time and (acid) tide can be seen the magic lantern figures of Bizzozero, Jaworski, Salomon, Edkins, Doenges, Freedberg, Palmer and a host of others as they evanescently enter and exit amidst the Nebel und Nacht of intellectual fashion. Their lines are faintly heard and then lost in the mêlée of dogma, doctrine and personal animus expressed by the audience (the medical majority). The looming figure of Warren (Lear-like in its majesty) stands stage left, almost silent and somewhat aloof, representing a belief in both a principle and a vision of a future as yet unacceptable to the proletariat (drug designers and prescribers). Amidst the clash of the dark armies of industry and academia (journal review and rebuttal), the brash young hero from a humble background strides to the front of the stage, but his unfettered, even arrogant, declamation of the truth is lost in the general outcry evoked by his novel assertions. Undaunted, even provoked, by the apparent rejection of his ideas, the hero pits himself against authority (editors and program chairpersons) and the guards (peer review and enshrined professorial deities). In an unfolding series of dramatic events, including arduous journeys (medical meetings), the proof of Koch's postulates and final acceptance, the populace slowly accept the dawning of a new day. From the background can be heard the slowly rising cadence of the chorus as the entrenched custodians of archaic thought join the rising tide of belief and seek to be the first to proclaim a new savior of the mucosa. An almost religious apotheosis of the organism is achieved in the minds of the converted (gastroenterologists of the acid religion) and the backdrop image changes to one of crusader-like intensity as the massed battalions of the corporations and their medical lieutenants sally forth to save the world from the organism now cast in the role of a Satan of the stomach. With a resurgent fanfare (thought leaders and trendsetters), both the specter of acid and the age-old traditions fade on the parchment of the past (the books of Bockus, Spiro, Sleisenger and Fordtran) as the new word of infective etiology is inscribed on the Mosaic tablets (acid suppressive medication) of gastrointestinal disease. In a dramatic coda to a long and arduous performance (All's Well that Ends Well) Barry Marshall and Robin Warren are both acclaimed heroes who have slain the dragon of a disease that was the scourge of almost every country and race on Earth.

This unusual and extraordinary book not only tells the story of Warren and Marshall's exquisite solution to the riddle of peptic ulcer disease, but also includes accounts by the individuals directly involved or of participants in the tale. Figura of Sienna documents the legendary contributions of Bizzozero of Italy, while Susumu Ito in Boston plumbs the depths of his own stomach to identify the organism. Freedberg attests to his early prescience in describing the organism, and Rigas documents in heartbreaking detail the contributions of John Lykoudis who in the late 1950s detailed (to the deaf ears of the world) a successful antibacterial therapy for ulcers. The Russian perspective is elegantly outlined by Morozov, while Sonnenberg, originally of Dusseldorf and Zurich, considers bacterial diseases from the perspective of a cohort phenomenon. Howard Steer describes the general medical skepticism that met his observations and with British reserve adumbrates those who assume the mantle of intellectual authority. Fukuda provides an interesting assessment of the history of *H. pylori*, in particular the Japanese contribution to the understanding of gastric bacteriology, noting the special contributions of Kasai and Kobayashi. O'Connor and O'Morain detail the Irish contribution and with Celtic grace harp the paean of Fitzgerald who proposed the importance of gastric ammonia in the pathophysiology of the stomach. Lieber, of the Mount Sinai School in New York, recounts the fascinating parable of antibiotic usage in uremic patients that led to the notion of gastric urease-producing organisms. Peterson and his colleagues in Dallas, Texas describe an epidemic of achlorhydria and reflect on their considerations as to a bacterial cause of this phenomenon. Similarly Lee of Sydney, Australia reminisces that a bacterium called 'Stubby' might indeed have been the Holy Grail sought by so many gastroenterologists and which even came so tantalizingly close to evading the outstretched hands of Marshall and Warren. Finally, Unge of Sweden interfaces the 19th and 20th century cultures of chemotherapy and microbiology so presciently defined by Pasteur, Bordet, Ehrlich and Koch.

Suffice it to say that this story is little less than a modern-day odyssey. The trials and tribulations of those who sailed the stormy waters of *H. pylori* research in the last century are beautifully detailed, with the sometime tragedy, heartbreak and even grandeur of their observations. The hurdles of fate, the petty animosities, the entrenched dogma of medical society and the prevailing winds of understanding all buffeted the lives of those who dedicated them-selves to the elucidation of gastric mucosal pathobiology. We learn that for many the journey itself was the pleasure and the destination a secondary con-sideration, but for others it was clearly much like the road to Thebes and their outcome no different to that of Beckett's 'Waiting for Godot'. Yet such is the chronicle of human experience and it is the duty of those who have under-taken such trials (prospective or retrospective) to record them so that others may learn from their experiences.

It is clear that Barry Marshall undertook a great journey and in so doing benefited all mankind. In its accomplishment he and Robin Warren have con-tributed to history and will live on in both the annals of medicine and the hearts of all those who practice the art of healing. This book, replete not only with facts, but also with poignant personal details of the human condition (From Malraux to Marshall), cannot fail to arouse admiration and a sense of the extraordinary personal and professional virtues of the many who con-tributed to the story. In the immortal words of Giorgios Seferiadis,

> *As pines keep the shape of the wind*
> *Even when the wind has fled and is no longer there*
> *So words*
> *Guard the shape of man*
> *Even when man has fled and is no longer there.*

Given the reflective nature of this book, which so beautifully describes not only the history of *H. pylori* research, but also the path to the future, one is almost obligated to close a commentary on such an extraordinary subject with the words of some previous great observers of the fields of human endeavor. The somewhat cynical assessment of Lucan might have been, 'Pigmei gigan-tum humeris impositi plusquam ipsi gigantes vident' [Pygmies, by standing on the shoulders of giants who have gone before, are enabled to see further], but probably even more appropriate to the final discovery of *H. pylori* are the immortal words of Julius Caesar, 'Veni, vidi, vici!' In the contemporary context this may be broadly interpreted as 'These intrepid physicians *came* to Perth, they *saw* the bacteria, and they set in motion a train of events that *conquered* it!'

In identifying the agent, defining the disease process and initiating the cure, Barry Marshall and Robin Warren in far-off Perth together crossed a distant Rubicon and forever changed the concepts of acid peptic ulcer disease and altered the die (Iacta alia est) of destiny. One can only hope that, like me, future generations of young physicians will read this chronicle of those events and not only learn from them, but be forever inspired.

Professor Irvin M Modlin
Yale School of Medicine, New Haven, Connecticut, USA

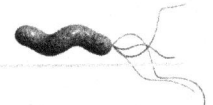

Preface

THE SEEDS FOR THIS BOOK were sown back in 1981 when Robin Warren and I first became aware of previous descriptions of gastric spiral bacteria, most notably, the image of Susumu Ito's own stomach biopsy, which adorns the cover. I wondered then who Susumu was, and who else had described these organisms. Then in 1983, like the re-opening of a time capsule, our initial report triggered a letter from Stone Freedberg, thanking us for acknowledging his publication of 1940. In the years since then, colleagues all over the world have added their friends, countrymen and mentors to my list of 'helicobacter pioneers', each with a unique story to tell and a fair claim to a part in the helicobacter discovery. When I visited Ireland in 1989 and obtained a copy of Oliver Fitzgerald's thesis from his widow, I realised that time was running out if I was to obtain the accounts of these pioneers. After that I began to correspond with and meet with them whenever possible. I finally met Stone Freedberg in Boston in 1995, and this year I discovered that Stone, now well into his nineties, is the personal physician to the much younger (82) Susumu Ito!

As the chapters arrived I was pleased to see that many were written by colleagues who had actually taken part in the studies, or who had firsthand knowledge of the pioneer. Some of the accounts literally brought tears to my eyes as I recognized a familiar pattern of medical conservatism, lack of resources, or merely making an important discovery in the wrong place at the wrong time.

As you will see, this book is not meant to be a textbook, but rather provides background and the human touch to a discovery process that took almost a century. I have no doubt that it will spark many more descriptions of important helicobacter pioneers and I hope those of you who know of such material will send it to me because if the new material warrants it, a second, expanded edition will likely be produced.

A volume as specialized as 'Helicobacter pioneers' cannot be expected to generate massive sales, so I am grateful to Janssen-Cilag and Eisai for sponsoring the first print run of the book. Unlike other books on H. pylori, 'Helicobacter pioneers' will never go out of date because it contains several original accounts that can never be embellished or duplicated. Thus, I expect to see it in medical history archives when I am Stone Freedberg's age (i.e. in 2045). Nevertheless, in order to also have some contemporary utility for readers, Peter Unge has written a special final chapter on past and current H. pylori therapy in which he refers also to Xiao's chapter where there are details of therapies that are useful in developing countries, or in penicillin allergic and difficult-to-cure patients.

I wish to express my gratitude to my long-suffering partner, Adrienne, for nourishing my H. pylori activities over many years and for adding her personal touch to my chapter. Thanks to Robin Warren and his late wife Win for their friendship and support since 1981, and thanks also to Professor Adrian Lee of the University of New South Wales for his friendship since 1983 and his encouragement of this endeavor. Finally, thanks to Susan Morrow, Debbie Smetherham and Helen Windsor for their editorial assistance, and to Chris Hum of Blackwell Science Asia for his enthusiastic support of the project.

The Helicobacter logo used on each new chapter is an original computer-aided design from Luke Marshall from whom high-resolution images can be obtained be sending an email to lmarshall@geniusswitch.com

Barry Marshall
30 September 2001

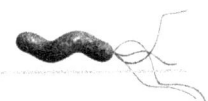

List of Contributors

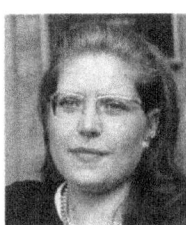

Laura Bianciardi, MD

Library of Medicine,
University of Siena, Italy

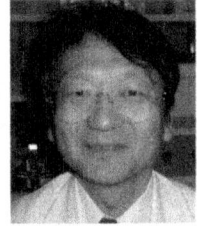

Yoshihiro Fukuda,
MD, PhD

Assistant Professor
Gastroenterology,
Hyogo College of
Medicine, Nishinomiya,
Hyogo, Japan

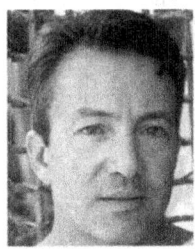

Natale Figura, MD

Institute of Internal
Medicine, University of
Siena, Italy

William Harford, MD

Professor of Internal Medicine, University of
Texas Southwestern Medical Center at Dallas
Staff Physician, Dallas Department of
Veterans Affairs Medical Center, Dallas,
Texas, USA

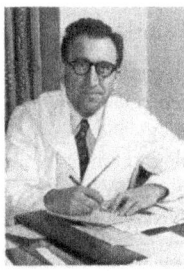

A. Stone Freedberg,
MD

Professor of Medicine
Emeritus, Harvard
Medical School
Physician to the
University Health
Service, Harvard
University
Honorary Consultant in
Medicine, Beth Israel
Hospital, Boston,
Massachusetts, USA

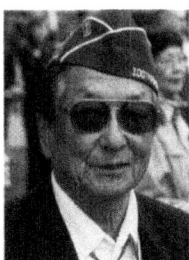

Susumu Ito, MD

James Stillman Professor
of Comparative
Anatomy
Emeritus Professor, Cell
Biology Department,
Harvard Medical
School, Boston,
Massachusetts, USA

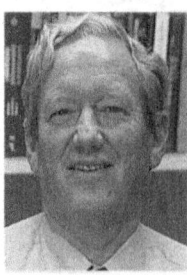

Adrian Lee, PhD

Professor of Medical
Microbiology, Pro-Vice
Chancellor (Education),
University of New
South Wales, Sydney,
NSW, Australia

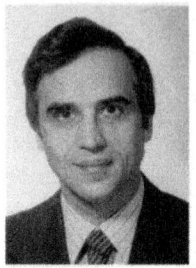

Charles S. Lieber,
MD, MACP

Professor of Medicine
and Pathology, Mount
Sinai School of
Medicine
Director, Alcohol
Research and Treatment
Center, Bronx VA
Medical Center, New
York, USA

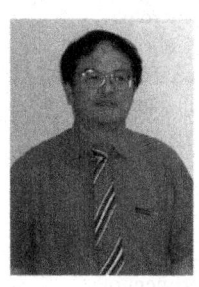

Wen-Zhong Liu, MD

Professor of Medicine,
Shanghai Second
Medical University
Vice Director, Shanghai
Institute of Digestive
Disease
Director, Division of
Gastroenterology, Renji
Hospital, Shanghai,
China

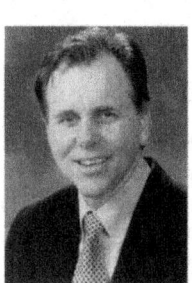

Barry J. Marshall,
FRACP, FAA, FRS

Clinical Professor of
Microbiology,
University of Western
Australia, Perth, WA,
Australia

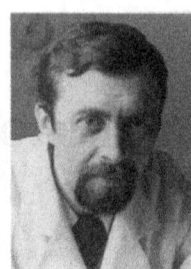

Igor A. Morozov,
MD, PhD, DSci

Professor, Central
Institute of
Gastroenterology,
Department of Clinical
and Experimental
Pathology
Honorary President,
Russian *Helicobacter
pylori* Study Group,
Moscow, Russian
Federation

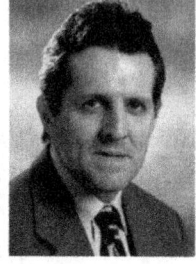

**Humphrey J.
O'Connor,** MD, FRCPI

Consultant
Gastroenterologist,
Department of
Gastroenterology,
Adelaide/Meath
Hospital, Dublin,
Ireland

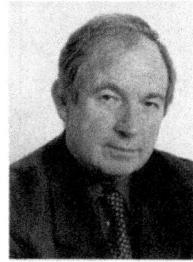

Colm A. O'Morain,
MD, MSc, DSc, FRCP,
FRCPI, FEBG, FACG

Consultant
Gastroenterologist,
Professor and Academic
Head, Department of
Medicine,
Adelaide/Meath
Hospital, Dublin,
Ireland

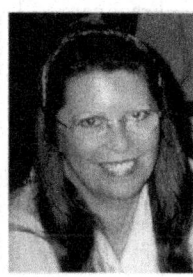

Jani O'Rourke, BSc

Senior Research
Scientist, School of
Microbiology and
Immunology, University
of New South Wales,
Sydney, NSW, Australia

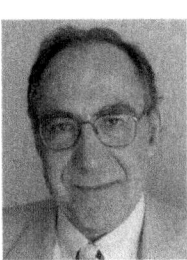

Efstathios D. Papavassiliou

Amalia Fleming Hospital, Athens, Greece

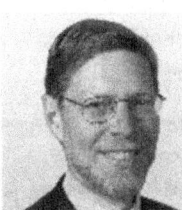

Walter L. Peterson, MD

Professor of Internal Medicine, University of Texas Southwestern Medical Center at Dallas Staff Physician, Dallas Department of Veterans Affairs Medical Center, Dallas, Texas, USA

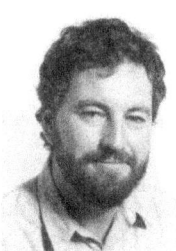

Michael Phillips, PhD

Ian Clunies Ross Laboratory, CSIRO Livestock Industries, Prospect, NSW, Australia

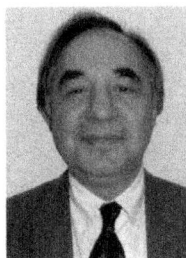

Basil Rigas

Sarah C Upham Division of Gastroenterology, New York Medical College, New York, USA

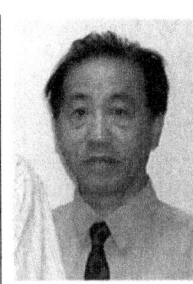

Yao Shi, MD

Professor of Pathology, Shanghai Second Medical University, Renji Hospital Chief, Department of Pathology, Shanghai Institute of Digestive Disease, Shanghai, China

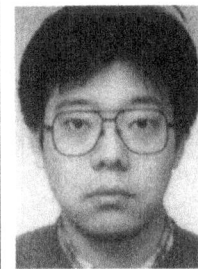

Tadashi Shimoyama, MD, PhD

Lecturer, First Department of Internal Medicine, Hirosaki University School of Medicine, Hirosaki, Aomori, Japan

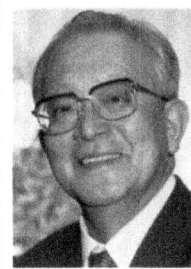

Takashi Shimoyama, MD, PhD

Director, Hyogo College of Medicine Professor of Medicine, Gastroenterology, Hyogo College of Medicine, Nishinomiya, Hyogo, Japan

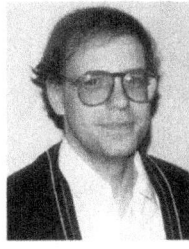

Amnon Sonnenberg, MD, MSc

Staff Physician, New Mexico Veterans Affairs Health Care System Professor of Medicine, Department of Medicine, University of New Mexico, Albuquerque, New Mexico, USA

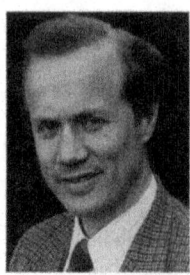

Howard W. Steer,
MA, BSc (Hons), PhD,
MBBS (Hons), FRCS

Consultant Surgeon,
Southampton General
Hospital, Southampton,
United Kingdom

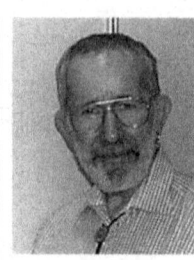

J. Robin Warren, MD,
FRCPA

Emeritus Consultant
Pathologist, Royal Perth
Hospital, Perth, WA,
Australia

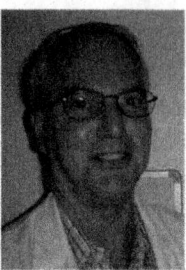

Peter Unge, MD

Senior Consultant,
Länssjukhuset Gävle
Sandviken,
Gävle sjukhus, Sweden

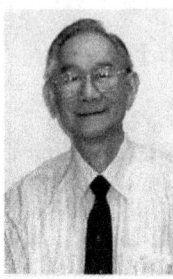

Shu-Dong Xiao, MD

Professor of Medicine,
Shanghai Second
Medical University,
Renji Hospital
Honorary Director,
Shanghai Institute of
Digestive Disease
President, Chinese
Society of
Gastroenterology
Editor-in-Chief, *Chinese
Journal of Digestive
Diseases*

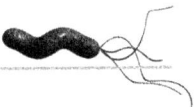

Acknowledgments

Natale Figura and Laura Bianciardi thank Professor Irvin M. Modlin, Yale School of Medicine, New Haven, Connecticut, USA, for permission to reproduce Figure 6, and Ms Chiara Bratto and the staff of the Accademia dei Fisiocritici Library for their help in the bibliography research.

Humphrey J. O'Connor and Colm A. O'Morain sincerely thank Dr Oliver Fitzgerald, son of Professor Oliver Fitzgerald and Consultant Rheumatologist at St Vincent's University Hospital Dublin, for his great help in providing reprints of his father's publications and the charming photograph, and Mrs Iris Martin for preparing the manuscript.

Amnon Sonnenberg was supported by a grant from the Centers for Disease Control and Prevention, Atlanta, Georgia, USA.

Basil Rigas and Efstathios Papavassiliou thank Evanthea and Nicholas Lykoudis, the widow and son, respectively, of John Lykoudis, for making accessible his archives and for sharing their recollections of his life and work on peptic ulcer disease. Thanks also to Mr Nicholas A. Rigas and Fr Ignatius Stavropoulos for providing information and photographs.

Walter L. Peterson and William Harford acknowledge the input of Cora Barnett and Drs John S. Fordtran, Charles T. Richardson, Edward J. Ramsey and Jerry Trier.

Professor Barry Marshall is supported by the Australian National Health and Medical Research Council (NHMRC) Burnet Fellowship.

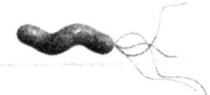

CHAPTER I

Helicobacters were discovered in Italy in 1892

An episode in the scientific life of an eclectic pathologist, Giulio Bizzozero

Natale Figura and Laura Bianciardi

Helicobacters come to light

... Ancora più curiosi sono degli spirilli che ho trovato costanti nello stomaco del cane e che, oltre all'essere numerosi nello strato di muco che riveste la mucosa, penetrano nel lume delle ghiandole tanto del piloro quanto del fondo ed arrivano talora fino al fondo del cieco terminale ...[1]

[... Even more exciting are certain spirilli I found constantly in the dog's stomach and that, in addition to being numerous in the mucus layer that covers the mucosa, penetrate into the gland lumen of both pylorus and fundus, and sometimes reach the bottom of glands ...]

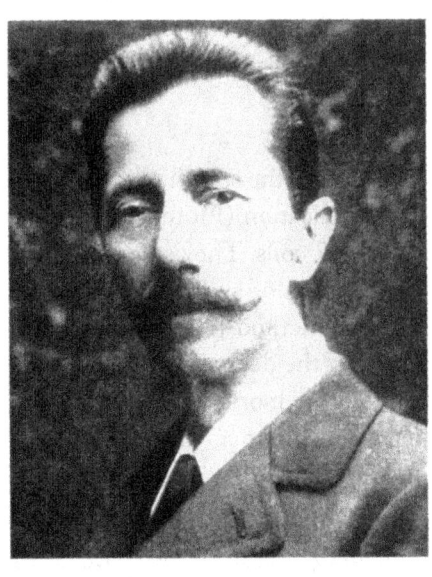

FIGURE I Giulio Bizzozero at age 35 years (*c.*1881).

With these words, more than one century ago, the Italian pathologist Giulio Bizzozero (FIGURE I) described for the first time the presence of helicobacters in the stomach of mammals (dogs) (FIGURE 2). Bizzozero presented his observations in an appendix (FIGURE 3) to the main publication that concerned the tubular glands of the gastroenteric tract and their relationship with the mucosal epithelial layer.[1] Bizzozero communicated his discovery during a meeting of the Turin Medical Academy on the 18th of March 1892. The

Sulle ghiandole tubulari del tubo gastro-enterico e sui rapporti del loro epitelio coll'epitelio di rivestimento della mucosa;

Nota settima del Socio GIULIO BIZZOZERO
(Con 1 Tavola).

FIGURE 2 Original title of the publication (1892).

APPENDICE

Sulla presenza di batteri nelle ghiandole rettali, e nelle ghiandole gastriche del cane.

FIGURE 3 Original title of the appendix.

description of the spirilli was accompanied by numerous illustrations, included in the publication (FIGURE 4): ... such spirilli are tiny, 3–8 μ [μm] long, and possess 3–7 coils. They stain intensely with fuchsin or safranin dissolved in a water solution of aniline followed by washing in alcohol. They de-stain with the Gram method [i.e. they were Gram negative]. They are usually in small number in the deepest parts of the gland: in the superficial parts, on the contrary, they are more abundant, so that, sometimes, disposed close or in succession to one another, they form a kind of bundle that lies in the axis of the gland lumen ...[1]

> Anche nelle ghiandole del fondo dello stomaco, che pure hanno lume così stretto, gli spirilli possono talvolta arrivare fino al fondo cieco della ghiandola ...[1]

> [Spirilli can get to the base of the fundic glands even though their lumen is so narrow. Such findings however, do not occur in all animals. Two in six dogs had spirilli down to the gland base, while four of the dogs had the spirilli confined to the superficial half or one-third of the glandular lumen. Even more interesting is the relationship between the spirilli and the cellular lining, in particular with the cells of the glandular neck. In all of the six dog stomachs that I have examined, a great number of the glandular neck cells contained 1–4 and even more spirilli in their protoplasm (figure 4 dell'annessa tavola) ...] (FIGURE 5).

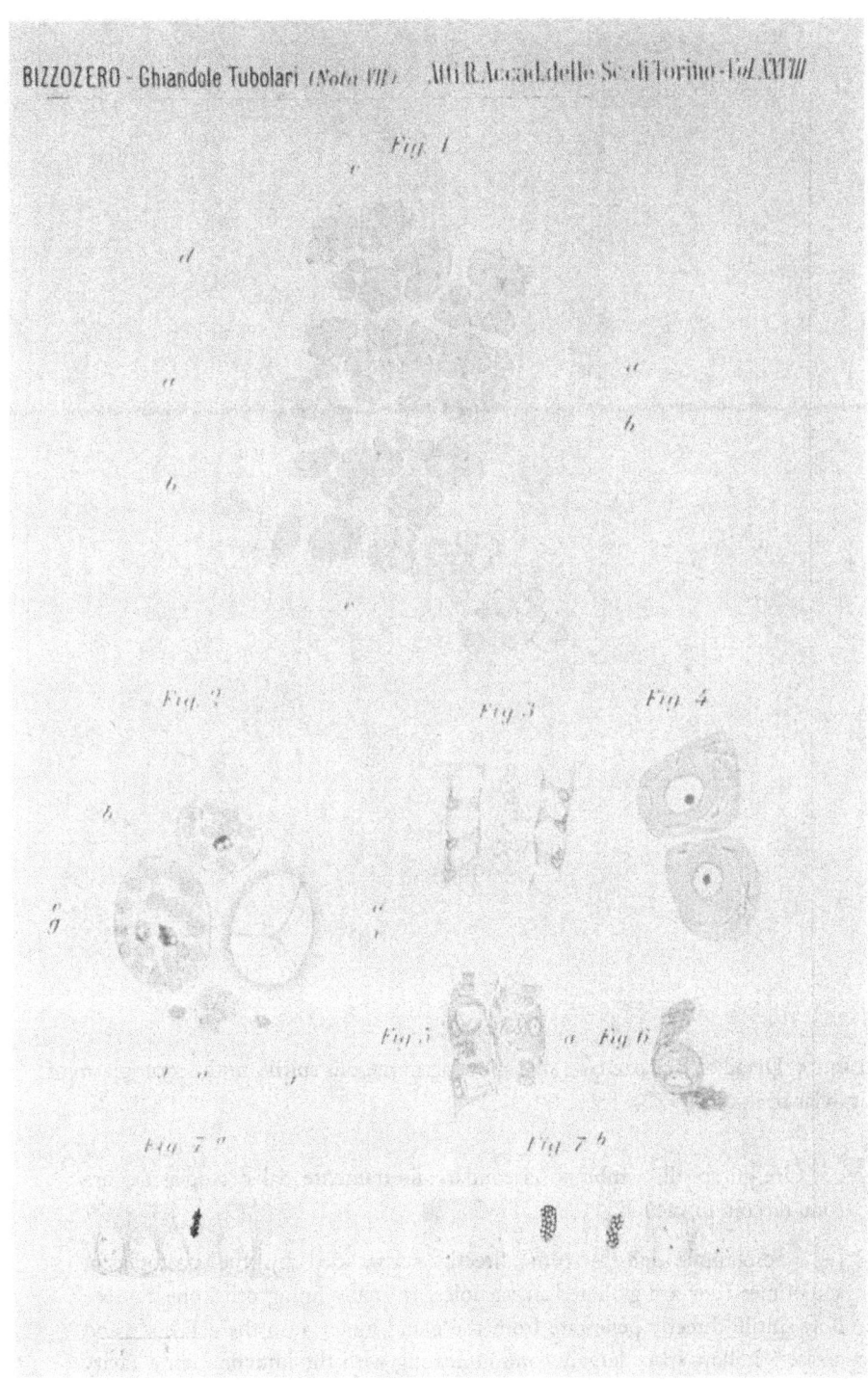

FIGURE 4 'Tavola' [Table] of Bizzozero's drawings of the dog gastric spirilli, showing their relationship with the glandular cells and gastric lumen.

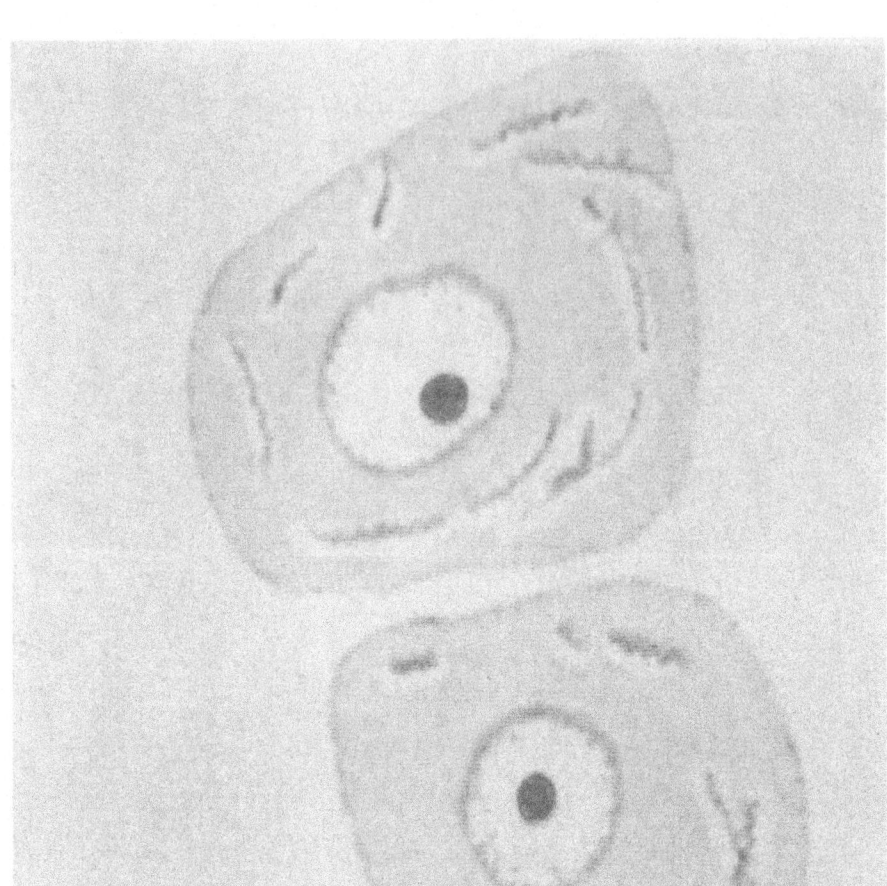

FIGURE 5 Detail of Bizzozero's Table showing numerous spirilli in the protoplasm of glandular neck cells (≈×3).

... Ora gli spirilli sembrano circondati direttamente dal protoplasma, ora sono raccolti in vacuoli . . .[1]

[... Sometimes spirilli seem directly surrounded by the protoplasm, sometimes they are gathered in vacuoles. In many lining cells, one can see how spirilli directly penetrate from the gland lumen into the cell body and create a hollow space largely communicating with the lumen. Such a cavity can be so large that the nucleus is pushed and compressed to the base of the gland, and the protoplasm does not represent more than a subtle marginal layer (figure 5) . . .][1] (FIGURE 6).

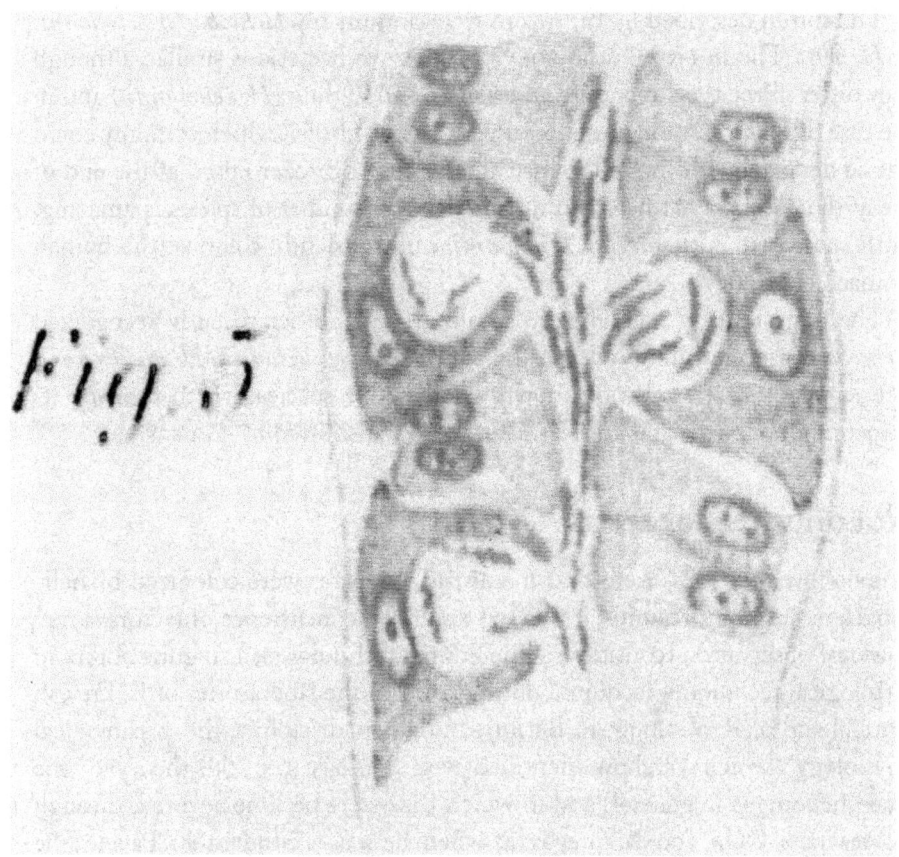

FIGURE 6 Detail of Bizzozero's drawing, showing spirilli free in the gastric gland lumen and gathered in vacuoles (≈×3).

It is not known whether Bizzozero realised that these spiral bacteria were not simply saprophytes. They particularly intrigued him because there was only one other description in the scientific literature at that time of the presence of bacteria ['*in elementi viventi*'] in cells of completely healthy animals.

> . . . Il primo venne scoperto contemporaneamente da me e da Ribbert, e riguarda la presenza normale di bacilli nelle cellule dei follicoli linfatici dell'intestino di coniglio . . .[1]

> [. . . The first example of this was revealed simultaneously by Ribbert and by me, and concerned the presence of bacilli in the lymphatic follicles of the healthy rabbit's intestine. Beyond the diverse bacterial species, however, there is a difference between the two cases: in the rabbit, bacilli stay in elements of mesodermic origin, which had probably phagocytosed them, while in dogs the spirilli reside in cells of endodermic origin which they had probably actively penetrated.]

The spirilli described by Bizzozero were presumably *Helicobacter heilmannii* or *H. felis*.[2] The *in vivo* morphology of these two bacteria is similar, although they differ in the type of coils (slender in *H. felis*, tight in *H. heilmannii*) and in the case of *H. felis*, in the presence of periplasmic fibrils,[2] which certainly could not be detected with the rough instruments that Bizzozero used at the end of the 19th century. That he could distinguish the number of spirals is amazing. Both species, in particular *H. heilmannii*, can transiently colonize the human stomach (FIGURE 7).

The dog stomach may also be colonized by another recently recognized *Helicobacter* species, morphologically similar to *H. heilmannii*: *H. bizzozeronii* (see Appendix 2).[2,3] It is not known whether this species, which received its name in honor of the Italian scientist, can be transmitted to humans.

Not only helicobacters

The discovery by Bizzozero that mammals' stomachs were colonized by helicobacters was not fortuitous; it was the result of a concurrence of factors: a rare power of observation (considering the limited technology), a singular ability in histological techniques (acquired during stints in the laboratories of E. Frey, in Zurich, and of R. Virchow, in Berlin), and a new discipline, the 'pathological physiology', which Virchow identified with 'biology' (i.e. the theory of the vital phenomena in general) and to which Bizzozera became devoted, through his teachers Oehl and Mantegazza, when he was a student in Pavia. The summa of the different determinants of Bizzozero's skilfulness was encompassed in his *Manuale di Microscopia Clinica* [Handbook of Clinical Microscopy], published in 1879 and translated into French, English and Russian. Through this handbook, Bizzozero hoped to promote the use of the microscope as a diagnostic instrument amongst physicians: it included a description of the microscope with instructions on its use, and various chapters dedicated to pathogenic bacteria and the examination of all the bodily fluids.

The discovery that dogs' stomachs can be colonized by spiral organisms, whose morphology confirms their identification with helicobacters, was a consequence of Bizzozero's interest in that organ. His profound knowledge of histological and microscopic techniques enabled him to differentiate the parietal cells from the chief cells, and to perceive that the neck cells generate both chief cells and surface epithelial cells. Bizzozero involved his favorite disciple, Camillo Golgi (best known for his discovery of the internal reticular apparatus of cells, called Golgi's apparatus), in his interest in the gastric glands. The collaboration was fruitful and lead to the understanding of the acid secretory function of gastric parietal cells and the morphological relationship of the gastric glands with the luminal channel (FIGURE 8).

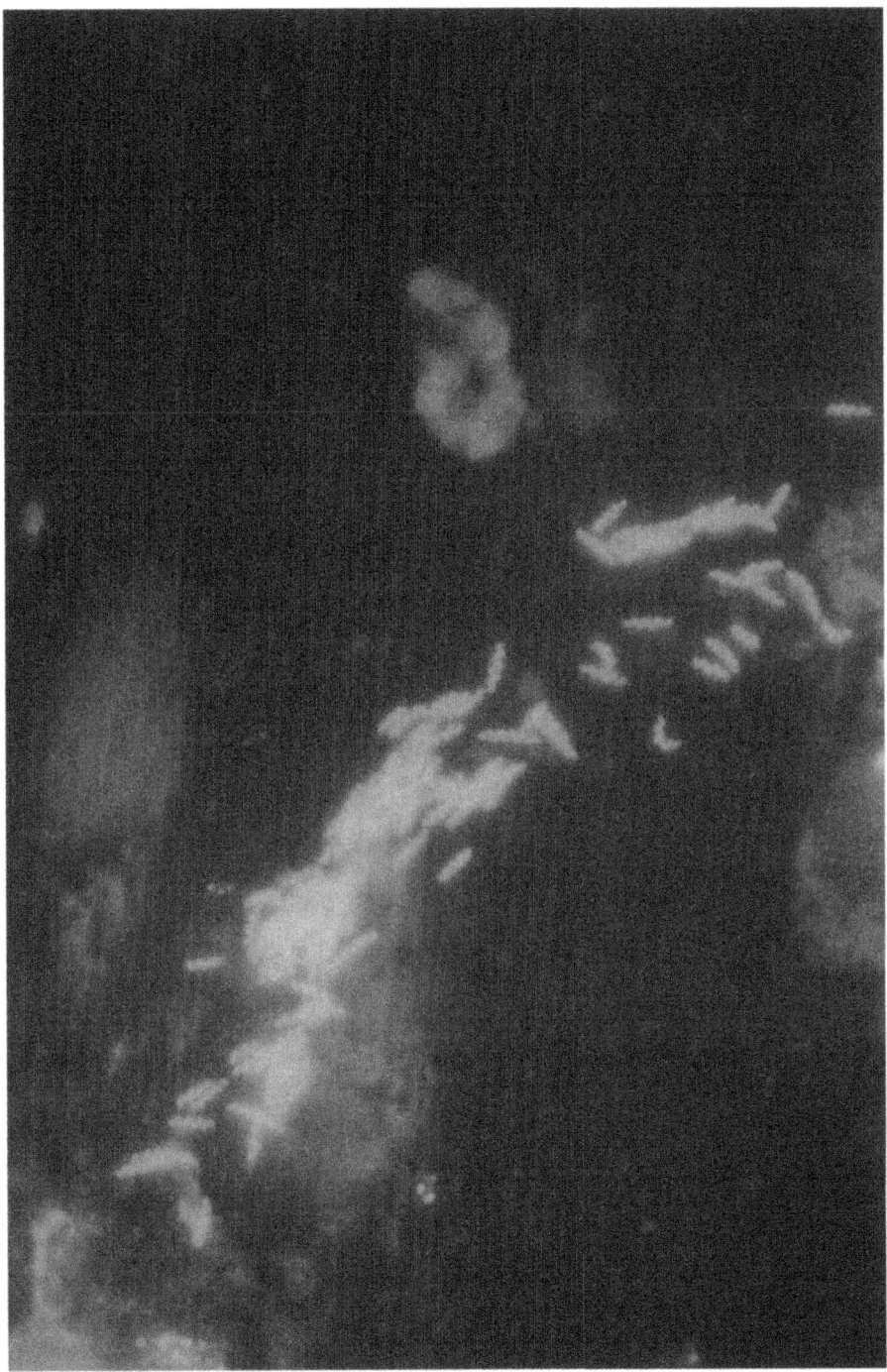

FIGURE 7 Bacteria resembling *Helicobacter heilmannii* in the stomach of a patient with dyspepsia (acridine orange; ×1000).

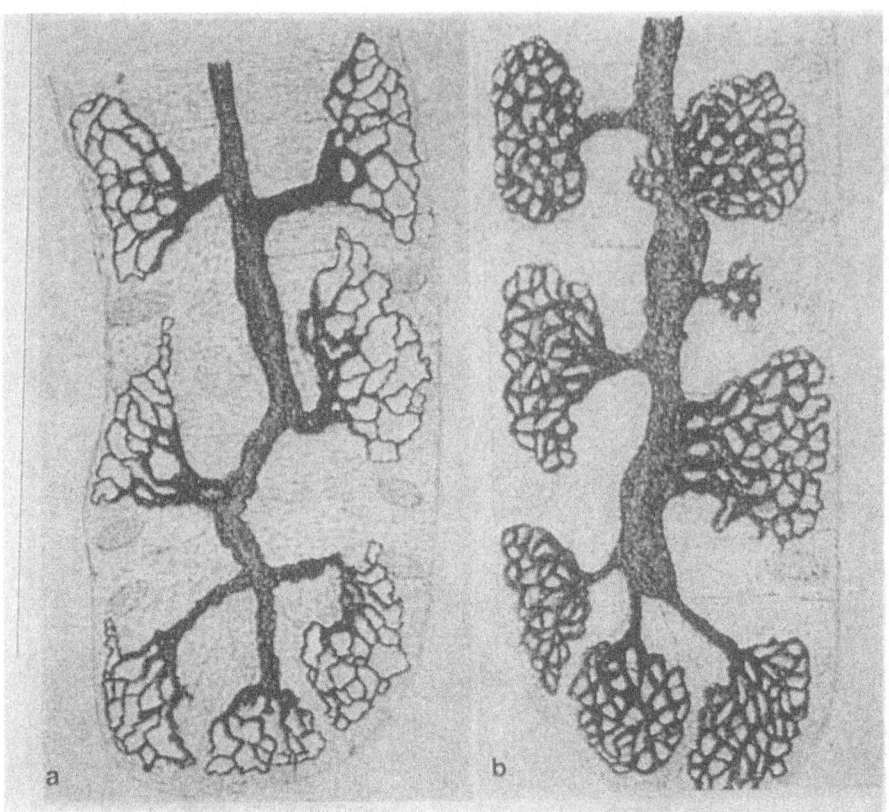

FIGURE 8 Reproduction of Golgi's original camera lucida drawing showing the expansion of the secretory canaliculi of parietal cells when they are stimulated. (a) Resting gastric glands, (b) secreting gastric glands. (Reproduced with the permission of Professor Irvin M. Modlin, Yale School of Medicine, New Haven, Connecticut, USA.)

Bizzozero was interested in many fields of medicine. The study of blood cells and the mechanism of coagulation were two contributions that have earned him a place in the history of medicine. His first original observations on bone marrow date back to the time when, as a student, he attended Mantegazza's laboratory at the Institute of General Pathology. In 1868–1869, he published a series of observations on the hematopoietic function of the bone marrow: 'Sulla funzione ematopoietica del midollo delle ossa. Due comunicazioni preventive sul midollo delle ossa', in which he confirmed the conjecture that bone marrow had a strong influence on hematopoiesis, described the different medullar elements and confuted the presumed metaplasia of white blood cells into red blood cells. He also started a systematic examination of bone marrow disorders.

In 1879, Bizzozero invented the chromocytometer, which is still used in clinical practice. In 1883–1884, he published his fundamental notes on 'le piastrine', the platelets: 'Di un nuovo elemento morfologico del sangue e della sua importanza nella trombosi'; 'Die Blutplaettchen im peptonisirtes Blute'; 'Sul terzo elemento morfologico del sangue'; 'Sulla preesistenza delle piastrine nel sangue normale dei mammiferi'. Fundamental to his discovery of platelets was a new type of experiment that he conceived: the study of the bloodstream in live animals. The microscopic observation of rabbit and Chinese hamster mesentery enabled him to claim that a third hematic morphological element circulated with the red and white blood cells.

> Esso è rappresentato da piastrine [platelets] pallidissime a forma di disco a superficie paralele, o, più di rado, di lente ovali o rotonde; di diametro uguale ad un terzo o alla metà di quello dei globuli rossi . . .

> [The third element is represented by platelets, very pale and disk-shaped . . . As a rule, they are separated from one another; however, this does not mean that they are never assembled in groups. Nonetheless, such phenomenon is already a sign of their alteration . . .]

His profound knowledge of histology made it possible for him to formulate, in 1887, a classification of tissues into labile, stable and perennial elements: 'labile cells have a short life, because, after they differentiate, they degenerate and die. The stable cells last for a lifetime and in certain cases can differentiate and multiply. Perennial cells, such as muscle and nervous tissues, last forever and never multiply.' This classification constituted the basis for the study of embryology and histology.

Bizzozero has also left his mark in the field of nephrology. In 1896 in Turin, C. Sacerdotti, another of his disciples, published his hypothesis of compensatory renal hypertrophy of the kidney after uninephrectomy. He postulated the existence of mediators released by the kidney, based on the observation that several mitoses occur in the renal epithelium (an expression of renal hypertrophy) when the kidneys of a normal dog received blood transfusions from uninephrectomized dogs (reported by Schena et al.[4]). Sacerdotti's observation was confirmed years later, and the mediators of which he predicted the existence belong to the family of proliferative peptides, which includes different growth factors.

Studies in the infective origin of tuberculosis (soon afterwards demonstrated by Koch in 1882), some aspects of inflammatory reactions and a description of the phagocytosis process (later demonstrated by Metchnikoff), have rewarded Bizzozero with the title of the father of Italian histology and recognition as one of the most important forerunners of preventive medicine.

Biography of Giulio Bizzozero

Giulio Bizzozero was born in Varese on the 20th of March 1846. The family name most probably derives from 'Bizzozzero', a locality close to Varese. He completed classical studies in Milan and attended the University of Pavia. In 1862, at the age of 16, as a student at the Institute of Experimental Physiology of E. Oehl, he completed his first work on microscopic anatomy and published a paper on the distribution of blood vessels. While he was a student at the Institute of General Pathology, he published many experimental works concerning normal and pathologic histology. In 1866, at the age of 20, he graduated in Medicine and earned the Matteucci award for passing all his exams with full marks.

Bizzozero was a leading spirit in scientific and social circles; his social and political commitments prompted him to support Garibaldi, the leader of the Italian war of independence. In 1867, he returned to Pavia where at the age of 21, in spite of the hostility of his colleagues for his extreme youth, and thanks to the intercession of the Minister of Education, the University of Pavia selected him for the position of Chief of General Pathology and Histology.

In Pavia, he dealt with subjects of normal and pathologic histology and furthered his education by spending time in the laboratories of the most important pathologists and histologists of the time: E. Frey in Zurich, where he became familiar with the histological techniques that he reported in his Manual; and R. Virchow in Berlin, where he studied Pathological Anatomy and Histology (a novel discipline in Germany), to whose principles he was introduced by E. Oehl, P. Mantegazza, A. Cantani, S. Tommasi and J. Moleschott.

In 1873, at the age of 27, he was elected to the Chair of General Pathology at the University of Turin, where he founded the Institute of General Pathology. His laboratory became a breeding ground for young scientists, and some of the greatest researchers in Italian medicine (e.g. C. Golgi (Nobel Prize for Medicine in 1906), P. Foà, E. Bassini etc.) collaborated with him.

At that time, he started a new interpretation of general pathology and inspired a new course of study based on a biological approach. He also devoted himself to publishing activity: the *Giornale di Scienze Fisiche e Naturali* [*The Journal of Physical and Natural Sciences*] and the *Archivio Italiano per le Scienze Mediche* [*The Italian Archives for Medical Sciences*], with two sections, *Rivista Bibliografica Italiana* and *Nuove Pubblicazioni*, which was recognized abroad as the authority on Italian experimental medicine. Bizzozero also implemented many civic initiatives in Turin, such as establishing the Laboratory of Hygiene and the hospital 'Amedeo d'Aosta', and modernizing the water supply and drainage system.

From 1884 onward, Bizzozero was the Director of the Veterinary High School of Turin, and in 1886, at the age of 40, he was made Chancellor of the University of Turin. From 1887, he was a member of the Italian Superior Council of Health, in 1888 he became a member of the Academy of Sciences of Berlin and in 1890 he was a senator of the Kingdom of Italy. In 1897, together with L. Pagliani, he took over the editorship of the *Rivista d'Igiene e Sanità Pubblica* [*Hygiene and Public Health Magazine*].

In the last years of his life, a serious bout of choroiditis obliged Bizzozero to give up any microscope research activity, but did not prevent him from taking part in the debate on public health problems, to which he had already contributed in 1879 with the work *Sui Provvedimenti Contro la Trichina* [*Measures against Trichinosis*].

He died in April 1901, at the age of 55, from acute bronchopneumonia.

References

1 Bizzozero G. Sulle ghiandole tubulari del tubo gastro-enterico e sui rapporti del loro epitelio coll'epitelio di rivestimento della mucosa. *Atti della Reale Accademia delle Scienze di Torino* 1892; **28**: 233–51.
2 Hänninen M-L, Happonen I, Saari S, Jalava K. Culture and characteristics of *Helicobacter bizzozeronii*, a new canine gastric *Helicobacter* sp. *Int J Syst Bacteriol* 1966; **46**: 160–6.
3 Fox JG, Lee A. The role of *Helicobacter* species in newly recognized gastrointestinal tract diseases in animals. *Lab Anim Sci* 1997; **47**: 222–55.
4 Schena FP, Strippoli GF, Wankelmuth P. Renal growth factors: past, present and future. *Am J Nephrol* 1999; **19**: 308–12.
5 MacAdoo TO. Proposed revision of Appendix 9, Ortography, of the International Code of Nomenclature of bacteria. *Int J Syst Bacteriol* 1990; **40**: 103–4.
6 Calonghi F. *Dizionario della Lingua Latina*, 3rd edn. Torino: Rosenberg & Sellier, 1960.

Appendix 1

Bibliography

Anonymous. A new part of blood: Giulio Bizzozero's 75th day of death. *Med Klin* 1976; **71**: 1344–5.

Bizzozero G. *Discorsi pronunciati in Senato nelle sedute del 15 e 16 giugno*. Roma: Forzani & C, 1891.

Bizzozero G. Il cittadino e l'igiene pubblica. *Nuova Antologia* Aprile 1898; **16**: 615–35.

Bizzozero G. *Contro la Tubercolosi*. Milano: Treves, 1899.

Bizzozero G. L'igiene pubblica in Italia. *Nuova Antologia* Aprile 16, 1900; 20–33; Maj 16: 220–37.

Bizzozero G. *La difesa della società contro le malattie infettive.* Torino: 1883.

Bizzozero G. Le macchine da scrivere dal punto di vista igienico. *Nuova Antologia* November 1, 1867; 45–68.

Bizzozero G. *Lezioni di patologia generale date nella r. Università di Torino: l'anno 1872–1873/da Giulio Bizzozero; riassunte dagli studenti Losio Scipione e Morra Emilio col consenso del professore.* Torino: Litografia Cassina Pietro.

Bizzozero G. Lo Stato e l'igiene pubblica. *Nuova Antologia* February 1, 1899; 385–408.

Bizzozero G. *Manuale di microscopia clinica: con aggiunte riguardanti l'uso del microscopio nella medicina legale/Giulio Bizzozero, 5th edn. Completamente Rifusa Ed Aumentata/Per Cura Di G. Bizzozero E C. Sacerdoti.* Milano: F. Vallardi, Pref. 1901.

Bizzozero G. *Manuale di microscopia clinica: con aggiunte riguardanti l'uso del microscopio nella medicina legale/per il dott. Giulio Bizzozero.* Milano: dottor Francesco Vallardi, 1880.

Bizzozero G. *Opere scientifiche di Giulio Bizzozero (Introduzione del Camillo Golgi).* Milano: Ulrico Hoepli, V 30 cm; 2: 1879–1896, bv.1bv: 1862–1879.

Bizzozero G. *Società piemontese d'igiene: discorsi pronunciati al Congresso nazionale d'igiene di Torino/da Giulio Bizzozero.* Torino: Stab. Fratelli Pozzo, 1899.

Bizzozero, Giulio. *Enciclopedia Italiana di Scienze, Lettere ed Arti.* Roma: Istituto Giovanni Treccani: [poi Istituto della Enciclopedia Italiana], 1929–.

Coller BS. Bizzozero and the discovery of the blood platelet. *Lancet* 1984; **8380**: 804.

Dianzani MU. Bizzozero and the discovery of platelets. *Am J Nephrol* 1994; **14**: 330–6.

Franceschini P. Giulio Cesare Bizzozero. *Dictionary of Scientific Biography* 1970, Vol. 2: 164–6.

Gravela E. *Omaggio a Giulio Bizzozero: fantasticare il vero: vecchi disegni e nuove immagini/testi di E. Giravela, di A. S. Balzala e di P. Mantovani.* Torino: Regione Piemonte, stampa 1991.

Gutt RW. On the 75th anniversary of the death of Bizzozero (20.3.1846–3.4.1901) and Marceli Nencki (15.1.1847–14.10.1901 (author's translation). *Przegl Lek* 1976; **30**: 882–84.

In Memoria Di Giulio Bizzozero Nel Primo Anniversario Della Sua Morte: la Famiglia. Torino: Stab. Fratelli Pozzo, 1901.

Lisi C, Bonincontro I. The archives of the section of history of medicine. *Med Secoli* 1998; **10**: 459–71.

Mazzarello P. Camillo Golgi's scientific biography. *J Hist Neurosci* 1999; **8**: 121–31.

Ottolenghi D. *I batteri patogeni in rapporto ai disinfettanti: tabelle pratiche/Donato Ottolenghi; con prefazione del Giulio Bizzozero.* Torino: Rosenberg & Sellier, 1899.

Pareti G. Giulio Bizzozero e la funzione ematopoietica del midollo osseo. *Nuncius* 1996; **11**: 563–80.

Scarani P, Zanarini P. A further object of controversy: Giulio Bizzozero and the discovery of platelets. *Pathologica* 1999; **91**: 412–13.

Appendix 2

On the correctness of the species name *Helicobacter bizzozeronii*

We think that the designation *Helicobacter bizzozeronii*, given to the newly recognized species of helicobacters that colonize the dog's stomach,[2] might not be completely grammatically correct. We would like to discuss this topic, as we cannot celebrate the discovery of helicobacters and maintain a supposedly incorrect bacterial name coined in honor of the scientist who first described them.

A taxonomic rule states that the species designation of all bacteria should be binomial and the names should be Latin or Latinized. The revised International Code of Nomenclature of bacteria recommends the suffix '*onii*' for any modern personal surnames that end in 'o' to produce the Latin genitive, and gives the example of 'Otto'.[5] However, the genitive of Latin names that end in 'o', such as 'Otto', should be '*Ottonis*', third declension; similarly, *sermo* (sermon, nominative), *sermonis* (genitive), *Scipio* (a Roman surname), *Scipionis* (genitive) etc., not '*Ottonii*' (second declension). The corresponding Latin name of Italian names that end in 'o' mainly end in '*us*' for a male name, or '*um*' for a neutral name (and '*a*' for a female name). The genitive of both gender names ends in '*i*' (second declension); for example, *numerus* (*i*) (number), *castrum* (*i*) (castle) etc. The corresponding Latin names of Italian proper names that end in 'o', such as Adriano, Carlo, Icaro etc., mostly belong to the second declension and end in '*i*': Hadrianus (i), Carolus (i), Icarus (i) etc.[6] Consequently, '*Bizzozerus*' (*i*), and therefore *Helicobacter bizzozeri*.

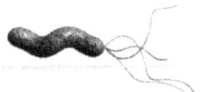

CHAPTER 2

Kasai, Kobayashi and Koch's postulates in the history of *Helicobacter pylori*

Yoshihiro Fukuda, Tadashi Shimoyama,
Takashi Shimoyama and Barry J. Marshall

Introduction

Helicobacter pylori is a Gram-negative bacterium with several flagella and a distinctive spiral shape from which its name is derived. Since its discovery, there has been increasing evidence of the etiopathologic role of this bacterium in several gastroduodenal diseases and today, *H. pylori* is clearly associated with chronic active gastritis and peptic ulcer disease (PUD), and is a well-recognized risk factor for the development of gastric cancer. Although *H. pylori* was first discovered and cultured in 1982, its historical origins begin in the late 19th century and this chapter introduces the Japanese contribution to that saga.

Prologue to the *H. pylori* discovery story

Helicobacter pylori induces gastritis, which then becomes a cause of PUD, but prior to the discovery of *H. pylori*, the cause of gastritis was uncertain and only symptomatic treatment could be provided. However, since the recognition that *H. pylori* is a cause of gastritis, the treatment strategies used in gastroenterology have changed drastically and eradication therapy is becoming popular worldwide, with the result that the number of patients who suffer from PUD is markedly decreasing. In addition, the incidence of gastric cancer is also decreasing and it is sure to become uncommon in the 21st century.

A similar epoch-making occurrence happened 200 years ago. In those days, smallpox was widespread in Europe and many people were disfigured or died. There were clinicians and researchers who knew that persons who had suffered from cowpox never acquired smallpox, but only one physician noticed that smallpox protection resulted when patients were accidentally or deliberately inoculated with cowpox. Edward Jenner, a physician from the United Kingdom consulted John Hunter, his teacher, about a trial of inoculations (vaccinations) with cowpox and Dr Hunter encouraged him, saying, 'Don't think, but try, be patient, be accurate. Why think, why not try the experiment?' Jenner inoculated some farmers with cowpox and none of those who received the vaccination with cowpox developed smallpox. He carefully observed the patients with cowpox and smallpox, and was able to prove his hypothesis about vaccination (FIGURE 1), but the public and the authorities would not accept his findings,

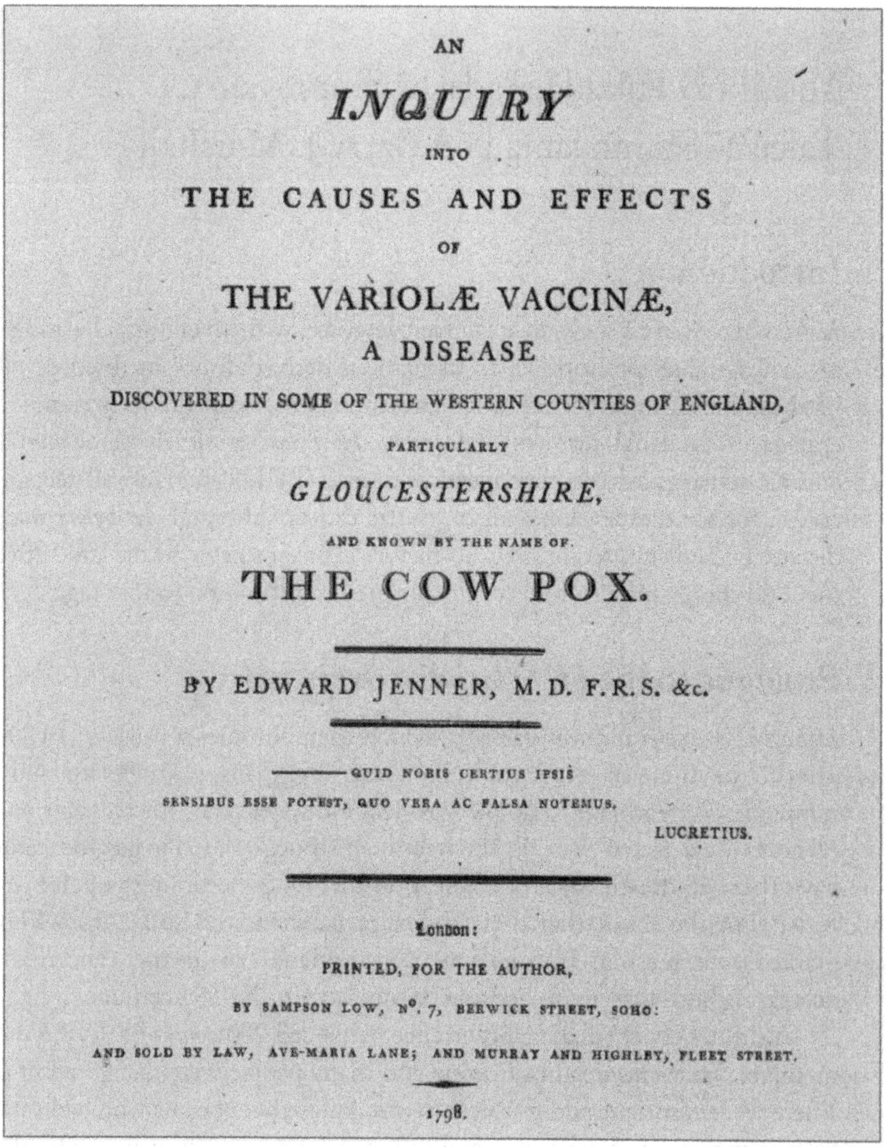

AN

INQUIRY

INTO

THE CAUSES AND EFFECTS

OF

THE VARIOLÆ VACCINÆ,

A DISEASE

DISCOVERED IN SOME OF THE WESTERN COUNTIES OF ENGLAND,

PARTICULARLY

GLOUCESTERSHIRE,

AND KNOWN BY THE NAME OF

THE COW POX.

BY EDWARD JENNER, M. D. F. R. S. &c.

——— QUID NOBIS CERTIUS IPSIS
SENSIBUS ESSE POTEST, QUO VERA AC FALSA NOTEMUS.

LUCRETIUS.

London:

PRINTED, FOR THE AUTHOR,

BY SAMPSON LOW, N°. 7, BERWICK STREET, SOHO:

AND SOLD BY LAW, AVE-MARIA LANE; AND MURRAY AND HIGHLEY, FLEET STREET.

1798.

FIGURE 1 Title page of Edward Jenner's hypothesis of smallpox vaccination.

and the cartoon of 'Vaccination with cowpox induces transformation into cattle' was widely published in the newspapers (FIGURE 2). However, Napoleon Bonaparte was interested in vaccination and encouraged its use. Finally, after 200 years of the use of Jenner's vaccine, the World Health Organization declared in 1977 that smallpox had been eradicated from the Earth. In that year, smallpox did not take a single precious life.

As with Jenner and smallpox, the hypothesis that PUD was caused by bacteria in the mucosa of the human stomach was rejected in 1954 by the major authority in American gastroenterology,[1] despite consistent information in the preceding 50 years of bacteria that adhered to the gastric mucosa (TABLE I). His words ensured that the development of bacteriology in gastroenterology would be closed to the world as if frozen in ice.

Nearly 30 years later, Robin Warren in Western Australia verified whether Palmer's stance was correct or not. Barry Marshall, who in those days was a medical resident, believed Warren's hypothesis and together they succeeded in culturing *H. pylori*, which had seemed impossible prior to 1982. The causal relationship between *H. pylori* and gastritis was proven by challenge with orally ingested *H. pylori*, but as in the time of Jenner, Marshall and Warren's reports in *The Lancet* were thought to be unusual, and did not lead to recognition from the health authorities.

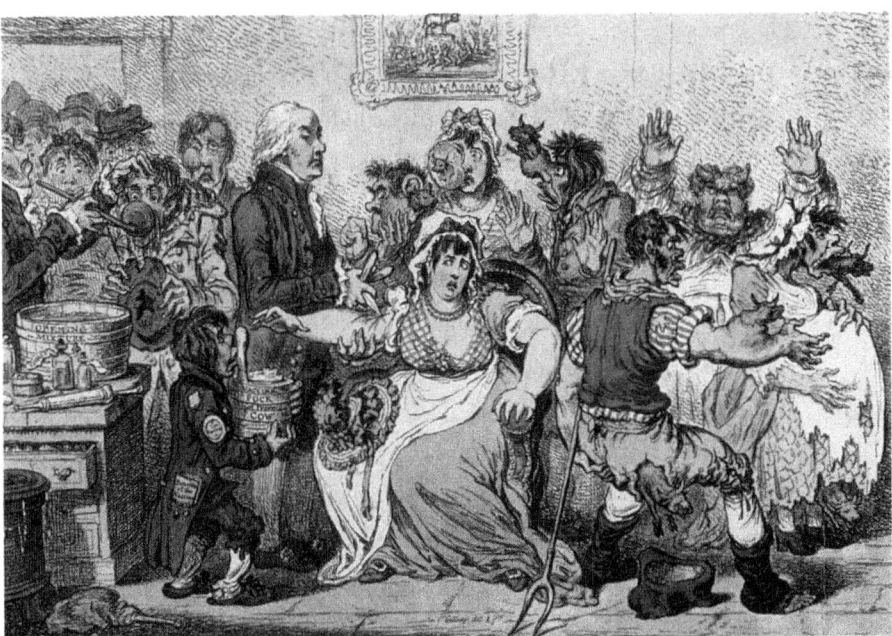

FIGURE 2 Cartoon of 'Vaccination with cowpox induces transformation into cattle'. (Reproduced with permission from The Welcome Trust.)

TABLE 1 History of the discovery of *Helicobacter pylori*

1875	Bottchet/Letulle	Bacteria in ulcer margin
1881	Klebs	Bacterial colonization and inflammation
1888	Letulle	*Staphylococcus aureus* induces acute gastritis in guinea pigs
1889	Jaworski	*Vibrio rugula* in the stomach
1893	Bizzozero	Spirochetes in dog stomach
1896	Salomon	Gastric spirochetes transmitted
1906	Krienitz	Spirochetes in the stomach with gastric cancer
1908	Turck	*Escherichia coli* induces gastric ulcer in the dog
1916	Rosenow	*Streptococcus* induces gastric ulcer
1917	Dragstedt	Bacteria do not induce gastric ulcer
1919	Kasai, Kobayashi	Gastric spirochetes transmitted
1921	Edkins	Experiment with *Spirilla regaudi* (*H. felis*)
1924	Luck	Urease activity in the stomach
1925	Hofman	'Hofmann's bacillus' induces ulceration
1930	Berg	Partial vagotomy inhibits secondary infections of ulcers
1938	Doenges	Spirochetes induce gastritis in monkeys and humans
1940	Freedberg/Barron	Gastric spirochetes are not pathogenic
1940	Gorham	Acidophilic bacteria induce gastric ulcer
1954	Palmer	No spirochetes detected using H&E in 1140 suction biopsies
1966	Aoyagi	Highest urease activity in the stomach
1975	Steer	*Pseudomonas aeruginosa* induces gastric inflammation in ulcer margin
1979	Warren	Spiral bacteria in the human stomach
1983	Warren	Gastric spiral bacteria associated with gastritis in humans
1983	Marshall	*H. pylori* isolated and cultured
1984	Inoue	First success in culturing *H. pylori* in Japan
1985–1987	Marshall/Morris	Inoculation with *H. pylori* proved Koch's 3rd postulate
1989	Goodwin	New spiral bacteria named *H. pylori*

Common threads in the *H. pylori* story are: (i) the hypothesis that over-turned common beliefs was proven; (ii) the authorities could not accept proven fact; (iii) the new treatment was carried out personally by the investigator; (iv) a great contribution to the health of mankind; and (v) the recognition of success was slow to arise. It gives me pleasure to recount the story of the many investigators (some of whom are included in this book) who reported spiral bacteria before Warren and Marshall.

Early investigations

In the latter half of the 19th century, Robert Koch, a German bacteriologist, developed the scientific theory that specific species of bacteria were the cause of certain diseases, and for the early gastric bacteriologists, to prove causative roles for certain foreign organisms was a task worthy of investigation. In 1881, Klebs, a German pathologist, noted the presence of bacilli-like organisms in the lumen of gastric glands, with corresponding inflammatory cell infiltration of the gastric mucosa (TABLE 1).[2] Bizzozero also observed bacterial colonization in the stomach during his studies in six dogs and in 1893 he reported that spirochete organisms were present in both the pyloric and fundic mucosa and were distributed from the base of the gastric glands to the surface epithelial cells.[3] Furthermore, following the report by Krienitz in 1906 of spirochete organisms in the gastric contents of a patient with gastric cancer, many other investigators in the early 20th century reported similar bacteria in the human stomach.[4] Luger showed that spirochete organisms were in the gastric juice,[5] and he also noted that these organisms were rarely seen in healthy subjects compared with patients with gastric cancer.[6] Using gastric autopsy specimens, Doenges found spirochete organisms in 43% of studied specimens, but he reported that the positivity of these organisms in human stomach was much lower than that in monkeys.[7] It was notable, however, that he found these organisms only in gastric and intestinal mucosa. Freedberg and Barron studied surgically resected gastric tissues and, using a silver staining method, demonstrated spirochete organisms in 53% of the stomachs with ulceration, but in only 14% of nonulcerated stomachs.[8] However, the fact that the frequency of these spirochete organisms in humans was lower than in other animals and also that these researchers could not transmit the organisms to show an etiopathologic role precluded them from concluding that the spiral bacteria were actually related to human gastric diseases.

In 1954, Palmer used a vacuum tube technique to obtain gastric mucosal specimens from 1140 subjects in order to investigate the presence of spirochete organisms in the human stomach.[1] However, he could not find any spirochete-like organisms histologically and concluded that bacteria could not live in the human stomach and that the findings of all previous studies were the result of contamination, mainly by the postmortem colonization of organisms from the oral cavity or within putrid ulcerations. He also suggested that spirochetes would normally be present in the gastric juice via the mouth. His study established the dogma that bacteria could not live in the human stomach, and as a result, investigation of gastric bacteria attracted little attention for the next 20 years.

The discovery of *H. pylori*

After great progress had been made in the use of fiberoptic endoscopy, reports suggesting the presence of bacteria in the human stomach began to reappear. In 1975, Steer studied the migration of polymorphonuclear leukocytes and lymphocytes through the gastric mucosa with the electron microscope, and found bacteria located close to the surface of the gastric epithelium, which suggested to him that there was a relationship between the cell migration and the bacterial colonization.[9] He also captured an electron microscopic image of the bacteria, which were consistent with what we now know as *Helicobacter*. Furthermore, he examined the epithelial differences between the normal stomach and that of 47 patients with gastric ulcers, and suggested the simultaneous occurrence of bacteria and gastric ulceration.[10] Unfortunately, Steer and his colleagues postulated that the bacterium was *Pseudomonas aeruginosa*, which they were able to culture, unlike *H. pylori*, which is microaerophilic. In 1979, Fung *et al.* also examined gastric biopsy specimens obtained from 29 patients and found a number of bacteria on the surface microvilli in the gastric pits of patients with chronic gastritis patients on scanning electron microscopy.[11]

Robin Warren, a histopathologist at Royal Perth Hospital in Western Australia, had noticed spiral bacteria in conventionally stained endoscopy gastric biopsy specimens since 1979. He and his young gastroenterology fellow, Barry Marshall, used the Warthin-Starry silver stain and revealed clearly the presence of numerous spiral bacteria, which were closely associated with active chronic gastritis that was notable for its infiltration with polymorphonuclear leukocytes.[12] In their first large consecutive study, they demonstrated that the bacteria were present in almost all patients with active chronic gastritis and duodenal ulcer or gastric ulcer, and thus suggested the new bacterium might be an important factor in the etiology of these diseases.[13] Their study fulfilled Koch's first postulate that 'The organism must always be found in the diseased animal but not in healthy ones'.

Koch's second postulate is 'The organism must be isolated from diseased animals and grown in pure culture away from the animal', and it was Marshall who first succeeded in culturing *H. pylori* using campylobacter isolation techniques in collaboration with a microbiologist, J. Pearman in Goodwin's laboratory.[14] After 34 failures, spiral bacteria were finally cultured on plates that had been left in the incubator over the Easter weekend. These bacilli were Gramnegative, flagellate and microaerophilic, and appeared to be a new species related to the genus *Campylobacter*. Initially they named the bacterium *C. pyloridis*,[15] but it was renamed *C. pylori* according to the grammatical rules of nomenclature.[16]

Koch's postulates

Although the first and second postulates of Koch had been fulfilled, there were two remaining postulates. Koch's third postulate requires that 'The organism isolated in pure culture must initiate and reproduce the disease when reinoculated into susceptible animals' and the fourth states that 'The organism should be re-isolated from the experimentally infected animals'. These postulates were fulfilled by several experiments in humans and monkeys.

After the successful isolation of *C. pyloridis*, Marshall himself, who had histologically normal gastric mucosa, ingested the bacteria.[16] A mild bout of acute gastritis developed, which lasted for 14 days, and histological gastritis was present on the 10th day after ingestion. A similar challenge was undertaken by Morris and Nicholson.[17] Morris, who had a histologically normal gastric mucosa, ingested the bacteria and three days later he developed moderate to severe attacks of epigastric pain. On day 11, *C. pyloridis* was cultured from both antral and fundal biopsies, which showed histological gastritis. Unfortunately, unlike Marshall, Morris's infection and gastritis persisted even after taking doxycycline for 28 days. Three years later, after 'triple therapy' with bismuth subsalicylate, his biopsies were culture negative and histologically only a minimal residual chronic gastritis was observed. The end result of these studies was that it appeared that *C. pyloridis* could cause acute upper gastrointestinal illness associated with histological gastritis.

It was studies in monkeys that enabled long-term investigation of *H. pylori* infection. Establishment of experimental animal models was definitely important because *H. pylori* infection causes chronic active gastritis. Fukuda and coworkers inoculated *H. pylori* isolated from humans into rhesus monkeys and observed the long-term changes in the gastric mucosa by endoscopy.[18] They demonstrated that *H. pylori* could colonize the monkey stomach and cause acute gastritis as well as histological active chronic gastritis. Fujioka and his colleagues also showed that inoculation of *H. pylori* caused gastritis in Japanese monkeys,[19] and demonstrated a decrease in the height of the antral glands in a 3-year follow-up study.[20]

Although many works have now fulfilled Koch's postulates for *H. pylori* infection, it is not widely known that the pathogenicity of gastric spiral bacteria had been already proven in Japan in 1919. Kasai and Kobayashi (FIGURES 3,4), Japanese microbiologists, transmitted spirochetes isolated from cats to rabbits and the inoculation successfully resulted in hemorrhagic erosions and ulceration of the gastric mucosa.[21] Histologically, the lesions were associated with colonization of spirochetes and were improved by 'eradication' treatment. Their results mean that Koch's postulates were already fulfilled for gastric spiral organisms more than 60 years before the official discovery of *H. pylori*.

Epilogue to the *H. pylori* discovery story

Although Marshall and Warren discovered *H. pylori* and the relevance to gastritis and peptic ulcer was emphasized, many gastroenterologists accepted the findings only after a very long period. Francis Bacon commented in Novum Organum that 'the human does not observe the fact which exceeded the

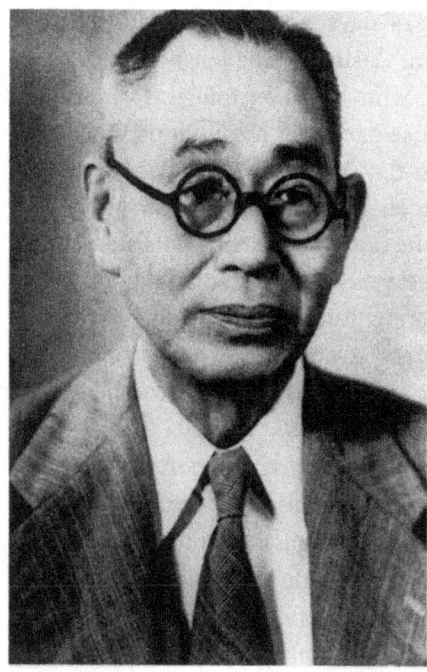

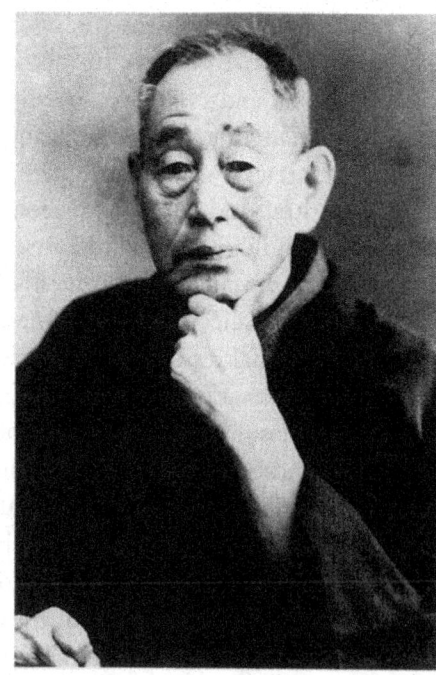

FIGURE 3 Dr Kasai.   FIGURE 4 Dr Kobayashi.

understanding of the self'. Many authorities did not believe that gastritis, peptic ulcer, lymphoma and cancer could be induced by small bacteria. Francis Bacon also said that it is necessary for scientists to observe carefully and report only the facts.

In 1989, *Campylobacter pylori* was recognized as not a true member of the genus and the new name *Helicobacter pylori* was given to this bacterium.[22] What is particularly interesting about the history of helicobacters, however, taking into consideration that an early Japanese study had shown the pathogenicity of gastric bacteria and that it was Australian scientists who believed in the presence of bacteria in the human stomach in spite of Palmer's theory, is that research into *H. pylori* started in Pacific countries.

References

[1] Palmer ED. Investigation of the gastric mucosa spirochetes of the human. *Gastroenterology* 1954; **27**: 218–20.

[2] Klebs C. Uber infectiose Magenaffectionen. *Allgemein Wien Med Z* 1881; 29–30.

[3] Bizzozero G. Uber die Schlauchformigen Drusen des Magendarmkanals und die Beziehungen ihres Epithels zu dem Oberflachenepithel der Schleimhaut. *Arch Mikr Anat* 1893; **42**: 82–152.

[4] Krienitz W. Uber das Auftreten von Spirochaeten verschiedener Form im Mageninhalt bei Carcinoma Ventriculi. *Dtsch Med Wochenschr* 1906; **22**: 872.

[5] Luger A. Uber Spirochaten und fusiforme Bazillen im darm, miteinem Beitrag zur Frage der Lamblien-enteritis. *Wein Klin Wochenschr* 1917; **52**: 1643–7.

[6] Luger A, Neuberger H. Uber Spirochatenbefunde im Magensaft und deren diagnostische Bedeutung fur das Carcinoma ventiriculi. *Z Klin Med* 1921; **92**: 54.

[7] Doenges JL. Spirochetes in the gastric glands of *Macacus rhesus* and of man without related disease. *Arch Pathol* 1939; **27**: 469–77.

[8] Freedberg AS, Barron LE. The presence of spirochetes in human gastric mucosa. *Am J Dig Dis* 1940; **7**: 443–5.

[9] Steer HW. Ultrastructure of cell migration through the gastric epithelium and its relationship to bacteria. *J Clin Pathol* 1975; **28**: 639–46.

[10] Steer HW, Colin-Jones DG. Mucosal changes in gastric ulceration and their response to carbenoxolone sodium. *Gut* 1975; **16**: 590–7.

[11] Fung WP, Papadimitriou JM, Matz LR. Endoscopic, histological and ultrastructural correlations in chronic gastritis. *Am J Gastroenterol* 1979; **71**: 269–79.

[12] Warren JR, Marshall B. Unidentified curved bacilli on gastric epithelium in active chronic gastritis. *Lancet* 1983; **1**: 1273–5.

[13] Marshall BJ, Warren JR. Unidentified curved bacilli in the stomach of patients with gastritis and peptic ulceration. *Lancet* 1984; **1**: 1311–15.

[14] Marshall BJ, Royce H, Annear DI *et al.* Original isolation of *Campylobacter pyloridis* from human gastric mucosa. *Microbiol Lett* 1984; **25**: 83–8.

[15] Marshall BJ, Goodwin CS. Revised nomenclature of *Campylobacter pyloridis*. *Int J Syst Bacteriol* 1987; **37**: 68.

[16] Marshall BJ, Armstrong JA, McGechie DB, Glancy RJ. Attempt to fulfil Koch's postulates for pyloric Campylobacter. *Med J Aust* 1985; **142**: 436–9.

[17] Morris A, Nicholson G. Ingestion of *Campylobacter pyloridis* causes gastritis and raised fasting gastric pH. *Am J Gastroenterol* 1987; **82**: 192–9.

[18] Fukuda Y, Tamura K, Yamamoto I *et al.* Inoculation of Rhesus monkeys with human *Helicobacter pylori*: a long-term investigation on gastric mucosa by endoscopy. *Dig Endosc* 1992; **4**: 19–30.

[19] Shuto R, Fujioka T, Kubota T, Nasu M. Experimental gastritis induced by *Helicobacter pylori* in Japanese monkeys. *Infect Immun* 1993; **61**: 933–9.

[20] Fujioka T, Kubota T, Shuto R *et al.* Establishment of an animal model for chronic gastritis with *Helicobacter pylori*: potential model for long-term observations. *Eur J Gastroenterol Hepatol* 1994; **6**(Suppl. 1): S73–8.

[21] Kasai K, Kobayashi R. The stomach spirochete occurring in mammals. *J Parasitol* 1919; **6**: 1–11.

[22] Goodwin CS, Armstrong JA, Chilvers T *et al.* Transfer of *Campylobacter pylori* and *Campylobacter mustelae* to *Helicobacter pylori* comb. nov. and *Helicobacter mustelae* comb. nov., respectively. *Int J Syst Bacteriol* 1989; **39**: 397–405.

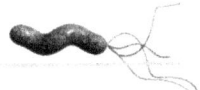

CHAPTER 3

An early study of human stomach bacteria

A. Stone Freedberg

IN 1939 I WAS a research fellow in a cardiology program at Beth Israel Hospital and Harvard Medical School, looking for evidence of reflex effects inducing coronary artery spasm,[1] as well as studying the cardiovascular response to fever and the relationship between changes in cardiovascular function during fever to the circulatory changes in infectious shock.[2-4] Both patients and animals were in short supply.

I had read about gastric mucosal hemorrhage and superficial ulcers, and other gastrointestinal changes, that occurred in infectious shock. There were also references to the presence of bacteria in the stomach and liver,[5-9] but I could not find a reference to their existence in the living tissue of humans.

A year spent in a pathology department had taught me, among much else, how to prepare tissues for sectioning, staining and mounting. I received permission from the Beth Israel Research and Publications committee to begin a study of human gastric tissue for the existence of bacteria. Dr Monroe J. Schlesinger, Professor of Pathology at Harvard Medical School and Head of Pathology at Beth Israel Hospital, graciously agreed to let me use the laboratory facilities after 5 pm and on weekends, with the stipulation that I leave the laboratory and the equipment in the condition in which I found it. He generously offered to review the slides. Mrs Edith Herman, Chief Technician, offered advice, free supplies and a space where I could work. My coworker, Dr Louis Barron, was a surgeon at Beth Israel and a medical school friend and he offered to persuade his surgical colleagues to give us specimens of resected stomachs. Approval of the patient was not required by existing standards.

When the specimens were obtained I prepared them, initially with hematoxylin–eosin staining. Not finding organisms, I explored other stains including silver stains. I still remember the surprise and good feeling I had when I first saw organisms in the superficial layers of the mucosa of some resected stomachs. Dr Schlesinger agreed that these were not artifacts. I decided to call the organisms 'spirochetes' because that was the term used in previous studies in animals and also because of the silver staining and the inability of bacteriologists to culture bacteria from human specimens. However, the organisms did not look like the spirilli seen in the dog stomach mucosa and illustrated in a published paper.[10] The organisms we saw seemed to have a flat end and an opposing curly end.

We studied more than 35 stomach specimens obtained from patients with duodenal ulcer, gastric ulcer or carcinoma of the stomach and we found organisms in 40% of cases. One specimen of gastric ulcer had many organisms, far more than was found in any other lesion and we wondered whether this was significant.

I submitted the paper to the Research and Publications Committee and they approved its publication. Dr Barron summarized the paper at the 1940 meeting of the American Society of Gastroenterology and I submitted it to the *American Journal of Digestive Diseases*, which accepted it.[11]

In discussion with Dr Frank Gorham of St Louis, Missouri, he noted that he gave Dr Cowdry 'some human stomachs' for study, but Dr Cowdry did not publish the results of his studies. Later, Doenges examined 42 well-preserved stomachs removed at autopsy and found spirochetes in some 43%.[10]

I heard that other investigators were not able to confirm our findings, but over the next few years I did not find any papers reporting negative results. Nor were there any confirmatory papers. I was most gratified when Dr Marshall called me from Australia and asked whether I was the author of the 1940 paper. I knew, of course, of his work and had wondered whether the organisms I saw were the same as those he drank.

Our paper was the result of my first independent work and the start of a career in academic medicine. Dr Barron left the Beth Israel Hospital in the early 1940s and had a successful career as a general surgeon in Lynn, Massachusetts. He died many years ago.

The primary laboratory books, the embedded blocks, the prepared slides and all the laboratory books accumulated during my 35 years at Beth Israel Hospital and Harvard Medical School were discarded in 1990, before Dr Marshall called me. Unfortunately, I was not informed that the hospital planned to use the storage space where my work was being kept.

References

1   Freedberg AS, Spiegi ED, Riseman JEFR. Effect of external heat and cold on patients with angina pectoris: evidence for the existence of a reflex factor. *Am Heart J* 1944; **27**: 411–22.
2   Altschule HD, Freedberg AS, McManus MJ. Circulation and respiration during an episode of chill and fever in man. *J Clin Invest* 1945; **24**: 278–389.
3   Freedberg AS, Altschule MD. The effects of infection on the circulation. *N Engl J Med* 1944; **233**: 560–7.
4   Freedberg AS, McManus MJ, Altschule MD. The electrocardiogram in man during an episode of chill and fever induced by the intravenous typhoid vaccine. *Am Heart J* 1947; **34**: 249–61.
5   Bizzozero G. Ueber die Schlauchformigen Drusen des Magendarmakanals und die Bezienhungen ihres Epithels zu dem Oberflachenepithel der Schleimhaut. *Arch Mikr Anat* 1893; **42**: 82–152.
6   Salomon H. Ueber das Spirillum des Saugetiermagens und sein Verhalten zu den Belegzellen. *Zentralbl Bakteriol* 1896; **19**: 433–42.
7   Kasai K, Kobayashi R. Stomach spirochetes occurring in mammals. *J Parasitol* 1919; **6**: 1–11.
8   Krienitz W. Ueber das Auftreten von Sprirochaten verschiedener Form im Mageninhalt bei Carcinoma Ventriculi. *Dtsch Med Wochenschr* 1906; **32**: 872.
9   Luger A, Neuberger H. Uber Spirochatenbefunde im Magensaft und deren diagnostische Bedeutung fur das Carcinoma ventriculi. *Z Klin Med* 1921; **92**: 54.
10 Doenges JL. Spirochetes in gastric glands of *Macacus rhesus* and of man without related disease. *Arch Pathol* 1939; **27**: 469–77.
11 Freedberg AS, Barron LE. The presence of spirochetes in human gastric mucosa. *Am J Dig Dis* 1940; **7**: 443–5.

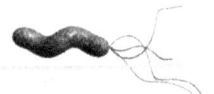

CHAPTER 4

Gastric urease in ulcer patients in the 1940s

The Irish connection

Humphrey J. O'Connor and Colm A. O'Morain

Introduction

Helicobacter pylori is unique as the only microorganism adapted to not only survive, but to thrive in the hostile environment of the human stomach. The key biochemical property of *H. pylori* that explains it's predilection for the stomach and its ability to cope with such an unusual microbiological niche is the possession of copious amounts of the enzyme urease. Urease hydrolyzes urea to carbon dioxide and ammonia, the latter acting as a buffer in the bacterial periplasm through the formation of ammonium and may also neutralize hydrogen ions further afield in the gastric juice.[1]

Recent research suggests that the urease system of *H. pylori* not only provides acid resistance for the organism, but is also necessary for colonization.[2] The urease proteins are synthesized constitutively by *H. pylori* and account for about 15% of its protein synthesis. At a clinical level, detection of urease has become a surrogate diagnostic test for *H. pylori* infection, using rapid urease tests such as the CLOtest on gastric biopsies, and the C13 or C14 urea breath test as the noninvasive test of choice.

In the light of what we now know about *H. pylori* and gastrointestinal disease, it is fascinating to look back at the history of gastric urease, focusing particularly on a unique Irish contribution to this body of knowledge. The name synonymous with this work is that of Professor Oliver Fitzgerald (1910–1987) (FIGURE 1). Throughout his illustrious career, Professor Fitzgerald was a gastroenterologist of international repute, a brilliant researcher and Professor of Therapeutics at University College Dublin. Incidentally, his brother Patrick, equally as gifted, was Professor of Surgery at University College Dublin at the same time, and together they made a formidable dynasty! Historically, the presence of ammonia in gastric juice was first described in 1852 by Bidder and Schmidt (cited by Fitzgerald and Murphy[3]), and Nencki in 1896[4] found that the gastric mucosa of dogs contained more free ammonia than any other tissue investigated. In 1924, James Murray-Luck in Cambridge showed that portal blood contained considerably more ammonia than systemic blood and that the ammonia content of gastric juice was 50–100 times more concentrated than that of arterial blood.[5] The following year, Luck and Seth were first to describe the presence of urease *in vivo* in the gastric mucosa of vertebrates.[6] They argued that the administration of urea in dilute hydrochloric acid in their experiments and the positive results they obtained following intravenous injection of urea showed that the observed effects could not be the result of urealytic bacteria that might be in the stomach, and that the enzyme was a constituent of the gastric cells. Interestingly, Luck and Seth also showed that urea was not hydrolyzed by preparations of intestinal mucosa. Fitzgerald probably came in contact with this work during his time in 1937 as a postgraduate student in the Physiology Laboratory at the University of Cambridge.

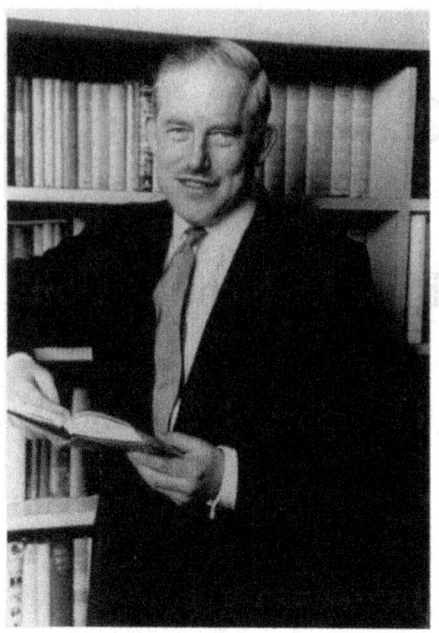

FIGURE 1 Professor Oliver Fitzgerald (1910–1987).

On his return to clinical and research work in Dublin, Fitzgerald and his colleagues at the Department of Physiology at University College Dublin set about their own research on gastric urease with specific reference to peptic ulcer disease (PUD).[3] They hypothesized, with admirable foresight, that the underlying problem in PUD involved an ill-adjusted interplay between gastric secretion, neutralization, and mucosal resistance. They also believed that the mechanisms underlying the production of ammonia by the gastric mucosa might be of 'great importance in the normal and pathological physiology of the stomach'.

Gastric urease across the species

Fitzgerald's initial investigations focused on demonstrating the existence of gastric urease across several species and on possible regional differences in the distribution of urease within the stomach. The methodology, which might seem quaint today, involved desiccating gastric mucosal specimens and preparing suspensions of mucosal powder in normal saline to which were added equal volumes of 1% urea solution. Urease activity was then measured by the amount of ammonia produced at intervals by this mixture. Human specimens were obtained after partial gastrectomy, the surgical treatment of choice at that time for PUD.

Fitzgerald and his coworkers found that gastric urease was widely distributed in all animal species tested, with larger amounts found in the stomach of humans, dogs and cats, compared with rabbits, pigs and rats. For instance, the average amount of urease present in the cat stomach was quite enough to release sufficient ammonia from urea to neutralize the usual amount of acid secreted by the cat. Within the stomach, enzyme activity was concentrated in the superficial rather than the deep part of the mucous membrane and high levels were found in the fundic and pyloric regions. Very little urease activity was found in the small intestine.

The Irish group also investigated possible ways of influencing the urease content of the mucosa.[7,8] In a series of animal experiments, cats fed on a high-protein meat diet showed a remarkable increase in the urease content of the gastric mucosa compared with milk-fed cats and there was no change in the urease content of the duodenal mucosa. Rats fed on a soya bean diet also showed a significant increase in urease content compared with rats fed on a standard laboratory diet. In the 1940s, concentrated pregnancy urine was considered a rich source of urogastrone and/or factors that might increase the mucosal resistance to ulceration in the experimental animal, and interestingly, rats injected with this substance had a higher level of gastric urease compared with the control group injected with distilled water. Finally, the group studied the possibility of influencing urease concentration by the use of a high urea intake. This was a logical next step given the fact that urea is the major end-product of protein metabolism and might be one of the ways through which a high-protein diet could affect urease concentration. Urea-fed rats showed a definite increase in mucosal urease content. These findings in animal experiments set the scene for later treatment studies in humans with PUD.

Urea and the acid content of gastric juice

Fitzgerald and his colleagues hypothesized that if the urea–urease system was important in the production of alkali in the gastric mucosa, increasing the system's substrate, urea, in the mucosa should lead to a decrease of gastric acid concentration. They examined this question in a series of elegant studies of 49 subjects, 'some normal subjects, some suffering from various forms of peptic ulcer'. The mainstay of their investigations was assessment of the gastric secretory response to subcutaneous histamine before and after subjects were given an oral solution of 15 g of urea in a solution of acacia, flavored with syrup of orange; that is, the double histamine test.[3]

There was a substantial fall in the amount of acid present in the gastric juice after urea was given, on average around 40 mEq, and this phenomenon was seen at all levels of acid secretion. The fall in acid content was not proportional to the basal level of acid secretion, indicating that the mechanism was probably not through direct interference with the formation of acid, but rather from neutralization of the acid after it had been formed. The average percentage fall in acid between the first and second histamine response was 34 for the normal stomach, 54 for gastric ulcer cases and 36 for duodenal ulcer cases. Individual differences in acid secretory capacity might have explained the variable response to urea, but Fitzgerald also speculated that individual variation in urease concentration might be responsible.

Blood urea levels were also measured during these experiments and there was a significant negative correlation between the level of gastric acid and blood urea concentration (FIGURE 2). They also found a negative correlation

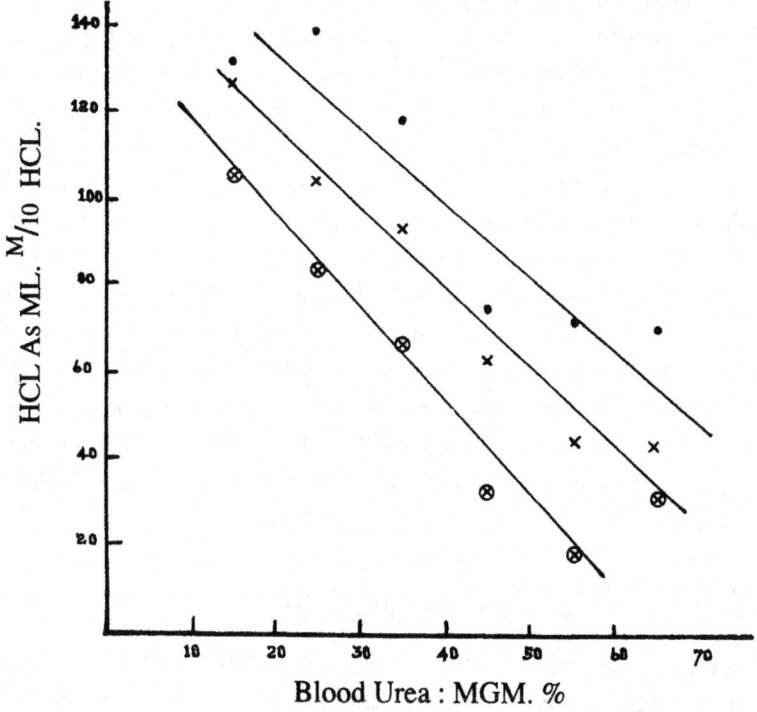

FIGURE 2 Negative correlation between intragastric acidity and blood urea concentration. (●) Duodenal ulcer patients, (+) gastric ulcer patients and normal subjects. (Reproduced with permission from Fitzgerald O, Murphy P. *Irish Med J* 1950; 292: 97–159.)

between the level of ammonia in gastric juice and intragastric acidity, but the rise in intragastric ammonia was often not sufficient to explain the decrease in acid in the gastric juice. The mean ammonia concentration in the gastric juice was higher in patients with gastric ulcer compared with those with duodenal ulcer or normal subjects. A strong positive correlation was found between the level of blood urea and the concentration of ammonia in the gastric juice (FIGURE 3), again supporting Fitzgerald's contention that 'gastric ammonia was derived from urea by its hydrolysis by intramucosal urease'.

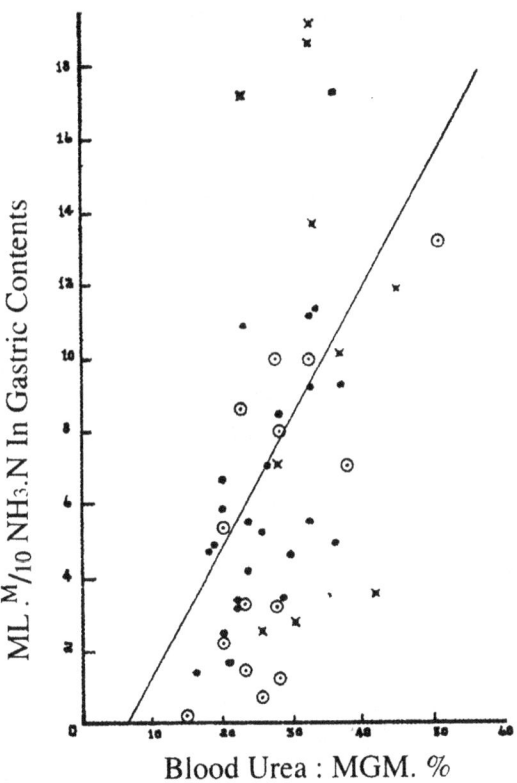

FIG. 3. Graph of ml. $\frac{M}{10}$ NH$_3$.N. in gastric contents plotted against the Fasting Blood Urea. The line has been inserted according to the regression equation
$$\times \text{ amm.} = 0.35 \times_B - 2.1.$$
⊙ = Normal subjects.
× = Gastric Ulcer Cases.
● = Duodenal Ulcer Cases.

FIGURE 3 Positive correlation between ammonia concentration in gastric juice and blood urea concentration. (Reproduced with permission from Fitzgerald O, Murphy P. *Irish Med J* 1950; **292**: 97–159.)

Two subjects underwent novel intravenous urea tests with infusion of a 5% solution of urea in normal saline and in both a substantial fall in acid was observed, but it was associated with a very slight rise in gastric ammonia concentration. Fitzgerald and his coworkers seemed troubled by the apparent discrepancy between the fall in gastric acid and the rise in intragastric ammonia and wondered whether neutralization by ammonia secreted into the stomach occurred mostly at the gastric wall, rather than in the lumen, and the neutralized contents then reabsorbed. To test this hypothesis, they performed a series of innovative neutralization experiments using the isolated cat stomach with sampling tubes tied into place through the stomach wall to concurrently sample the gastric contents in the lumen and at the surface of the mucosa after infusion of a dilute hydrochloric acid solution through a filling tube (FIGURE 4). In all these experiments, the tube from the mucosal surface gave a lower acid content than the tube from the depths of the gastric contents. No urea was administered in any of these experiments, but again, the intragastric level of ammonia was usually not sufficient to explain the degree of neutralization achieved.

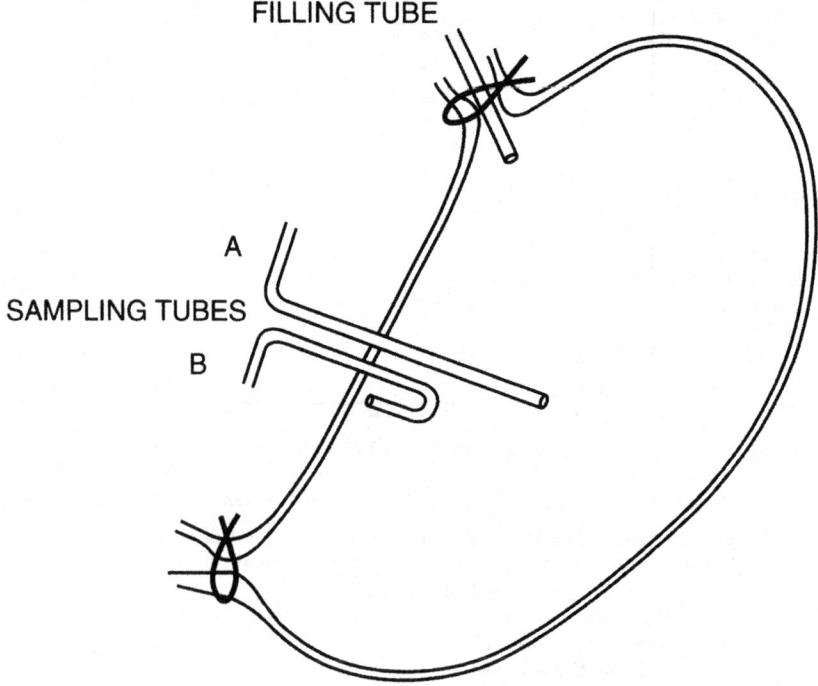

FILLING TUBE

A

SAMPLING TUBES

B

FIGURE 4 Isolated cat stomach with sampling tubes in place. (Reproduced with permission from Fitzgerald O, Murphy P. *Irish Med J* 1950; **292**: 97–159.)

Urea in peptic ulcer therapy

Medical treatment of PUD in the 1940s was unsatisfactory, largely consisting of prolonged bed rest and milk alkali diet. Oliver Fitzgerald was first and foremost a clinician and his research work on gastric urease was essentially driven by the prospect of finding a new treatment for PUD. The experimental work in animals and humans raised the possibility that the urea–urease system, a constituent part of the gastric mucosa as Fitzgerald's group saw it, could be activated for therapeutic purposes in peptic ulcer to protect the mucosa and neutralize acid.[9,10] It is ironic indeed that the ultimate medical cure for peptic ulcer should prove to be elimination, not activation, of gastric urease by eradicating *H. pylori* and that this seminal discovery should also take place in Dublin more than 40 years later.[11]

By administering oral urea, Fitzgerald and his colleagues aimed to increase the levels of intragastric and blood urea, which would then be available as a substrate for gastric urease. The solution of urea used contained 15 g of urea in syrup of acacia flavored with orange or lemon. 'This made a fairly palatable mixture, but certainly not a solution which could ever be described as elegant'! Some patients found the solution difficult to take, but the great majority had no particular difficulty with it. A series of 62 patients with a mixture of gastric, duodenal, and anastomotic ulcers were studied and were ambulant at all times during treatment.[3] Every patient was assessed by a barium meal examination and those with gastric or anastomotic ulcers underwent gastroscopy, performed by Oliver Fitzgerald himself. Given that the requirement for urea could be upwards of 500 g/week per case, there was sometimes a problem with supply, and this came to a head in 1949 when, at a time of truculent trade relations, there was an embargo on the export of urea from Great Britain to Ireland!

A survey of the results is shown in TABLE I. Approximately 80% of the patients were relieved of their symptoms by administration of urea and quite a number were entirely relieved of symptoms. Urea appeared to produce quicker relief of the symptoms of gastric ulcer than in cases of duodenal ulcer, and anastomotic ulcers seemed to respond in general more like cases of gastric ulcer. The acid response to urea in the double histamine test described earlier gave a good idea of the hopefulness of urea therapy, though a few patients gave very encouraging double histamine test results and yet did not do well on treatment. Fitzgerald cited complicating factors such as psychoneurosis and spastic colon as possibly responsible for these clinical aberrations.

The most common dosage of urea administered was 15 g five times daily, but on occasions a larger dose was used if the symptoms proved intractable. Attempts were also made to control the dosage by measuring fasting blood

TABLE 1 Summarized results of urea treatment of 62 patients suffering from various forms of peptic ulcer

Diagnosis	Excellent	Good	Fair	Poor
Gastric ulcer	8	5	3	0
Anastomotic ulcer	3	1	0	1
Duodenal ulcer	24	10	5	2
Total	35	16	8	3

Excellent, patient is symptomless either on continued treatment or with none at all; Good, patient definitely improved, but not free of symptoms; Fair, some temporary relief of symptoms with the urea mixture; Poor, no relief of any importance.

urea concentrations, with the aim of maintaining the concentration between 60 and 80 mg per cent; side-effects such as headache, nausea and loss of appetite tended to occur at concentrations greater than 80 mg per cent. Conscious of the relapsing nature of PUD, urea therapy was continued for at least six months, though the treatment was not evaluated as regards its usefulness for the prevention of ulcer recurrences.

Fitzgerald candidly acknowledged that if urea therapy was to be proved of value, controls were imperative.[7] For a variety of reasons, suitable controls were not employed in the group's series. The patients included tended to be the more intractable cases who had already been through other forms of treatment, and a suitable control substance for urea was difficult to find, especially in regard to taste. They tried quinine, but that was a gastric irritant and proved unsuitable. They also acknowledged the practical disadvantages of urea therapy, such as the difficulty in determining the dose required, the frequency of dosage, its relative unpalatability, and the necessity for blood urea measurement. With commendable humility, Fitzgerald and his colleagues concluded that urea therapy was unlikely to become routine treatment for PUD.

The origin of gastric urease: Mucosal or bacterial?

Fundamental to Fitzgerald's hypothesis on the role of gastric urease in health and disease was the belief that the enzyme system was an inherent function of the vertebrate stomach, and not the result of infection with urealytic bacteria. If gastric urease proved to be bacterial in origin, their whole hypothesis vis-a-vis gastric urease providing mucosal protection and neutralization would be rendered null and void. In the early 1950s, a number of papers were published that suggested gastric urease might indeed be bacterial in origin. Dintzis and Hastings introduced large doses of penicillin, terramycin and sulfaguanidine into the gastrointestinal tract of mice and found that the gastric mucosa was clear of urease in just over two days.[12] Similarly, Kornberg and Davies abolished the growth of bacteria in the gastrointestinal tract of the cat and at the same time removed gastric urease activity using large doses of antibiotics administered as a mixture of penicillin, terramycin and sulfaguanidine.[13]

In what appears like a spirited response to these reports, Conway, Fitzgerald and coworkers went on to perform a detailed assessment of the location and origin of gastric urease using a mouse model.[14] In their experiments, microcannulas were used to cannulate gastric mucosal cells and withdraw samples of protoplasm, which were then examined for urease activity and cultured. Gastric, oral and esophageal washings were also cultured for urease-containing bacteria. The results of these experiments seemed to show that urease in the gastric mucosa was contained within the surface epithelial cells, which did not contain bacteria. The amount of urease in the gastric mucosa of the mouse was relatively large and 'would require so great a bulk of bacteria to supply it that a bacterial origin for such urease appears untenable'. The detection of the presence of fetal gastric urease by Cardin,[15] and the normal paucity of gastric flora, were also cited by Conway et al. as supportive evidence for the nonbacterial origin of gastric urease.

Conclusions

Ultimately, we now know that gastric urease is bacterial in origin, and the raison d'etre in the treatment of peptic ulcer is not, as Fitzgerald thought, to enhance urease activity, but to completely suppress it. In the 1980s, Oliver Fitzgerald maintained a keen interest in the rapidly evolving *H. pylori* saga, and his wry sense of deja vu was obvious in personal contacts and correspondence that we had with him on the subject. Perhaps it helped that, coincidentally, both of us are graduates of University College Dublin, and one of us (H.J. O'C) had the privilege, during postgraduate training, of working on his team. With the benefit of hindsight, cynics might dismiss the work of the Fitzgerald group, but their ideas on peptic ulcer are as relevant today as they were 50 years ago. We are still striving to readjust the 'ill-adjusted interplay' between secretion, neutralization and mucosal resistance in the dyspeptic patient. The discovery of *H. pylori* has simply made the task a lot easier.

References

1 Sachs G, Shin JM, Munson K *et al.* The control of gastric acid and *Helicobacter pylori* eradication (Review). *Aliment Pharmacol Ther* 2000; **14**: 1383–401.

2 Weeks DL, Eskandari S, Scott DR, Sachs GA. H$^+$-gated urea channel the link between *Helicobacter pylori* urease and gastric colonization. *Science* 2000; **287**: 482–5.

3 Fitzgerald O, Murphy P. Studies on the physiological chemistry and clinical significance of urease and urea with special reference to the stomach. *Irish J Med Sci* 1950; **292**: 97–159.

4 Nencki M, Pawlow JP, Zaleski J. Ueber den Ammoniakgehalt des Blutes und der Organe und die Harnstoffbildung bei den Saugethieren. *Arch Exp Pathol Pharmacol* 1896; **37**: 26–51.

5 Luck JM. Ammonia production by animal tissues *in vitro*. *Biochem J* 1924; **18**: 814–24.

6 Luck JM, Seth TN. The physiology of gastric urease. *Biochem J* 1925; **19**: 357–65.

7 Fitzgerald O. Urease in the gastric mucosa and its increase after a meat diet, soya bean flour diet or urogastrone injections. *Nature* 1946; **158**: 305–6.

8 Fitzgerald O, Murphy P. Role of gastric urease. *Nature* 1948; **162**: 896–7.

9 Fitzgerald O, Murphy P. The function of gastric urease. *Lancet* 1949; **2**: 1107–10.

10 Fitzgerald O. The urea–urease mechanism as a factor in the depression of gastric acidity and the protection of the mucosa against acid-pepsin. *Gastroenterologia* 1950; **76**: 85–8.

11 Coghlan JG, Gilligan D, Humphries H *et al. Campylobacter pylori* and recurrence of duodenal ulcers: a 12 month follow-up study. *Lancet* 1987; **2**: 1109–11.

12 Dintzis RZ, Hastings AB. The effect of antibiotics on urea breakdown in mice. *Proc Natl Acad Sci USA* 1953; **39**: 571–8.

13 Kornberg HL, Davies RE. Gastric urease. *Physiol Rev* 1955; **35**: 169–77.

14 Conway EJ, Fitzgerald O, McGeeney K, Geoghegan F. The location and origin of gastric urease. *Gastroenterology* 1959; **37**: 449–56.

15 Cardin A. L'ureasi nella mucosa gastrica del feto. *Arch di Sci Biol* 1933; **19**: 76.

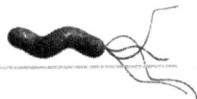

CHAPTER 5

How it was discovered in Belgium and the USA (1955–1976) that gastric urease was caused by a bacterial infection

Charles S. Lieber

Introduction

My training in gastric physiology and pharmacology started as a junior investigator in the Department of Pharmacology, University of Brussels (1951–1956) working on experimental and clinical studies of inhibitors of gastric acid secretion.[1,2] When I became a resident (1955–1956) and then a Research Fellow in Internal Medicine and Gastroenterology (1956–1958) at the Medical Service and the Queen Elizabeth Medical Research Foundation, University Hospital Brugmann, Brussels, (Figure 1), I participated in the care of 23 patients who were suffering from acute anuria and were undergoing hemodialysis in the hospital. Nine of them developed gastroduodenal ulceration with severe upper gastrointestinal bleeding, which was lethal in six.[3] Several possible explanations were considered, one of which was based on the fact, known already at that time, that blood urea, when it diffuses into the stomach, is converted into ammonia by a gastric urease. Several authors had shown that the concentration of ammonia in gastric juice is roughly proportional to the blood urea level[4-7] and consequently one could expect the concentration of gastric ammonia in patients with uremia to be very high. Therefore, I raised the hypothesis that this ammonia could neutralize the gastric acid and that with the decrease in the urea concentration after dialysis, the ammonia would disappear and the acid reappear, provoking the bleeding of a mucosa the defenses of which against acid-peptic digestion had been weakened by the chronic renal insufficiency. Furthermore, because various microorganisms, including spirochete-like ones, had been described on the human gastric mucosa, I wondered if they might provide the urease responsible for splitting the urea into ammonia.[8,9] The nephrologists involved in the cases agreed to include my hypothesis in their written account of these patients[3] and they included in the list of authors not only my name but also that of my coworker, Andre Lefèvre (FIGURE 2), then still a medical student. We could not, however, test this hypothesis directly in the hemodialyzed subjects, but we were allowed to continue studying patients with chronic renal failure, despite the general skepticism at that time concerning the possibility that bacteria might reside in the stomach. In fact, Luck and Seth had already found urease in the stomach, in 1924, but they believed it to be an enzyme intrinsic to the mucosal cells and this had become the prevailing view.[10]

Bacterial origin of gastric urease and the role of gastric ammonia in the hypoacidity of uremic patients

Antibiotics were of course unknown in 1924, but when they became available, Andre and I used them to assess the possibility that the gastric urease might be of bacterial origin. Accordingly, we measured ammonia, urea, free and total acid, and chlorides in basal and post histamine secretions in five nonuremic and six uremic patients who received oral oxytetracycline (20 mg per kg daily) for 4–7 days.[11,12] The subjects were fasted for 16 hours and gastric juice was collected by a Levine tube with the patients placed in the left lateral position, as proposed by Henning,[8] to facilitate the quantitative recovery of gastric secretions.[13] After a 45-minute period of stabilization, gastric juice was aspirated

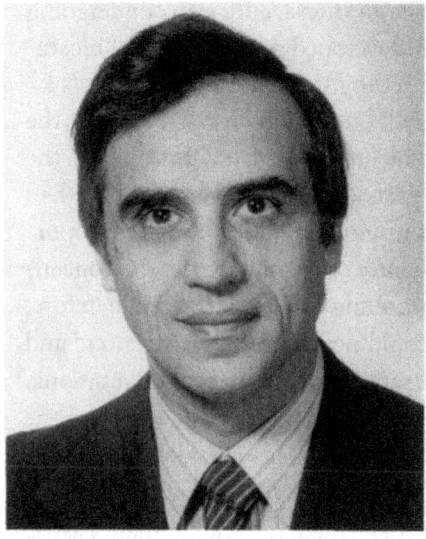

FIGURE 1 Charles S. Lieber (*c*.1958).

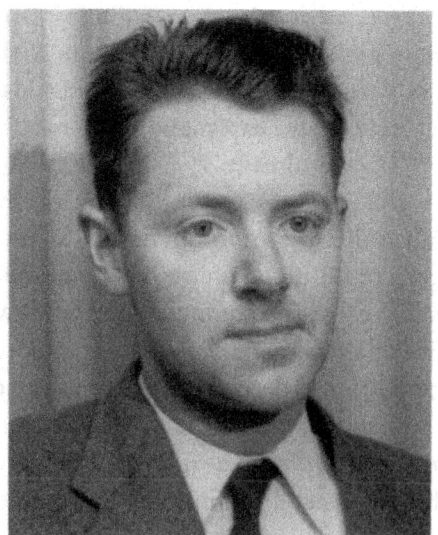

FIGURE 2 Andre Lefèvre (*c*.1957).

every 15 minutes and collected for examination. Basal secretion was studied in the four specimens collected during the first hour. At the end of this period, 0.005 mg/kg histamine dihydrochloride was administered subcutaneously, and the effect of this drug on the volume and composition of gastric secretions was determined in the four specimens collected during the second hour. This procedure was performed before and after antibiotic treatment. Mean ammonia concentrations of the basal and posthistamine gastric secretions were found to be much higher in uremic than nonuremic subjects and they were lowered in all instances by the antibiotic. The reduction in ammonia concentration was about 80% and the urea concentration was increased by an equivalent amount. In nonuremic subjects, the gastric acidity was not altered, but in five of the six uremic patients, both basal and posthistamine acidity was initially low, but increased after oxytetracycline administration. Hypo- and anacidity were known to occur in patients with uremia, but had remained unexplained, and these studies revealed, for the first time, the striking decrease by an antibiotic (oxytetracycline) of the capacity of human gastric juice to convert urea into ammonia. From these results we concluded that the most likely explanation for the suppression of gastric ammonia (and its replacement by unsplit urea) after oxytetracycline was the eradication of urease-producing microorganisms in the stomach.[14]

These results were presented at the first World Congress of Gastroenterology in Washington in 1958, together with the data showing that the increased ammonia production from urea in uremic subjects could explain the gastric hypoacidity observed with uremia by its neutralization of the juice.[15] However, the international community did not believe that this urease activity had an infectious basis because the dogma was that bacteria could not survive in an acid environment. The most common argument used against our interpretation of the results of the antibiotic tests was the hypothesis that the tetracycline may not have been acting as an antibiotic, but rather in some direct chemical way; for instance, as a pharmacologic agent inhibiting the activities of a 'constitutive' urease present in the gastric cell.

To address this, we next used not only oxytetracycline, but also other structurally unrelated antibiotics. Our prior investigations were extended and expanded: a total of 50 hospitalized subjects were studied, 24 without evidence of renal dysfunction, 25 with uremia caused by chronic renal disease, and 1 patient with azotemia from obstructive uropathy. Oxytetracycline (20 mg/kg) was given orally for 4–7 days to 5 nonuremic and 6 uremic subjects; 300 mg of the same drug was injected intramuscularly daily for 3–8 days to 3 nonuremic and 3 uremic subjects. The blood urea concentration in the patients with uremia varied from 46 to 174 mg nitrogen/100 mL (N%) with an average of 114 mg N%, as compared with a mean of only 19 mg N% in the nonuremic patients. Five uremic and five nonuremic subjects received 20 mg/kg chloramphenicol orally for 4–7 days, and six nonuremic and five uremic subjects were treated similarly with 20 mg/kg erythromycin. Chemical measurements were carried out as described for the earlier studies. Increased blood urea concentration was again associated with high gastric ammonia concentration in uremic patients (FIGURE 3) compared with nonuremic subjects (FIGURE 4), in both the basal state and after administration of histamine. The mean ammonia concentrations of the basal and posthistamine gastric secretions were lowered significantly ($P < 0.05$) in the patients treated with oral oxytetracycline (FIGURES 3,4) and comparable effects were observed with erythromycin. The urea concentration in the gastric juice increased in association with the decrease in ammonia and both changes were of the same order of magnitude.

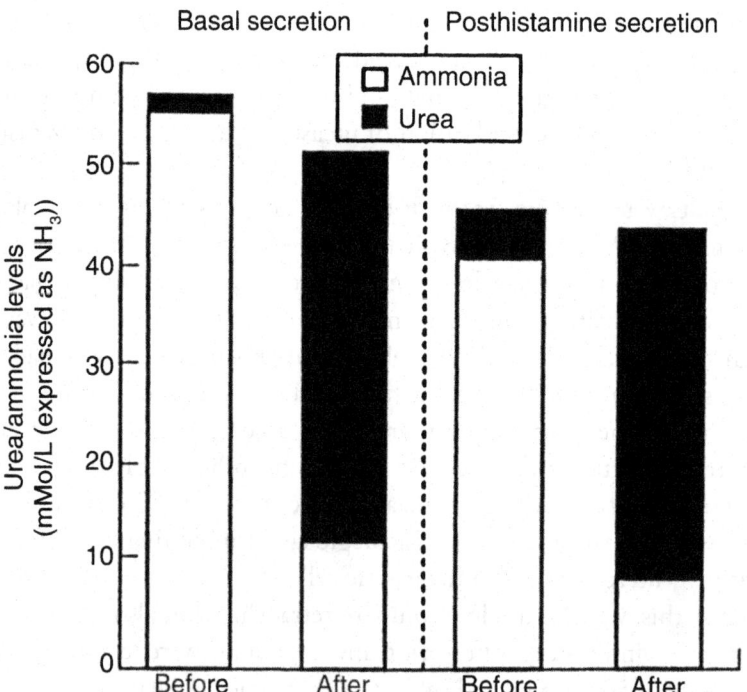

FIGURE 3 Mean gastric ammonia and urea concentrations in six uremic patients in their basal and posthistamine secretions before and after one week of treatment with oxytetracycline (20 mg/kg per day p.o.), which produced approximately 80% reduction in the level of gastric ammonia ($P < 0.05$), replaced by an equivalent amount of unsplit urea, illustrating the suppression of gastric urease activity. (Data from Lieber CS, Lefèvre A, *CR Soc Biol (Paris)* 1957; **151**: 1038–42 and *J Clin Invest* 1959; **38**: 1271–7.)

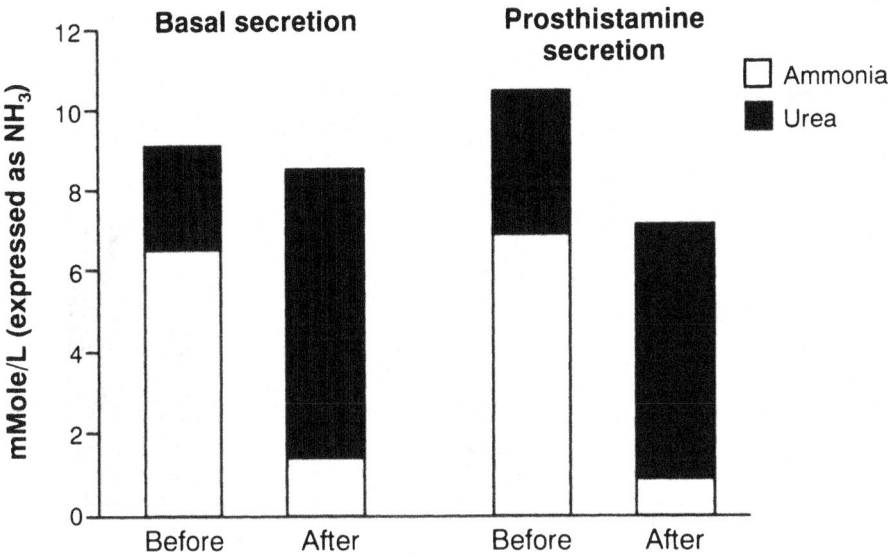

Figure 4 Mean gastric ammonia and urea concentrations in five nonuremic subjects in their basal and posthistamine secretions before and after one week of treatment with oxytetracycline (20 mg/kg per day p.o.), which resulted in a significant decrease in gastric ammonia and a corresponding increase in urea. (Data from Lieber CS, Lefèvre A, *CR Soc Biol (Paris)* 1957; **151**: 1038–42 and *J Clin Invest* 1959; **38**: 1271–7.)

In the patients with uremia, the decrease in ammonia was accompanied by a rise in total acidity with the appearance of free acid, which had been absent before (Figure 5), whereas in subjects without renal dysfunction, no change in acidity was detectable. Similar results were obtained when the values were calculated on the basis of hourly gastric output. No change in either chloride content or the volume of gastric juice was observed. Oxytetracycline was less effective when administered intramuscularly than when given by mouth, both in reducing gastric ammonia concentration and in increasing acidity. The levels of gastric ammonia, acid or chlorides were not significantly influenced by chloramphenicol.

The observed effects of the antibiotics on gastric secretion were reversible. In patients with uremia in whom the gastric ammonia concentration had been reduced by antibiotics, it increased again after cessation of the treatment. The relationship between the changes in gastric ammonia and acid concentrations was also studied in the one patient in whom the azotemia caused by obstructive

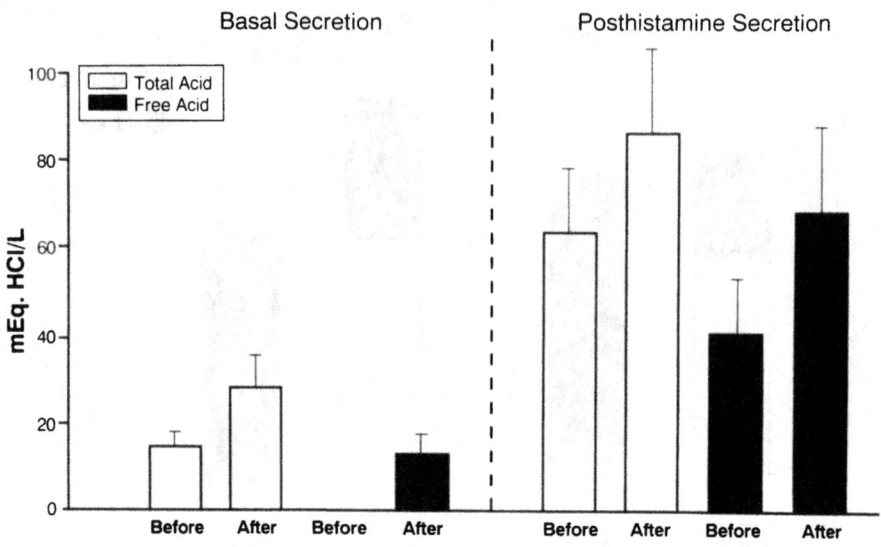

FIGURE 5 Total and free acid concentrations in the stomachs of the six uremic subjects of FIGURE 3. The suppression of ammonia was associated with a restoration of free acid, as well as an increase of total acid in the basal secretion and corresponding changes in the posthistamine response. (Data adapted from Lieber CS, Lefèvre A, *J Clin Invest* 1959; **38**: 1271–7.)

uropathy had been relieved by cystostomy. In that patient, the gastric ammonia content was lowered and gastric acidity rose in parallel with the fall in blood urea (FIGURE 6).

In eight patients with uremia caused by chronic glomerulonephritis in whom no change in blood urea concentration occurred during the period of investigation, administration of antibiotics also resulted in a significant decrease in gastric ammonia and a significant increase in gastric acidity.[16]

Because erythromycin exerted effects on urease activity and acidity similar to those of tetracycline, these results again strongly supported the bacterial hypothesis. After I received a fellowship to Harvard where I joined Charles S. Davidson and Rudi Schmid, they encouraged me to submit these observations to the *Journal of Clinical Investigation* in March 1959 and the report was accepted the same month;[16] the editor was obviously convinced, unlike many other people. Subsequently, when I moved to New York and the Mount Sinai School of Medicine, I carried out similar experiments in 21 normal and 15 azotemic subjects, but used other antibiotics, namely ampicillin (administered

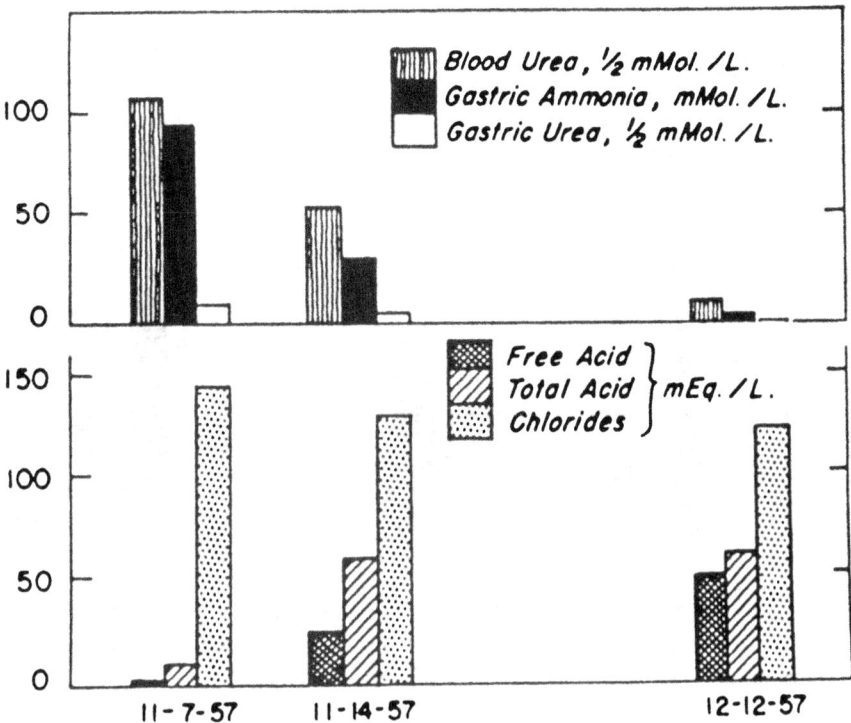

FIGURE 6 Effects of a decrease in blood urea on gastric ammonia content and acidity
(posthistamine secretion) in the patient with azotemia, caused by obstructive
uropathy, that was relieved by cystostomy. The gastric ammonia content lowered
proportionally to the blood urea and gastric acidity rose with the decrease in blood
urea. (Data reprinted with permission from Lieber CS, Lefèvre A, *J Clin Invest* 1959;
38: 1271–7.)

either p.o. or i.m.) or oral neomycin, and stimulated gastric acid secretion with
betazole instead of histamine.[17] The results (FIGURE 7) were similar to those
observed previously with oxytetracycline (FIGURE 4). Again, the ammonia produced from the urea was shown to be responsible for the gastric hypo- or
anacidity in the uremic subjects, whereas in individuals with normal blood
urea, there was not sufficient ammonia to affect the gastric acid.

Thus, the results of studies conducted in an aggregate of 68 patients in
whom four antibiotics as structurally different as oxytetracycline, erythromycin, neomycin and ampicillin had similar effects on gastric urease activity strongly supported the initial hypothesis that this effect was of an
antibacterial nature rather than caused by some pharmacologic inhibition of
enzyme activity.[14–16] We did not succeed, however, in culturing the bacteria.

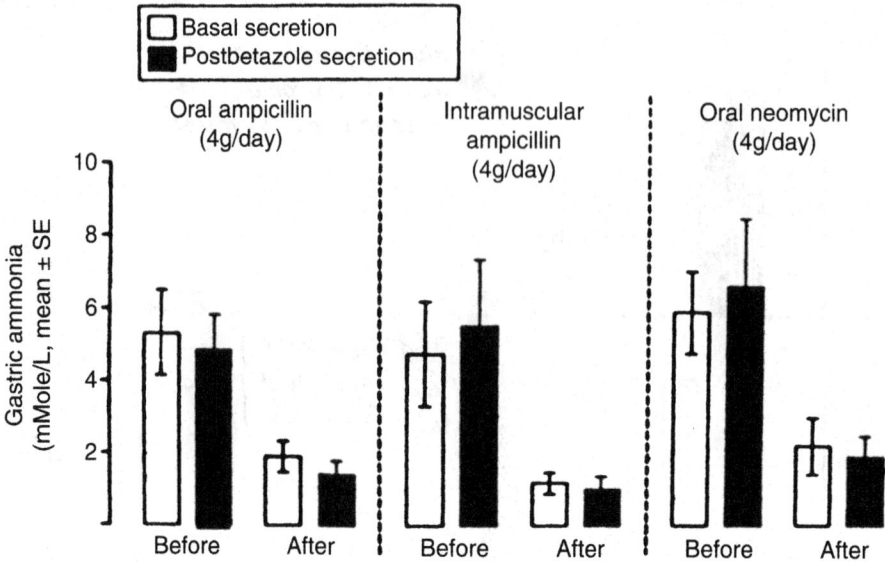

FIGURE 7 Effect of antibiotic treatment (7 days) on gastric ammonia concentration. The mean ammonia concentration in basal and postbetazole gastric juices is shown for 21 normal subjects before and after administration of the antibiotics. (Data reprinted with permission from Meyers S, Lieber CS, *Gastroenterology* 1976; **70**: 244–7.)

Because ammonia is a toxic compound, a long-standing debate started on its other possible pathogenic effects in the stomach, including gastritis, especially in conjunction with alcohol.[18] Gastric ammonia was also studied as a possible exacerbating factor in hepatic encephalopathy, especially in patients with uremia.

Role of gastric ammonia in hepatic encephalopathy

The tolerance of patients with liver disease to exogenous nitrogenous substances, including urea, was known to be poor.[19,20] Indeed, it had been established that oral administration of urea to patients with cirrhosis induced hepatic coma or precoma, and it was known that the ingested urea is split into ammonia by intestinal urease.[19,21] Because the ammonia resulting from the splitting of exogenous urea is reabsorbed into the bloodstream, urea administration increases the blood ammonia concentration[20] and this ammonia had been shown to be detrimental to the patient, thus explaining the adverse effects of urea ingestion.[19,22,23]

It became apparent that endogenous urea follows a similar catabolic pattern[24] and it was quantified by the administration of radioactive urea to normal subjects in whom it was demonstrated that at least 25% of the total urea produced in the body is converted to ammonia in the gastrointestinal tract.[25] The human body produces 23–46 g of urea daily, so the average amount of gastrointestinal ammonia formed is equivalent to about 4 g of nitrogen.[25] Similar studies have not been carried out in uremic patients and they would be difficult to do, as a steady state is unusual in uremia. It has been shown, however, that the urease mechanism has a high capacity; even in severe uremia, the proportion of gastric urea split into ammonia is the same as in normal subjects; for instance, in a case with blood urea levels as high as 174 mg N%, most of the gastric urea (85%) was split into ammonia.[14–16] It was therefore reasonable to assume that in patients with uremia, gastrointestinal ammonia production increased roughly in proportion to the blood urea level and thus, in subjects with a four-fold increase in blood urea, not uncommon in patients with uremia, gastrointestinal ammonia formation might reach very high levels, with about a four-fold increase of the 24-hour ammonia production (from 4 to 16 g). In patients with uremia, but normal liver function, the blood circulation levels of ammonia remain normal because of the high capacity of the normal liver to reconvert ammonia to urea.[26] However, in patients with liver disease, an ammonia load of 16 g nitrogen, an amount equivalent to that produced from at least 100 g of protein, is known to precipitate neurological disturbances, with precoma and coma in patients with serious liver disease, in association with an increase of arterial blood ammonia concentration.[19,26,27] Thus uremia, even of a moderate degree, appeared to be a potential danger for patients with liver disease and this entity was named the 'renal–hepatic syndrome', to differentiate it from the 'hepatorenal syndrome'.[28] Indeed, liver and kidney diseases often occur together, and this association had been hitherto characterized by the term 'hepatorenal syndrome'[29] because most clinical and experimental investigators interested in the hepatorenal syndrome had been concerned with the possible mechanism by which various hepatic diseases may alter renal function. The reverse possibility, namely, the effect of renal failure in patients with liver disease (i.e. the renal–hepatic syndrome) had been overlooked. We pointed out, however, that in patients with liver disease, the occurrence of even mild renal decompensation is often accompanied by the appearance or aggravation of symptoms usually attributed to failure of liver function (i.e. mental confusion, flapping tremor, and other signs of precoma or coma).[28] We postulated that a major mechanism for this 'renal–hepatic syndrome' was the increased ammonia production resulting from the uremia.

Patients with liver disease were studied to test the hypothesis that ammonia produced in the stomach could play an important role as a precipitant factor of hepatic encephalopathy. To that effect, antibiotics were given to patients with cirrhosis and we observed that the disappearance of the ammonia from the stomach (FIGURE 8) was indeed paralleled by a clinical improvement of their encephalopathy.[26] Thus, reduction of gastric ammonia with oxytetracycline was achieved not only in normal subjects and in patients with uremia, but also in those with cirrhosis.[26] The exacerbation by the ammonia derived from urea of the encephalopathy in patients with underlying liver disease, especially when renal insufficiency developed, and the success of antibacterial treatment in alleviating symptoms were clearly attributable to the fact that 'these antibiotics prevent urea splitting by interfering with urease activity of bacterial origin'.[28] Therefore, based on our prior case reports of successful therapeutic use of oxytetracycline in cirrhotic subjects with encephalopathy, shown to be

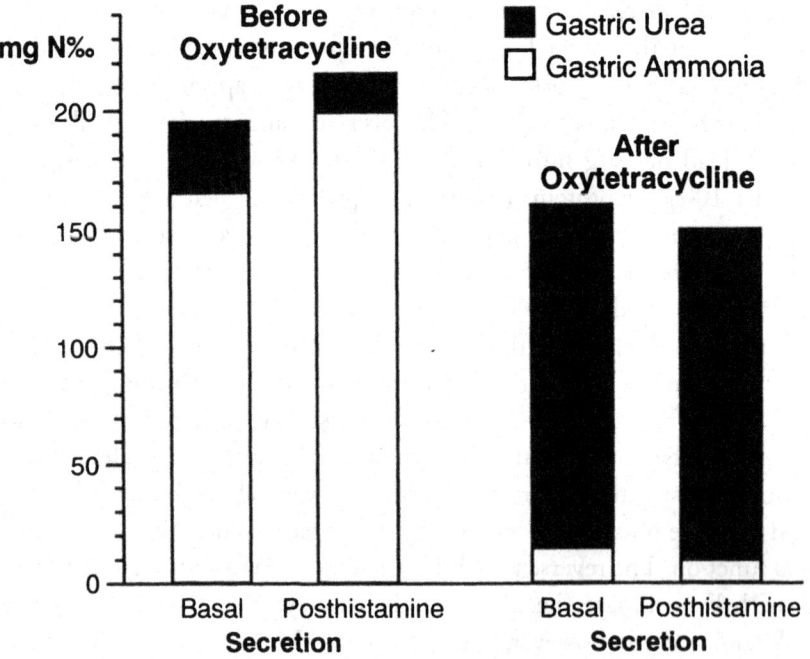

FIGURE 8 Effect of oxytetracycline on gastric ammonia and urea levels in a patient with liver cirrhosis. After 5 days of antibiotic treatment (20 mg/kg per day), there was a striking decrease in the gastric ammonia concentration. (Data from Lieber CS, Lefèvre A, *Acta Clin Belg* 1958; **13**: 328–57.)

associated with a striking inhibition in the production of ammonia from gastric urease, it was suggested that antibiotics be used to prevent this complication (FIGURE 8).[26] Because some antibiotics are excreted by the kidney and thus may be retained in uremia, the need for judicious selection of the antibiotics was emphasized.[28] The call for antibiotic therapy against bacterial gastric urease came from Boston and Harvard[16] (and not from Brussels), but it was still generally ignored, and it was another 26 years after our original description of the effects of antibiotics on human gastric urease[14] for the medical fraternity to eventually be convinced by Warren and Marshall that there were indeed pathogenic bacteria in the stomach after they had successfully cultured *Helicobacter pylori*.[30]

Forty years after those original studies, I returned to my original interest in gastric ammonia and encephalopathy, and confirmed the initial studies using a more modern approach to the eradication of *H. pylori* (amoxicillin with omeprazole), verified the disappearance of *H. pylori* and quantified the encephalopathy with a Number Connection Test, thus documenting quantitatively the role of gastric bacterial infection in the pathogenesis of encephalopathy.[31]

Summary and conclusions

The clinical studies (started in the 1950s) showed that various antibiotics given to volunteers resulted in a striking decrease of the gastric ammonia content, stoichiometrically replaced by urea. The results were explained by the fact that when urea diffuses from the blood into the gastric secretion, it is split by a gastric urease, ostensibly of bacterial origin in view of its elimination by various structurally unrelated antibiotics, such as oxytetracycline, erythromycin, ampicillin and neomycin. This gastric urease had a high enzymatic capacity because even in patients with uremia, most of the urea reaching the stomach was split into ammonia. As a consequence, in patients with renal insufficiency, gastric ammonia levels were found to be extremely high and capable of neutralizing gastric acid, thereby accounting for the previously unexplained observation that patients with uremia often suffer from gastric hypo- or anacidity. Indeed, the anacidity was fully reversed by antibiotic treatment. This resurgence of gastric acidity in patients with a gastric mucosa weakened by chronic uremia also explained the relative frequency of acute gastrointestinal bleeding observed in such patients when they underwent dialysis. In subjects with underlying liver disease, the increased gastric ammonia production resulting from uremia was shown to also be associated with increased blood levels of ammonia, which aggravated the encephalopathy. The latter was found to respond to antibiotic treatment and its associated decrease in the gastric ammonia produced from endogenous urea. Thus, ammonia formed from endogenous urea by bacterial gastric urease was found to have several negative effects; namely, gastric hypo- or anacidity in patients with uremia, and exacerbation of encephalopathy in patients with underlying liver disease when they developed uremia. The recognition of the bacterial origin of the gastric urease and its eradication by antibiotics resulted in the elimination of these untoward effects. The most important consequence of gastric infection with *H. pylori* is, of course, its adverse effects on gastroduodenal ulcer disease, which, following the pioneering work of Warren and Marshall[30] on the pathogenesis of gastroduodenal ulcer and the importance of antibacterial treatment, is now widely accepted, but its involvement in gastritis is still debated;[18] hopefully, it will now take less than three or four decades for the role of *H. pylori* in the pathogenesis (and hence treatment) of this condition to be accepted as well.

References

1   Lieber CS. Study of inhibitory effects of parasympatholytic drugs on the gastric secretion in the rat. *CR Soc Biol (Paris)* 1956; **150**: 600–3.
2   Lieber CS. Inhibitory effect of atropine and two synthetic parasympatholytic agents on gastric posthistamine secretion in man. *Acta Gastroenterol Belg* 1956; **19**: 399–408.
3   Verbanck M, Toussaint C, Lieber CS, Lefèvre A. Gastroduodenal bleeding complicating acute anuria during treatment by artificial kidney. *Acta Gastroenterol Belg* 1957; **20**: 798–809.
4   Simici D, Vladesco R, Popesco M. Recherches sur l'urée et l'ammoniac des liquides gastriques a l'état pathologique. *CR Soc Biol (Paris)* 1929; **101**: 202–4.
5   Fitzgerald O, Murphy P. Studies on the physiological chemistry and clinical significance of urease and urea with special reference to the stomach. *Irish J Med Sci* 1950; **292**: 97–159.
6   Von Korff RW, Ferguson DJ, Glick D. Role of urease in gastric mucosa. III. Plasma urea as source of ammonium ion in gastric juice of histamine-stimulated dog. *Am J Physiol* 1951; **165**: 695–700.
7   Bessman SP, Staufer JC. Factor affecting the appearance of ammonia in the gastric juice (Abstract). *J Clin Invest* 1957; **36**: 874.
8   Henning N. Die Bakterien Besiedlung des gesunden Magens und Kranken. *Arch F Verdauungs kr* 1930; **47**: 1–59.
9   Doenges JL. Spirochetes in the gastric glands of *Macacus rhesus* and of man without related disease. *Arch Pathol* 1939; **27**: 469–77.
10   Luck JM, Seth TN. Gastric urease. *Biochem J* 1924; **18**: 1227–31.
11   Conway EJ. *Microdiffusion Analysis and Volumetric Error*. London: Crosby, Lockwood & Son, Ltd, 1957.
12   Schales O, Schales SS. A simple and accurate method for the determination of chloride et al. in biological fluids. *J Biol Chem* 1941; **140**: 879–84.
13   Kimbel KH, Kinzlmeier H. Quantitative intragastrale Bestimmung der Saureproduktion des gesunden und kranken Magens. *Gastroenterologia* 1954; **81**: 193–206.
14   Lieber CS, Lefèvre A. Effect of oxytetracycline on acidity, ammonia and urea in gastric juice in normal and uremic subjects. *CR Soc Biol (Paris)* 1957; **151**: 1038–42.

[15] Lieber CS, Lefèvre A. Effects of antibiotics on gastric juice in normal and uremic subjects: Ammonia as source of hypoacidity in uremic patients. In: *Proceedings of the World Congress of Gastroenterology*, Vol. 1. Baltimore: Williams & Wilkins Co., 1959; 117–18.

[16] Lieber CS, Lefèvre A. Ammonia as source of gastric hypoacidity in patients with uremia. *J Clin Invest* 1959; **38**: 1271–7.

[17] Meyers S, Lieber CS. Reduction of gastric ammonia by ampicillin in normal and azotemic subjects. *Gastroenterology* 1976; **70**: 244–7.

[18] Lieber CS. Gastritis in the alcoholic: Relationship to gastric alcohol metabolism and *Helicobacter pylori. Addiction Biol* 1998; **3**: 423–33.

[19] Phillips GB, Schwartz R, Gabuzda GJ Jr, Davidson CS. The syndrome of impending hepatic coma in patients with cirrhosis of the liver given certain nitrogenous substances. *N Engl J Med* 1952; **247**: 239–46.

[20] Webster LT, Davidson CS. Sources of blood ammonium after feeding protein to patients with hepatic cirrhosis. *J Clin Invest* 1956; **35**: 742–3.

[21] Dintzis RZ, Hastings AB. The effect of antibiotic on urea breakdown in mice. *Proc Natl Acad Sci USA* 1953; **39**: 571–8.

[22] Van Caulaert C, Deviller C, Halff M. Troubles provoqués par l'ingestion de sels ammoniacaux chez l'homme atteint de cirrhose de Laenne C. *CR Soc Biol (Paris)* 1932; **111**: 739–40.

[23] Sherlock S, Summerskill WHJ, White LP, Phear EA. Portal-systemic encephalopathy. *Lancet* 1954; **2**: 453–7.

[24] Webster LT Jr, Gabuzda GJ. Relation of azotemia to blood ammonium in patients with hepatic cirrhosis. *Arch Intern Med* 1959; **103**: 15–22.

[25] Walser M, Bodenlos LJ. Urea metabolism in man. *J Clin Invest* 1959; **38**: 1617–26.

[26] Lieber CS, Lefèvre A. Ammonia and intermediary metabolism in hepatic coma: Value of the determination of blood ammonia in the diagnosis and management of cirrhosis. *Acta Clin Belg* 1958; **13**: 328–57.

[27] Summerskill WHJ, Davidson EA, Sherlock S, Steiner RE. The neuropsychiatric syndrome associated with hepatic cirrhosis and extensive portal collateral circulation. *Q J Med* 1956; **25**: 245–66.

[28] Lieber CS, Davidson CS. Complications resulting from renal failure in patients with liver disease. *Arch Intern Med* 1960; **106**: 749–52.

[29] Davidson CS. Hepatic Coma. In: Schiff L (ed.) *Diseases of the Liver*. Philadelphia: JB Lippincott Co., 1956; 234.

[30] Warren JR, Marshall B. Unidentified curved bacilli on gastric epithelium in active chronic gastritis. *Lancet* 1983; **1**: 1273–5.

[31] Dasani BM, Sigal SH, Lieber CS. Analysis of the risk factors for chronic hepatic encephalopathy: The role of *Helicobacter pylori* infection. *Am J Gastroenterol* 1998; **93**: 726–31.

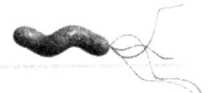

CHAPTER 6

A personal history of giving birth to the cohort phenomenon of peptic ulcer disease

Amnon Sonnenberg

Introduction

In my lifetime, aside from many small encounters with *Helicobacter pylori*, I experienced two major ones early in my career. I did not appreciate them at the time, and even now I still do not understand all of their meaning. The first occurred during my gastroenterology fellowship in Zürich in 1978, when I tried to implement a technique for measuring intragastric pH. In these experiments, I was helped by an American medical student, John Bartmess, who had met a Swiss girl he planned to marry and he wanted to combine his visit to Switzerland and her family with a 2-month research clerkship in our gastroenterology laboratory. John tested the pH measuring equipment diligently on several patients, many of the laboratory technicians, and most frequently on himself. After three weeks he came down with flu-like symptoms that included nausea and epigastric pain for three days. When he resumed his experiments one week later, he had become achlorhydric. On upper gastrointestinal endoscopy, he was found to have a small antral ulcer and severe acute gastritis on all biopsies, which were evaluated by both the state-of-the-art techniques at our own hospital, including electron microscopy, and several other well-known gastrointestinal pathologists. Except for a massive infiltration of the gastric mucosa with polymorphonucleocytes, nothing out of the ordinary was described by the many pathologists who looked at the biopsies. In a subsequent publication of the case, we speculated that John had become infected by some unknown pathogen that had led to a transient achlorhydria.[1] Dr Walter Peterson reports elsewhere in this book about his larger series of similar cases that were later identified as instances of acute infection with

H. pylori transmitted through pH probes, so I will not dwell on this event any longer, except for using this first encounter with *H. pylori* as a reminder of the fact that most people, including pathologists, see and accept only what they already know and fail to recognize what they do not understand.

Susser and Stein: Birth-cohort patterns in peptic ulcer disease

After my fellowship, I joined the Gastroenterology Division at the University of Düsseldorf as a junior faculty member. In addition to continuing my experiments on the physiology of the upper gastrointestinal tract, I became increasingly more interested in the epidemiology of peptic ulcer disease (PUD). During a research project devoted to the socioeconomic impact of PUD, we analyzed the time trends of mortality from peptic ulcer in Germany and the mortality data were subsequently published as a separate article.[2] Looking at the German data, we wondered whether they would reveal a birth-cohort phenomenon, as previously described in mortality data from England and Wales. In a landmark paper written by Mervyn Susser and his wife Zena Stein,[3] it was shown that the temporal trends of peptic ulcer were more closely related to the time of birth of individual patients than to the time when they developed their ulcer and died from it (FIGURE 1). When the original paper was published in *The Lancet* in 1962, the overall frequency of both gastric and duodenal ulcer was still rising in the British population, and the British birth-cohorts born between 1870 and 1890 carried the highest risk of developing gastric and duodenal ulcer, respectively. As these cohorts grew older and their general age-related mortality increased, the overall number of deaths associated with bleeding and perforated peptic ulcers was still rising in the population. Susser and Stein speculated that eventually, as these high-risk cohorts grew older and their proportion in the population declined, the occurrence and mortality of peptic ulcer would start to fall again, and in fact from their birth-cohort analysis of peptic ulcer mortality in England and Wales between 1900 and 1959, they were able to correctly predict the future decline of PUD 10–20 years prior to its actual occurrence.

Birth-cohort analysis was introduced by Wade Hampton Frost[4] and others[5,6] to study the time trends of tuberculosis in the USA, and the method also proved useful in linking rubella embryopathy with the periods of birth following rubella epidemics in Australia. Although it constitutes an established technique in the armamentarium of epidemiologists, the birth-cohort analysis is not well explained by most textbooks and it takes additional time and effort to be fully understood. I have wondered why, despite these

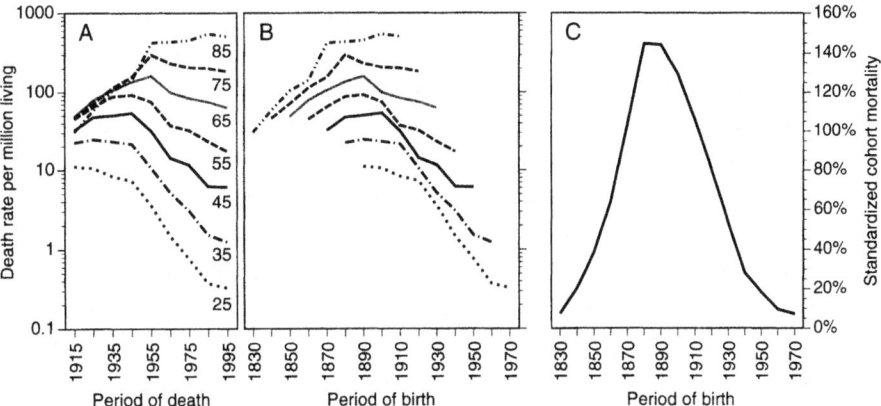

FIGURE 1 Age-specific death rates from duodenal ulcer in England and Wales between 1911 and 1998 plotted as period–age contours (panel A), as cohort–age contours (panel B), and as standardized cohort mortality ratio (panel C). The different lines (full, dashed, dotted etc.) refer to the same ages in both panels A and B. Ten-year age groups are labeled by their central age; for instance, 25 instead of 20–29, 35 instead of 30–39 etc. Similarly, periods of death or birth are labeled by their central year; for instance, 1915 instead of 1911–1920. Men and women are analyzed jointly.

obstacles, the paper in *The Lancet* has always remained part of the common knowledge among investigators interested in PUD. The obvious reason, of course, was its publication in a widely distributed medical journal. The second reason was that people liked the article for the wrong reasons, as it was assumed to provide evidence for the psychosomatic nature of peptic ulcer. Susser and Stein speculated that the stress associated with urbanization in England around the turn of the century led to strong and lasting mental or physical imprints in subjects born during this transitional period of English history. These imprints rendered subjects susceptible to PUD for the remainder of their life. When stress and psychological factors were still much in vogue to explain peptic ulcer, the influence of 'urbanization' seemed one of the strongest arguments in favor of such a hypothesis.

The ubiquity of the birth-cohort phenomenon

Germany did not seem a good country to re-examine the birth-cohort phenomenon of peptic ulcer because of the disruptions wrought by two world wars on the size and composition of its population, the repeated changes to its land area, as well as the lack of mortality statistics clearly separating gastric from duodenal ulcer prior to 1950. For the reasons, I was concerned that the German statistics would yield a poor example for re-visiting the birth-cohort pattern of peptic ulcer in order to convince a critical reviewer of its general occurrence. Switzerland, in contradistinction, had managed to remain a neutral country and keep out of all armed European conflicts since 1848. Its population had remained largely stable, and well-maintained health statistics were available for peptic ulcer since 1921. The data showed a clear-cut birth-cohort phenomenon very similar to the data from England and Wales.[7] Although Switzerland, as with most European countries, had experienced an industrial revolution at the beginning of the 19th century and a resultant expansion of its urban population throughout the remainder of the 19th century, the socioeconomic changes and their impact on public health and culture, population growth and political climate were less dramatic than in England. Urbanization suddenly seemed a far less valid explanation for the birth-cohort pattern of both gastric and duodenal ulcers. The risk for gastric ulcer peaked in generations born 10–20 years prior to those affected most by duodenal ulcer (FIGURE 2), and although this phenomenon is clearly visible in Susser and Stein's original data, those authors did not take pains to explain it. However, the occurrence of a similar time lag between the development of gastric and duodenal ulcers in Switzerland and in Germany could no longer be ignored. Urbanization lost its explanatory appeal even more, as it could not account for such obvious differences in the behavior of the two ulcer types.

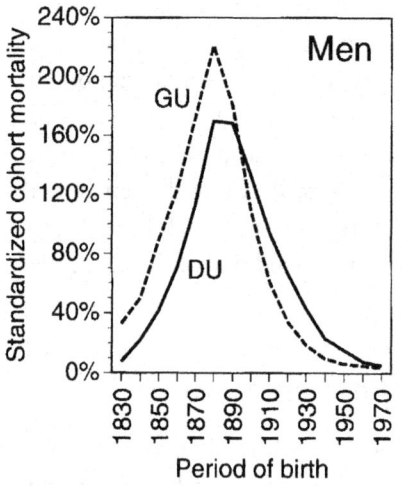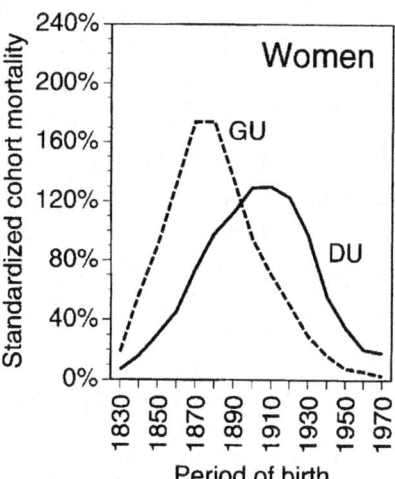

FIGURE 2 Standardized cohort mortality ratio of gastric ulcer (GU) and duodenal ulcer (DU) analyzed separately for men and women from England and Wales.

For me, it was an almost breathtaking experience to key-in large amounts of data reflecting populations and ulcer deaths from distant countries and times long ago, and after many and lengthy manipulations suddenly see clear-cut patterns emerge. Almost magically the curves of age-specific death rates would align themselves to form a single hyperbola and give rise to a unique birth-cohort phenomenon. Despite the confidence gained from the consistency and uniformity of the observed patterns, I wanted to ascertain that I had not been fooled by a systematic bias or some mistake that an experienced epidemiologist would be able to identify immediately. Since the publication of their original paper, the Sussers had moved from England to the USA to work in the Department of Epidemiology at Columbia University in New York. Although their interests had shifted from peptic ulcer to neuro-epidemiology, they still maintained their interest in general epidemiology. During a visit for a job interview at the Mount Sinai Hospital in New York in 1984, I also took the opportunity to visit the Sussers at their home in Hastings on Hudson. After going over my plots of birth-cohorts from various countries, Mervyn Susser reassured me about the validity of my data analyses.

The presence of a birth-cohort pattern in three separate countries, that is, England, Germany and Switzerland, suggested that the birth-cohort might be a general phenomenon underlying all ulcer mortality. Mervyn Susser indicated that he had also considered testing the birth-cohort phenomenon in other countries besides England, but for various reasons the project had never gotten started. After publishing the data from Switzerland, I tried to systematically accumulate ulcer data from all countries with a central office of health statistics. At the time of the analysis, mortality data broken down by age, sex and ulcer type were only available from countries in Western Europe, North America, Australia, New Zealand and Japan. The data from countries for which vital statistics covered sufficiently long time periods revealed similar trends (FIGURES 3,4). In all the statistics alike, the time of birth exerted a stronger and more obvious influence on ulcer mortality than the time of ulcer occurrence. Peptic ulcer mortality was highest among birth-cohorts born before the turn of the 19th century, with similar patterns observed in men and women. The peak of gastric ulcer preceded that of duodenal ulcer by 10–20 years in most countries, and nowhere did duodenal ulcer precede gastric ulcer.[8,9]

The meaning of the birth-cohort phenomenon

Because genetically determined mechanisms stay unchanged during historical time periods, the marked temporal trends of gastric and duodenal ulcer disease indicated that their occurrence was largely influenced by exogenous risk

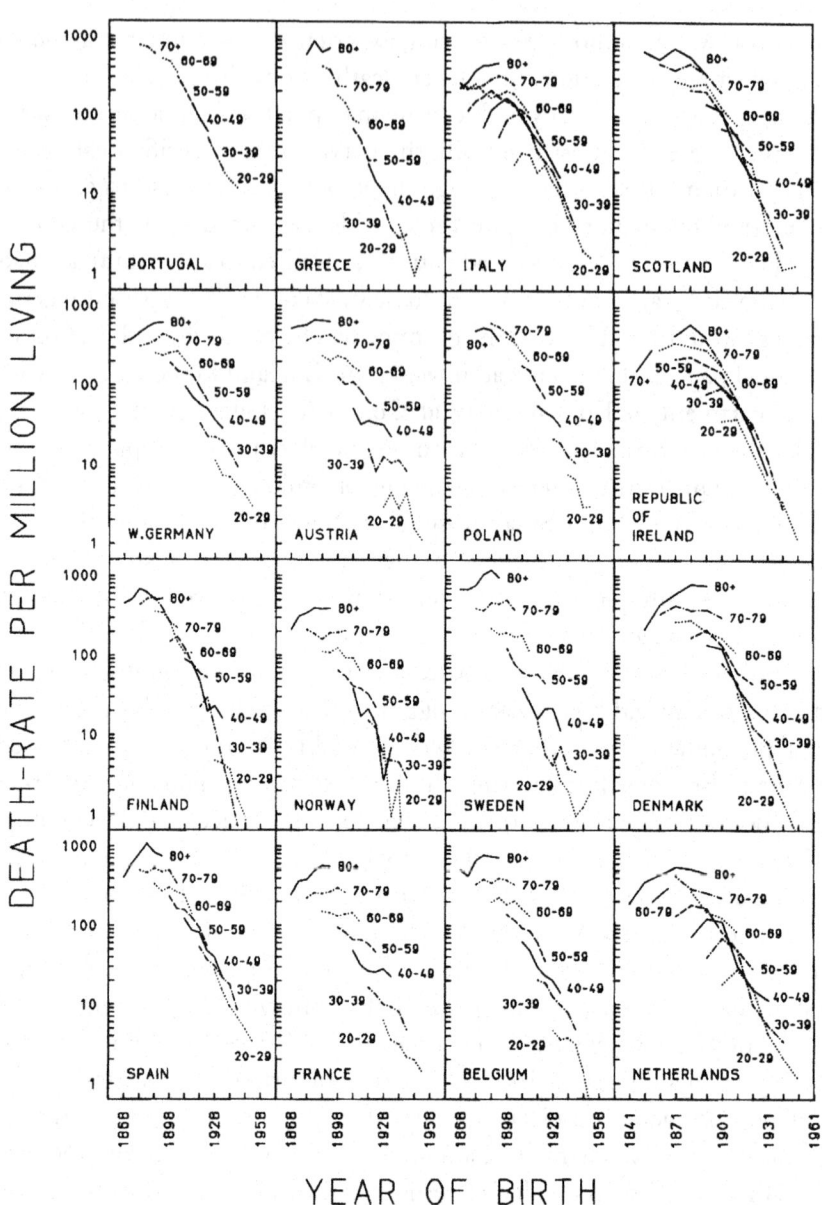

FIGURE 3 Cohort–age contours of gastric ulcer among men from different countries.

factors. The simpler and more consistent pattern obtained by considering the patients' period of birth rather than death implies that influences during or shortly after birth are very important. A birth-cohort pattern suggests that exposure to the relevant risk factors of the disease occurs during early life

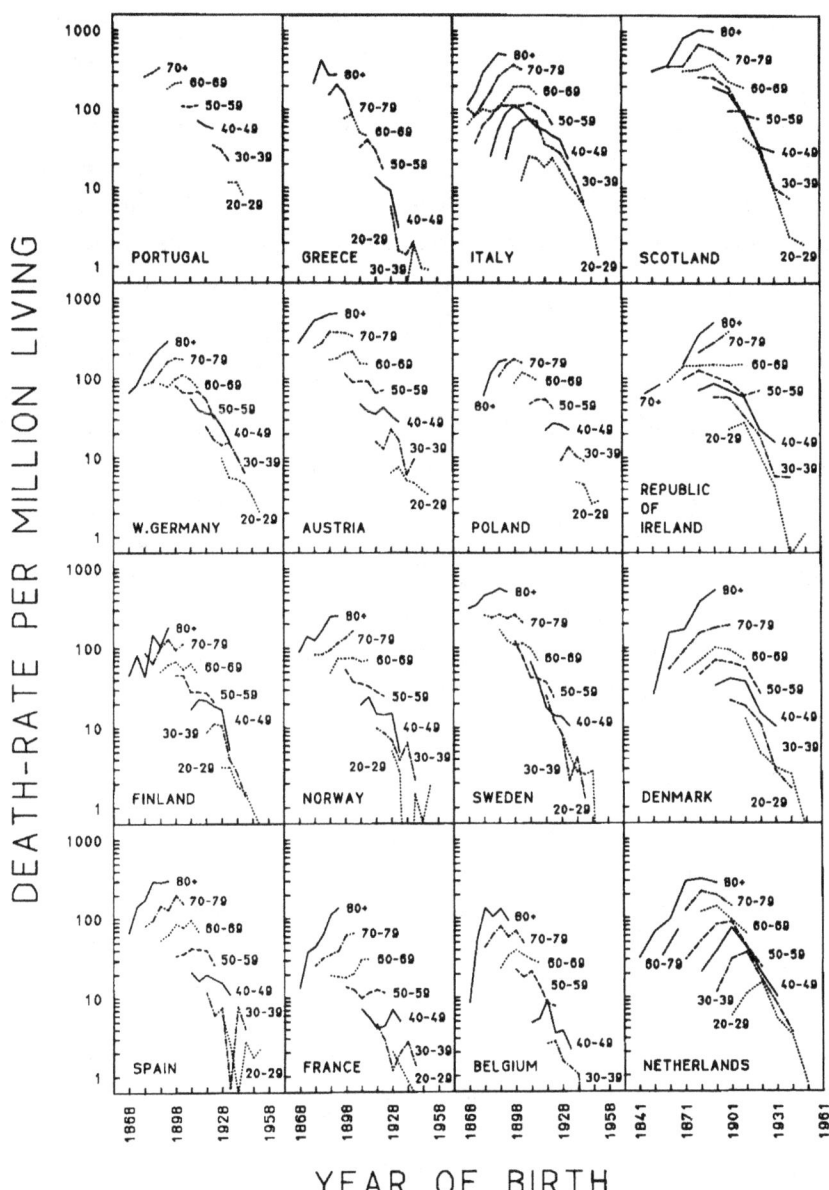

FIGURE 4 Cohort–age contours of duodenal ulcer among men from different countries.

between the prenatal period and adolescence. The risk factors must exert their effect within a limited time interval and the amount or type of exposure must be changing with time, otherwise successive generations could not exhibit rapidly varying rates of disease occurrence. As the exposure to the risk factor(s) changes over time, consecutive generations, that is, birth-cohorts, come to reflect its varying influence on the risk of developing the disease.

The occurrence of a birth-cohort phenomenon indicated that environmental factors were important in the etiology of gastric and duodenal ulcers. In order to learn about the nature of these factors, I believed that it would be important to pinpoint more precisely the age at which the environmental influences start becoming effective. When I embarked on these studies, *H. pylori* had not been discovered. Because PUD and its resultant mortality have always been rare events in childhood, no representative patterns could be obtained by analyzing the data from any individual country. To overcome the problem of small numbers in the young age groups, I pooled the mortality data from 18 different countries in which vital statistics with respect to peptic ulcer covered at least the time since 1951. Age-specific death rates were calculated as the weighted averages from 16 European countries, the USA and Japan. Two independent types of analyses suggested that for both ulcers the environmental factors started exerting their influence before the age of 15 years.[10] In the case of gastric ulcer, the parallelism in the geographic distribution of the disease and between the curves of successive age groups started at the age of 5 years. In duodenal ulcer, the parallelism did not start before the age of 15 years.

Dealing with journals and reviewers

Except for the very first paper that had analyzed the birth-cohort phenomenon in Switzerland, it proved very difficult to get any of the subsequent studies published, and many of the articles languished in various editorial offices for years. The birth-cohort analysis predicted that the incidence and prevalence of PUD would drop in the general population. First and foremost, it was difficult for reviewing gastroenterologists to accept the idea that one of their major and favorite diseases was about to fade into nonexistence. Gastric ulcer had given the profession part of its name. The reviewers tried to concoct all kinds of complicated schemes that would explain away the obvious time trends.

The period–age contours of peptic ulcer are characterized by the simultaneous occurrence of rising and falling mortality rates in old and young patients, respectively. The seeming discrepancy and discontinuity in the age-specific death rates only become resolved if the same type of data are plotted vagainst the year of birth (FIGURE I). Without paying much attention to the age-specific trends, however, some reviewers contended that initially the improvement in diagnosis through the introduction of X-rays had given rise to the detection of more peptic ulcers. Subsequently, the diagnostic precision added by fiberoptic endoscopy had led to weeding out unspecific dyspepsia and to a virtual decline in the number of cases. Different versions of this argument suggested that changes in physicians' awareness regarding peptic ulcer or in the coding practices used by the International Classification of Disease were responsible for the trends. Others tried to explain the recent decline as the results of medical improvements in the management of complicated ulcers, such as aseptic surgical conditions, intensive care units, blood transfusions and antibiotics. Some would even incriminate the introduction of histamine-2 receptor antagonists, although these became clinically available only in 1977 and could have affected only one data point, at best, representing a 5- or 10-year time period in an analysis that covered 50–80 years overall. More sophisticated reviewers assumed that recent changes in treatment (or diagnosis) had benefited young patients more than the old and had, thus, contributed to the differential time trends. Such arguments failed to account for the fact, however, that in some countries with far-reaching vital statistics, the rise and fall of peptic ulcer could be appreciated even in a single age-group (FIGURE 1).

By plotting peptic ulcer death rates against the year of birth, one is given the opportunity to seemingly open a window and view most of the 19th century, even if the data themselves were generated during the 20th century. An occasional reviewer dismissed any data 'that were more than 100-years-old'. Some reviewers failed to understand the time shift between periods of death and periods of birth. They admonished the author that the cohort-age contours covered time periods only until 20 years ago and requested to see 'more recent data'. Many argued that, considering a case-fatality rate of less than 5%, mortality was an unreliable parameter to assess the time trends of PUD, and they wanted mortality to be replaced by similarly far-reaching incidence data. The vital statistics are particularly suited to analyze temporal trends of diseases, because they have been recorded for the longest time periods and because they are available from many different countries. Subsequent studies showed that a birth-cohort pattern shaped the time trends of various other parameters of ulcer morbidity besides mortality, such as hospitalization, disability pensions and perforations.[11–14]

Lastly, reviewers questioned the uniqueness of the birth-cohort phenomenon in PUD. They suggested that it stemmed from some foggy and complicated means of data manipulation that would yield similar patterns in any other type of disease or that the birth-cohort phenomenon represented a general characteristic of all mortality. The truth is that the time trends of the vast majority of diseases do not reveal any underlying birth-cohort phenomenon. Only a few other diseases besides peptic ulcer are characterized by a cohort pattern, such as celiac disease, tuberculosis, laryngeal cancer and lung cancer. In both laryngeal and lung cancer, it can be related to the acquisition of smoking habits during adolescence. And not all birth-cohort patterns are alike. In lung cancer, for instance, the ascent and decline occur more slowly and the peak appears much broader than in peptic ulcer. Generations born around 1920 are the ones most affected, and the rise and fall of lung cancer exists only in men, not in women.[15] The only other gastrointestinal disease that I have found to present a clear-cut birth-cohort pattern is ulcerative colitis.

The review system is based on the idealized concept that one's scientific colleagues will objectively assess the merits of new data and that by a friendly exchange of opposing arguments the common truth will be agreed upon. It is usually impossible to counter all arguments raised with hard evidence, because they often reflect beliefs, judgments or conclusions that defy objective verification or falsification. The critiques may represent a different interpretation of identical data or stem from a different way of seeing and summarizing the evidence. Many comments regarding the birth-cohort phenomenon reflected the deeply held belief that the practice of medicine (through diagnosis and therapy) exerted a major influence on the time trends of disease. If this argument held true, however, epidemiology as a serious research endeavor could be easily dismissed because all its results would depend primarily on the success, and occasional mistakes, of physicians. Reviewers would also, in various forms, blame the vital statistics for their apparent imperfection. They argued that these data dealt with death, contained no means of ascertaining diagnostic accuracy, and relied on varying standards of certification, to name just a few points of criticism. Although such a line of thought may appear valid on the surface, it actually fails to acknowledge that all scientific advance is ultimately based on inherently imperfect data. Perfect data only become available after the scientific problem has been solved and the issue under investigation has become trivial. Every hospital laboratory, for instance, can now prove the presence of *H. pylori* in patients with duodenal ulcer.

Reviewers and editors alike failed to understand that the possibility of other explanations did not necessarily invalidate the investigator's own interpretation. The mere presence of some complicated theoretical construct to explain the data by other means does not automatically refute the birth-cohort assumption, and the onus of proving or disproving all seemingly competing hypotheses should not be placed exclusively on the author. Ockham's razor suggests that natural phenomena are best explained by the smallest number of the least complicated hypotheses. A single hypothesis, such as a birth-cohort phenomenon, appears far more probable than a complicated theory that involves multiple assumptions about the interacting changes in the practices of coding, diagnosis, therapy and their simultaneous and ubiquitous occurrence all over the globe.

Risk factors to explain the birth-cohort patterns

Shortly after discovering the birth-cohort patterns in almost all types of ulcer statistics, I started an investigation of the possible environmental risks contributing to its occurrence. The search for risk factors included, among many others, consumption of aspirin and other non-steroidal anti-inflammatory drugs (NSAID), smoking, physical exercise and occupational workload.[16]

- Aspirin was first introduced in Germany in 1899 when peptic ulcer had already started its descent among consecutive generations.
- Cohort analysis of lifetime cigarette consumption revealed a birth-cohort phenomenon with a peak consumption occurring among male generations born around 1920. When I did the study in 1984, smoking was still rising in consecutive female cohorts.[17] The birth-cohort patterns of cigarette consumption match those of lung cancer, but not peptic ulcer.[15]
- There is some preliminary physiological evidence to suggest that physical exercise stimulates acid secretion.[18–20]
- Several epidemiologic studies show a correlation between occupational workload and the prevalence of peptic ulcer.[21–23] Workload appeared to be a stronger risk factor for duodenal ulcer.[22] Cumulative lifetime energy expenditure is characterized by a birth-cohort phenomenon that resembles that of peptic ulcer.[24] Although there is a rise during the 19th century followed by a marked decline during the 20th century, the match between energy expenditure and peptic ulcer disease is far from perfect. I think that gender-related differences in occupational workload could explain some of the male predominance with respect to duodenal ulcer.

During a wide-ranging search for potential risk factors I also came across dietary salt as a potential risk factor for gastric cancer and gastric ulcer, but less so for duodenal ulcer.[25,26] However, I could not accumulate enough age-specific data on dietary salt during different time periods to conduct a rigorous analysis of cumulative lifetime salt consumption among consecutive birth-cohorts. I believe that aspirin, occupational workload and dietary salt consumption are important risk factors in the development of peptic ulcer, but I no longer believe that they are primarily responsible for its underlying birth-cohort pattern.

Based on the results of these analyses, I could not convince myself that I had found the main culprit for the birth-cohort pattern. I began to entertain the possibility that some childhood infection, as in the rubella paradigm, might have been responsible. I was also familiar with an article, published by Simon Rune and his coworker in *The Lancet*, that suggested that gastrointestinal infection by herpes simplex might be responsible for the occurrence of peptic ulcer.[27] My wife worked as a diabetologist with insulin pumps and had established a collaboration with scientists at the national laboratories of the Medical Research Council (MRC) in Mill Hill, London. Building on these connections, in 1983 I visited the virologists at the MRC to obtain some ideas on how to pursue an infectious etiology. I could not imagine that a bacterium would have been missed by the hundreds of previous ulcer researchers. The advices were as useful as many others given subsequently by basic scientists consulted: develop an 'animal model' or raise highly specific monoclonal antibodies against *Herpes simplex* and most other viruses known to mankind.

The appearance of *Helicobacter pylori*

The discovery of *H. pylori* has changed our concepts of PUD and gastric cancer. In developing countries with high prevalence rates of *H. pylori*, the infection is acquired during early childhood, and by the age of 20 years, over 80% of the population have become infected.[28] Because the immune system is unable to rid the body of *H. pylori*, any infection acquired during early childhood remains a lifelong event. The rise and fall of peptic ulcer could, thus, represent the historic scars of rising and falling infection rates experienced during early childhood by large fractions of the population, as in a birth-cohort phenomenon.[29] The marked decline in the occurrence of peptic ulcer during the past two decades is matched by a steep decline in the infection rates with *H. pylori* in all Western countries.[30] Urbanization and the crowded living conditions of the expanding cities during the beginning of the industrial revolution at the onset of the 19th century probably meant a decline in hygiene for large fractions of the population with a concomitant rise in exposure to *H. pylori*. Subsequently, the increase in knowledge about the importance of hygiene in preventing the spread of diseases led to various governmental and municipal efforts to improve sanitation and supply clean water to urban residents, efforts that probably resulted in a decline in the *H. pylori* infection rate.[29] Throughout the 20th century, peptic ulcer has affected lower social classes of unskilled workers with low income more frequently than the higher social classes comprising professionals and families with high incomes.[21,31] A relationship between living conditions, standards of hygiene and social class could also have contributed to the socio-demographic distribution of peptic ulcer. Numerous studies have revealed that peptic ulcer affected the lower social classes more frequently than the higher social classes. Lastly, the geographic variation of peptic ulcer could also reflect in part underlying infection rates with *H. pylori*.[29]

For a long time the prevailing paradigm of peptic ulcer pathophysiology held that a disruption in the delicate balance between aggressive and protective influences at the mucosal level was primarily responsible for the development of acute ulceration. If at any given point in time the integrity of the gastric and duodenal mucosa was the result of an ongoing battle between good and bad, how could any factors from a long-gone childhood possibly affect it? The discovery of *H. pylori* provided a paradigm to conceptualize the potential role of childhood factors, and it rekindled the interest in the birth-cohort phenomenon. The general acceptance of *H. pylori* as a major contributing factor to the etiology of peptic ulcer made it, for a short while, easier to publish studies of the birth-cohort phenomenon. Childhood infection with *H. pylori* and its persistence until adulthood provided a mechanism to explain this seeming discrepancy that had remained one major obstacle to the acceptance of the birth-cohort phenomenon. On a personal level, things were further helped along by Mervyn Susser becoming the editor of the *American Journal of Public Health*.[32–34]

Unresolved issues

Even if the decline in peptic ulcer during the second half of the 20th century can be explained by improvements in hygiene and a reduction in *H. pylori* transmission, it remains unresolved why the incidence of peptic ulcer rose so suddenly 100 years earlier.[35] Most epidemiologic evidence suggests that *H. pylori* has been a human pathogen for thousands of years. Other *Helicobacter* species reside in the stomachs of many mammals.[36] Proteins specific to *H. pylori* have been identified by enzyme-linked immunosorbent assay in the stomach of a 7000-year-old mummy from Peru.[37] The worldwide distribution of *H. pylori*, even among remote populations, on four continents also supports the contention that *H. pylori* was not recently acquired by humans, especially those in Western or industrialized countries.[38] Gastric cancer is actually the only disease in which the trends vary in the time-dependent fashion that would be expected from a well-behaved *H. pylori*-related disease.[32] It remained stable among consecutive generations until the turn of the 19th century and has declined ever since. The decline in the infection rate with *H. pylori* may also be responsible for an increase in the occurrence of gastroesophageal reflux disease (GERD) in Western societies.[39] As the prevalence of *H. pylori*-induced gastritis decreased in the general population, the average amount of gastric acid output increased and more subjects became susceptible to acid reflux.[40]

The rise in the occurrence of gastric and duodenal ulcer during the 19th century is difficult to explain utilizing *H. pylori* as the sole explanation. The strange behavior of peptic ulcer from an *H. pylori* perspective has caused the birth-cohort phenomenon to fall into disfavor again. When gastroenterologists speak nowadays of the cohort pattern of PUD, they usually refer only to its well-explained decline, but tend to ignore its mysterious rise during the 19th century.[41]

Others have tried to explain the initial rise of peptic ulcer based on a set of complex interactions among various modes of *H. pylori* acquisition, dietary factors, and other childhood infections.[42,43] Malnutrition and weakening of the immune system by infectious diarrhea or other concurrent infections may render the host more susceptible to persistent gastric colonization with *H. pylori*. Healthy, well-nourished children may be more capable of fending off an early invasion by *H. pylori*. Subjects who become infected with *H. pylori* at a young age are more likely to develop chronic or atrophic gastritis with a subsequent reduction of acid secretion that protects them from developing duodenal ulcer. Such gastritis is associated with development of gastric ulcer, as well as gastric cancer. In contrast to gastric ulcer, duodenal ulcer seems to develop primarily in subjects who contract *H. pylori* infection at the end of childhood or later. Acquisition of *H. pylori* at an older age may less affect the parietal cell mass, and specifically in duodenal ulcer patients, the levels of acid secretion are maintained above a threshold MAO of 15 mEq/h despite the ongoing inflammation.[44] The 10–20-year time lag between the birth-cohorts with peak mortality from gastric and duodenal ulcers seems to be consistent with this hypothesis. The age-dependent parallelism of ulcer mortality from different countries starting at ages 5 and 15 in gastric and duodenal ulcer, respectively, would also support such a contention.

The high and low infection rates of *H. pylori* infection in developing and developed countries, respectively, during the first half of the 20th century were not matched by a similar distribution of PUD. Marked variations in the occurrence of duodenal ulcer are observed even within a single country that appears to be characterized by a uniformly high prevalence of *H. pylori* infection.[45] Again, such discrepancies indicate that additional factors besides *H. pylori* are needed to cause gastroduodenal ulceration, increased consumption of dietary salt being probably only one among other risk factors for the gastric mucosa.[16] Mental stress and physical workload are exogenous risk factors that possibly promote duodenal ulceration by stimulating acid secretion, and smoking appears to exert its action independently of gastric acid.[16] Occupational workload and cigarette consumption could also serve as partial explanations for the higher morbidity and mortality of gastric, and especially duodenal, ulcer in men as compared with women.

My own reservation towards all these explanations stems from their complexity and the ever increasing number of factors necessary to explain the few characteristic features of ulcer epidemiology. I find it difficult to envisage how a multitude of individual risk factors, each one characterized by its own temporal, spatial and demographic variations, could align in many different countries at the same time to cause a unique, clear-cut and sharp rise and fall of ulcer risk among consecutive human generations. The contribution of several factors should have caused at least some blurs or spread of the cohort pattern, which is not observed. William of Ockham again comes to mind and his quest for the most parsimonious use of hypotheses in explaining a single natural phenomenon.

In the birth-cohort analyses from all countries alike, identical male and female generations were affected by the risk for developing peptic ulcer. The generational time lag of 10–20 years between gastric and duodenal ulcer development is also displayed similarly by male and female cohorts (FIGURE 2). A birth-cohort analysis is focused on the relative changes in disease occurrence over time affecting consecutive generations. It is less suited to study the temporal variation of PUD in terms of the absolute number of subjects affected by the disease. Apart from a few cases of peptic ulcer mentioned in the early medical literature from the preceding centuries, PUD began almost like an epidemic in Europe during the early 19th century. It presented itself as acute perforations of gastric ulcers in young girls. The disease had a dramatic course with sudden onset of severe pains, abdominal rigidity, and subsequent death within 24–48 hours. Necropsy would reveal a hole with sharp margins in the gastric wall. Later, gastric ulcer became more common in men than women. At the end of the 19th century the incidence of duodenal ulcer started to rise first in men and then in women. The time trends are documented in hospital statistics throughout Europe and have been recorded in numerous publications.[46–49] During the first half of the 20th century, duodenal ulcer occurred almost four-fold more often in men than women and gastric ulcer occurred about twice as often in men. It is only recently that both types of peptic ulcer have become equally common in both genders. These temporal changes in the prevalence of peptic ulcer represent yet another well-described fact from history that we tend to ignore because it does not fit our current understanding of *H. pylori* and its role in peptic ulcer.

A strange link with inflammatory bowel disease

Similar to PUD, the epidemiology of ulcerative colitis and Crohn's disease is also characterized by marked sociodemographic, geographic and temporal variations, which point unmistakably to the existence of some yet undefined environmental influences that must be shaping the occurrence of both types of inflammatory bowel disease (IBD). For a gastrointestinal epidemiologist, the huge enigma surrounding the etiology of IBD was a scientific temptation that was hard to resist. I entered the field of IBD with some warm-up epidemiologic exercises analyzing the geographic and temporal distribution.[50,51] In showing a parallelism between the published prevalence and incidence data on the one hand and the mortality data on the other, I also hoped to give more credence to the mortality data and potentially avert some future arguments about their validity.[51] To the eye trained by years of looking at the time trends of peptic ulcer, a quick glance at the period–age contours of ulcerative colitis revealed the characteristic fan-like behavior of age-specific death rates, with rising and falling trends in the younger and older age groups, respectively (FIGURE 5). In ulcerative colitis, the cohort–age contours aligned to a clear-cut hyperbola with its peak located around 1890,[52] and subsequent analyses confirmed similar birth-cohort patterns in the time of ulcerative colitis in most Western countries.[53]

The time trends of Crohn's disease revealed a very peculiar pattern. Ever since its inclusion into vital statistics in 1950 until about 1970, mortality from Crohn's disease had been rising, but then started to fall upon reaching the level of ulcerative colitis (FIGURE 6). It appeared as if mortality associated with Crohn's disease failed to continue its rise above the level of mortality associated with ulcerative colitis.[52] This pattern was discernible in each age group, in each gender and, as subsequently shown, in different countries alike.[54] As usual, the initial article dealing with the time trends of IBD proved a very tough sell, and after its eventual acceptance by *Digestive Diseases and Sciences* it 'fell still-born off the press' as no one seemed to have paid it much attention.[52]

Although the time trends of Crohn's disease were very different from anything hitherto described, I was actually disappointed to discover a birth-cohort phenomenon of ulcerative colitis. Throughout my academic career I tried to tell my fellow scientists that the birth-cohort pattern of peptic ulcer represented a peculiar and specific characteristic that merited further investigation and that it held the key to solving the puzzle of peptic ulcer. Suddenly I found myself confronted with an almost identical pattern in a completely different and seemingly unrelated disease. Would that not invalidate the ulcer data and rubber-stamp me as the 'mad scientist' who discovers birth-cohort phenomena wherever he goes? I decided to focus my attention on other aspects of IBD epidemiology, and I left its time trends unattended for a decade. Only recently did I start again to analyze the trends of ulcerative colitis in a more systematic fashion and openly address the similarity between the birth-cohort patterns of ulcerative colitis and peptic ulcer.[53–55] The data suggest that in many countries, ulcerative colitis and duodenal ulcer share a very similar birth-cohort pattern that affects exactly the same generations, with a peak occurring around 1890 (FIGURE 7). The overlap between duodenal ulcer and ulcerative colitis is the more striking because it does not involve gastric ulcer, gastric cancer or, as far as I know, any other disease. To me it suggests that the etiologies of ulcerative colitis and duodenal ulcer share some common pathway and that this pathway

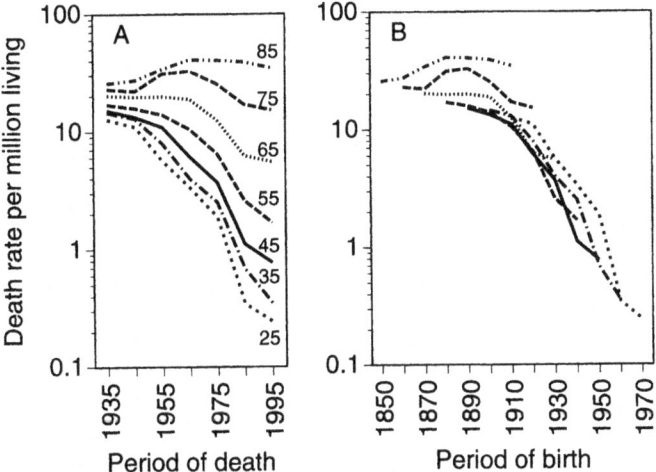

FIGURE 5 Age-specific death rates from ulcerative colitis in England and Wales between 1931 and 1998 plotted as period–age contours (panel A) and as cohort–age contours (panel B). The different lines (full, dashed, dotted etc.) refer to the same age groups in both panels A and B. Male and female rates are analyzed jointly.

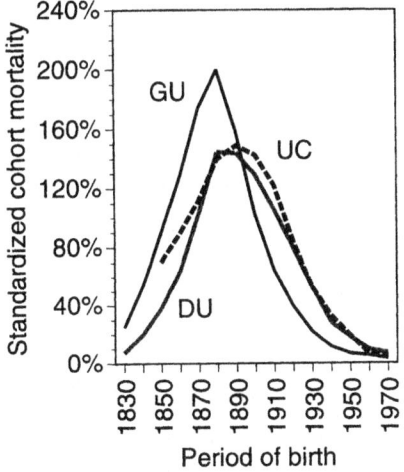

FIGURE 6 Standardized cohort mortality ratio of ulcerative colitis (UC), gastric ulcer (GU) and duodenal ulcer (DU) in England and Wales; male and female data analyzed jointly.

relates to some environmental exposure before or during childhood. As gastric ulcer is obviously linked to duodenal ulcer, and Crohn's disease is linked to ulcerative colitis, there appears to be some single mechanism that influences a large portion of gastroenterology's most important diseases.

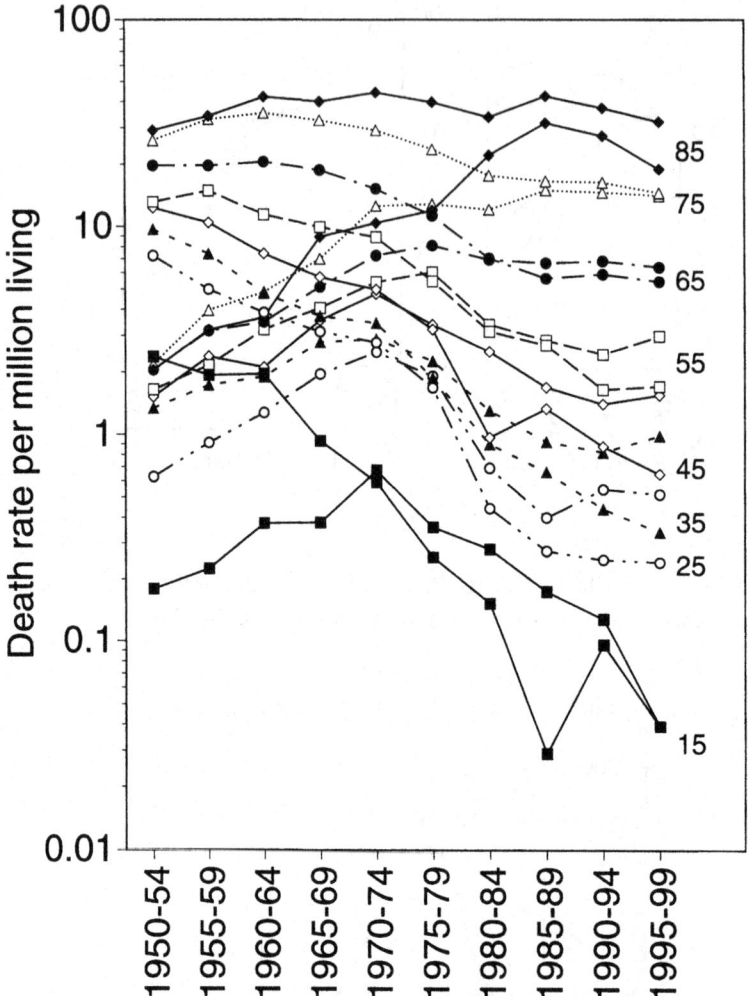

FIGURE 7 Superimposed curves of age-specific death rates from ulcerative colitis and Crohn's disease from England and Wales between 1950 and 1998. Death rates from ulcerative disease show a decline that is more pronounced in younger than older age groups. For each separate age group, death rates from Crohn's disease show an initial rise, but then fail to continue to rise above the level of mortality associated with ulcerative colitis. Age groups are labeled by their central age; for instance, 25 instead of 15–24, 35 instead of 25–34 etc. Each point represents the average death rate of a 5-year period.

Conclusion

It would be nice to be to be able to present at the end a grand unifying theory, but, fortunately or unfortunately, I have not reached this point as yet. I still do not know how to interpret the variety of my encounters with peptic ulcer, the birth-cohort phenomenon and *H. pylori*. One possible hypothesis holds that another *Helicobacter* species may be responsible for ulcerative colitis. The birth-cohort phenomenon could stem from an underlying variation in the as yet poorly understood infection mode of *Helicobacter* species. Rather than *H. pylori* itself, some unknown carriers or modes of transmission could vary among populations in a birth-cohort fashion. The birth-cohort phenomenon could also result from the superimposition of one major declining trend and several, possibly interrelated, rising trends (FIGURE 8). The combined influence of opposing time trends would give rise to the succession of peaks affecting consecutive generations with gastric ulcer, duodenal ulcer, ulcerative colitis, and lastly

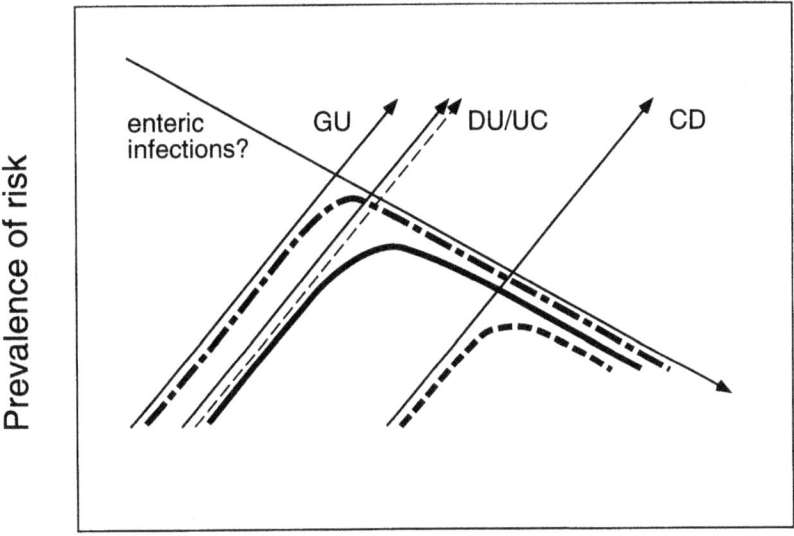

FIGURE 8 Hypothetical scheme to explain the linked rise and fall of four gastrointestinal diseases, that is, gastric ulcer (GU), duodenal ulcer (DU), ulcerative colitis (UC) and Crohn's disease (CD). In all diseases, the peculiar time trends could stem from the interaction of two risk factors, one rising and another falling. Although each disease must be characterized by its own specific risk factor, all four diseases may also depend on the presence of at least one additional shared risk factor the prevalence of which has declined during the 20th century.

Crohn's disease. It may be that, similar to the pre-*H. pylori* era when we tried to explain all of peptic disease by variations in acid secretion alone, we now fail to account for one or several major factors in PUD besides *H. pylori*.

With respect to the already available epidemiologic evidence, clinicians and investigators involved in solving the puzzle of IBD are at a similar stage of denial as were the ulcer researchers prior to 1985.[56] In spite of irrefutable data, they still ignore the birth-cohort phenomenon of ulcerative colitis, its association with Crohn's disease, and the marked temporal trends of both IBD. It amazes me that even today books are still written about peptic ulcer without even mentioning its underlying birth-cohort phenomenon.[57] It may reflect a difficulty in understanding complex temporal patterns that defy a simple explanation by a quick scientific sound bite. Rather than giving a conclusive answer, it keeps pointing at the persistent existence of a big gap in our understanding of PUD and IBD. Once resolved, the enigma of the birth-cohort phenomenon also carries the potential for finding some profound link among these seemingly heterogeneous diseases that may explain in one fell swoop (if one includes GERD) almost half of all gastroenterology.

References

1   Sonnenberg A, Bartmess J, Kern L, Siebenmann RE, Joris F, Blum AL. Hypochlorhydria in acute gastritis. *Dtsch Med Wochenschr* 1979; **104**: 1814–16 (in German).
2   Sonnenberg A, Fritsch A. Changing mortality of peptic ulcer disease in Germany. *Gastroenterology* 1983; **84**: 1553–7.
3   Susser M, Stein Z. Civilization and peptic ulcer. *Lancet* 1962; **1**: 115–19.
4   Frost WH. The age selection of mortality from tuberculosis in successive decades. *Am J Hyg (Section a)* 1939; **30**: 91–6.
5   Case RAM. Cohort analysis of mortality rates as an historical or narrative technique. *Br J Prev Soc Med* 1956; **10**: 159–71.
6   MacMahon B, Terry WD. Application of cohort analysis to the study of time trends in neoplastic disease. *J Chron Dis (J Clin Epidemiol)* 1958; **7**: 24–35.
7   Sonnenberg A. Occurrence of a cohort phenomenon in peptic ulcer mortality from Switzerland. *Gastroenterology* 1984; **86**: 398–401.
8   Sonnenberg A, Müller H. Cohort and period effects in peptic ulcer mortality from Japan. *J Clin Epidemiol* 1984; **37**: 699–704.
9   Sonnenberg A, Müller H, Pace F. Birth-cohort analysis of peptic ulcer mortality in Europe. *J Clin Epidemiol* 1985; **38**: 309–17.
10 Sonnenberg A. Causative factors in the etiology of peptic ulcer disease become effective before the age of 15 years. *J Clin Epidemiol* 1987; **40**: 193–202.
11 Hoogendoorn D. Opmerkelijke verschuivingen in het epidemiologische patroon van het ulcus pepticum. *Ned Tijdschr Geneeskd* 1984; **128**: 484–91.
12 Sonnenberg A. Disability pensions due to peptic ulcer in Germany between 1953 and 1983. *Am J Epidemiol* 1985; **122**: 106–11.
13 Svanes C, Lie RT, Kvale G, Svanes K, Søreide O. Incidence of perforated ulcer in western Norway, 1935–90: cohort- or period-dependent time trends? *Am J Epidemiol* 1995; **141**: 836–44.

14 Monson RR, MacMahon B. Peptic ulcer in Massachusetts physicians. *N Engl J Med* 1969; **281**: 11–15.

15 Office of Population Censuses and Surveys. *Cancer Statistics: Incidence, Survival and Mortality in England and Wales.* Studies on Medical and Population Subjects No. 43. London: HMSO, 1981; xii–xiii.

16 Sonnenberg A. Factors which influence the incidence and the course of peptic ulcer. *Scand J Gastroenterol* 1988; **23**(Suppl. 155): 119–40.

17 Sonnenberg A. Smoking and mortality from peptic ulcer in the United Kingdom. *Gut* 1986; **27**: 1369–72.

18 Øktedalen O, Guldvog I, Opstad PK, Berstad A, Gedde-Dahl E, Jorde R. The effect of physical stress on gastric secretion and pancreatic polypeptide levels in man. *Scand J Gastroenterol* 1984; **19**: 770–8.

19 Markiewicz K, Cholewa M, Gorski L, Chmura J. Effect of physical exercise on gastric basal secretion in healthy men. *Hepatogastroenterology* 1977; **24**: 377–80.

20 Markiewicz K, Cholewa M, Lukin M. Gastric basal secretion during exercise and restitution in patients with chronic duodenal ulcer. *Hepatogastroenterology* 1979; **26**: 160–5.

21 Sonnenberg A, Sonnenberg GS. Occupational mortality from gastric and duodenal ulcer. *Br J Ind Med* 1986; **43**: 50–5.

22 Sonnenberg A, Sonnenberg GS. Occupational factors in disability pensions for gastric and duodenal ulcer. *J Occup Med* 1986; **28**: 87–90.

23 Sonnenberg A, Haas J. The joint effect of occupation and nationality on the prevalence of peptic ulcer in German workers. *Br J Ind Med* 1986; **43**: 490–3.

24 Sonnenberg A, Sonnenberg GS, Wirths W. Historic changes of occupational work load and mortality from peptic ulcer in Germany. *J Occup Med* 1987; **28**: 756–61.

25 Sonnenberg A. Dietary salt and gastric ulcer. *Gut* 1986; **27**: 1138–42.

26 Sonnenberg A. Concordant occurrence of gastric and hypertensive diseases. *Gastroenterology* 1988; **95**: 42–8.

27 Vestergaard BF, Rune SJ. Type-specific herpes-simplex-virus antibodies in patients with recurrent duodenal ulcer. *Lancet* 1980; **1**: 1273–4.

28 Pounder RE, Ng D. The prevalence of *Helicobacter pylori* infection in different countries. *Aliment Pharmacol Ther* 1995; **9**(Suppl. 2): 33–9.

29 Sonnenberg A. Temporal trends and geographic variations of peptic ulcer disease. *Aliment Pharmacol Ther* 1995; **9**(Suppl. 2): 3–12.

30 Parsonet J. The incidence of *Helicobacter pylori* infection. *Aliment Pharmacol Ther* 1995; **9**(Suppl. 2): 45–51.

31 Jones FA. Clinical and social problems of peptic ulcer. *Lancet* 1957; **1**: 786–93.

32 Sonnenberg A. The US temporal and geographic variations of diseases related to *Helicobacter pylori*. *Am J Public Health* 1993; **83**: 1006–10.

33 Sonnenberg A, Wasserman IH. Associations of peptic ulcer and gastric cancer with other diseases. *Am J Public Health* 1995; **85**: 1252–5.

34 Sonnenberg A, Everhart JE. The prevalence of self-reported peptic ulcer in the United States. *Am J Public Health* 1996; **86**: 200–5.

35 Blaser MJ. *Helicobacter*s are indigenous to the human stomach: duodenal ulceration is due to changes in gastric microecology. *Gut* 1998; **43**: 721–7.

36 Fox JG, Lee A. The role of *Helicobacter* species in newly recognized gastrointestinal tract diseases of animals. *Lab Anim Sci* 1997; **47**: 222–55.

37 Correa P. *Helicobacter pylori* in pre-Columbian mummies. *Gastroenterology* 1998; **114**: A956.

38 Mégraud F. Epidemiology of *H. pylori* infection. *Gastroenterol Clin North Am* 1993; **22**: 73–88.

39 El-Serag HB, Sonnenberg A. Opposing time trends of peptic ulcer and reflux disease. *Gut* 1998; **43**: 327–33.

40 El-Serag HB, Sonnenberg A, Jamal MM, Inadomi JM, Crooks L, Feddersen RM. Corpus gastritis is protective against reflux esophagitis. *Gut* 1999; **45**: 181–5.

41 Roosendaal R, Kuipers EJ, Buitenwerf J *et al. Helicobacter pylori* and the birth cohort effect: evidence of a continuous decrease of infection rates in childhood. *Am J Gastroenterol* 1997; **92**: 1480–2.

42 Lee A, Veldhuyzen van Zanten S. The aging stomach or the stomach of the ages. *Gut* 1997; **41**: 575–6.

43 Graham DY. *Helicobacter pylori* is the primary cause of gastric cancer. *J Gastroenterol* 2000; **35**(Suppl. 12): 90–7.

44 Baron JH, Logan RPH. Infection by *Helicobacter pylori* is the major cause of duodenal ulcer. *Proc R Coll Physicians Edinb* 1994; **24**: 21–36.

45 Holcombe C. *Helicobacter pylori*: the African enigma. *Gut* 1992; **33**: 429–31.

46 Jennings D. Perforated peptic ulcer: Changes in age-incidence and sex-distribution in the last 150 years. *Lancet* 1940; **1**: 444–7.

47 Kucsko L. Das Verhalten der Ulkuskrankheit auf Grund der Sektionsprotokolle des Wiener pathologischen Institutes in den letzten 100 Jahren. *Schweiz Z Pathol Bakteriol* 1958; **21**: 433–7.

48 Brinton W. *On the Pathology, Symptoms and Treatment of Ulcer of the Stomach* (Facsimile of the Original 1857 edition). Oxford: Oxford Historical Books, 1990.

49 Wulff RH. *Rational Diagnosis and Treatment*, 2nd edn. Oxford: Blackwell, 1981; 62–3.

50 Sonnenberg A. Mortality from Crohn's disease and ulcerative colitis in England–Wales and the US from 1950 to 1983. *Dis Colon Rectum* 1986; **29**: 624–9.

51 Sonnenberg A. Geographic variation in the incidence of and mortality from inflammatory bowel disease. *Dis Colon Rectum* 1986; **29**: 854–61.

52 Sonnenberg A, Koch TR. Period and generation effects on mortality from idiopathic inflammatory bowel disease. *Dig Dis Sci* 1989; **34**: 1720–9.

53 Delcò F, Sonnenberg A. Birth-cohort phenomenon in the time trends of mortality from ulcerative colitis. *Am J Epidemiol* 1999; **150**: 359–66.

54 Delcò F, Sonnenberg A. Commonalities in the time trends of Crohn's disease and ulcerative colitis. *Am J Gastroenterol* 1999; **94**: 2171–6.

55 Delcò F, Sonnenberg A. Exposure to risk factors for ulcerative colitis occurs during an early period of life. *Am J Gastroenterol* 1999; **94**: 679–84.

56 Sonnenberg A. Geographic and temporal variations in the occurrence of peptic ulcer disease. *Scand J Gastroenterol* 1985; **20**(Suppl. 110): 11–24.

57 Modlin IM, Sachs G. *Acid Related Diseases: Biology and Treatment*. Konstanz, Germany: Schnetztor-Verlag, 1998.

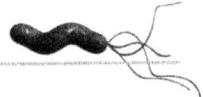

CHAPTER 7

John Lykoudis

The general practitioner in Greece who in 1958 discovered the etiology of, and a treatment for, peptic ulcer disease

Basil Rigas and Efstathios D. Papavassiliou

Introduction

The etiology of peptic ulcer disease (PUD), a major medical enigma for more than a century, occupied the minds and efforts of many clinicians and basic scientists,[1,2] which is not surprising, because until recently PUD caused significant morbidity and mortality. Elucidation of its etiology was expected, justifiably, to lead to a successful treatment, which, in the era of etiological conjecture, was largely empirical, not to say arbitrary. It is instructive to recall that successive generations of investigators, some of them truly talented, endeavored more or less along the principle that hydrochloric acid and the vagus nerve were at the center of PUD pathogenesis. Early in the 20th century Moynihan summarized the prevailing concept when he ascribed duodenal ulcer to 'the digestion of the duodenal mucosa by the hyperacid gastric juice'.[3] Virtually everyone stayed within the confines of this medical orthodoxy until Marshall and Warren established *Helicobacter pylori* as the dominant cause of PUD,[4] revolutionizing the therapeutic approach to the disease.

The number of investigators who entertained the possibility of an infectious etiology was very small indeed.[1,5,6] The 'bacterial hypothesis' for the etiology of PUD was articulated as early as 1875, but only very few attempted to document a causative role of the microorganisms that were observed in or around peptic ulcers. Some, including Kussmaul in 1868 and Gorham in 1940, advocated the use of bismuth compounds to treat ulcers and, as was recently reported, in 1946 Constance Guion at The New York Hospital in Manhattan's elegant Upper East Side used to prescribe the antibiotic aureomycin for PUD.[7] These isolated efforts, however, received scant attention and were quickly forgotten.

It is therefore totally astonishing that in the 1950s John Lykoudis (FIGURE 1), a general practitioner in a small, isolated town in Greece, prompted by a single clinical observation, developed on his own the concept that PUD and gastritis had an infectious etiology. As if this was not enough, this most unlikely student of PUD proceeded to devise an apparently effective treatment, based on the antibiotics of his time.[7] His heroic saga, because this is what it was, is chronicled here.

A brief biography

John Lykoudis was born in 1910 in the Greek town of Missolonghi, about 70 miles west of Delphi, the site of the famed oracle and, according to the ancients, the center of the Earth. Missolonghi, situated on the shore of a vast lagoon, with less than 10 000 inhabitants in 1960 and about 15 000 nowadays, occupies a special place in Greek history. It is also quite familiar to the English-speaking world, for here died on 19 April 1824 the greatest Romantic poet, Lord Byron.

During the Greek war of independence (1821–1828) Missolonghi was a major stronghold of the Greek insurgents and had to endure three sieges by forces of the Ottoman Empire. On 30 December 1823 Lord

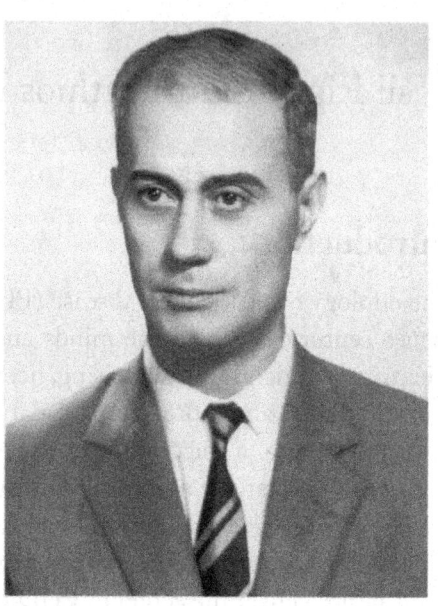

FIGURE 1 Dr John Lykoudis (1910–1980).

Byron came to Missolonghi and as Commander-in-Chief, he inspired the defenders with his enthusiasm and dedication. He died the following April before the beginning of the final siege, during which several idealistic European philhellenes (Italians, Swedes, French, Poles, Swiss and Germans among them) gave their lives for the cause of freedom. The heart of the English bard is still buried there, at the base of his statue in the Garden of the Heroes.

Lykoudis, born to a poor family of farmers, was the third of four children. His father died when Lykoudis was 8 years old and he had to work at a shoemaker's store to supplement the family's meager finances. Always a top student, he enrolled in the Military Medical School, graduating in 1934 with high honors. Assigned to a remote mountainous post, he reached the rank of first lieutenant, but four years later, he developed pulmonary tuberculosis and had to resign from the military. For reasons likely related to his health he opted not to pursue a medical residency in Athens and in 1938 started his medical practice in Missolonghi, where by all accounts he was a very successful practitioner. Lykoudis married in 1945 and had three children, the second of whom became a physician, currently an internist at Missolonghi General Hospital.

Early in his medical career, Lykoudis showed a strong social conscience, being remembered to this day as the physician of the underprivileged. During the difficult years of World War II, malaria became endemic in Missolonghi and in response to the great public health need, Lykoudis formulated the anti-malarial quinacrine for intramuscular administration, with which he achieved better results because of enhanced absorption and higher compliance (some patients were avoiding taking quinacrine because of its bitter taste). In 1952 Lykoudis ran as an independent for mayor of Missolonghi and was elected twice for successive four-year terms (1952–1960). Although not wealthy, he gave his mayor's salary to a local pharmacy, so that the poor could obtain free medicines.

In 1961, having already developed his ideas on PUD, Lykoudis relocated to Athens, where he continued his practice, becoming known as the 'ulcer doctor'. He retired in 1978 transferring his practice, which was by then centered on PUD, to his son. However, both father and son gave up on the novel PUD treatment in 1980, because of their failure to gain official approval of the treatment and because some of the ingredients had become unavailable. Lykoudis died the same year of a heart attack while visiting his beloved Missolonghi where he is now buried.

Lykoudis' work on peptic ulcer disease

Lykoudis himself suffered for years from PUD, complicated by several episodes of gastrointestinal bleeding. In 1958 he had an attack of hemorrhagic gastroenteritis for which he treated himself with antibiotics. The treatment not only cured his gastroenteritis, but also led to a sustained remission of his PUD symptoms, which prompted Lykoudis to consider that a microbial agent caused PUD.

Lykoudis repeated his own treatment in several of his patients, with encouraging results. In an effort to devise as effective a cure for PUD as possible, Lykoudis experimented with various combinations of antibiotics, his last formulation including two quinoleines. 8-Hydroxyquinolines were used clinically for their amoebicidal action, but apparently had some broader effectiveness against gut flora. His reasoning was that oral nonabsorbable antibiotics would be the most efficacious as they would achieve high concentrations against the infectious agent residing in the stomach and duodenum. Another (commonsense) concern of Lykoudis' was to use compounds with limited side-effects. He also included vitamin A 'to enhance epithelial repair in the stomach and duodenum'.

The optimal combination, according to Lykoudis, was 5,7-diiodo-8-oxyquinoleine (0.125 g), 5-iodo-7-chloro-8-oxyquinoleine (0.125 g), phthalylesulfathiazole (0.3 g), streptomycin sulfate (0.075 g), and vitamin A (10 000 IU), to be taken 6–8 times per day for 10 days. On 16 November 1961, Lykoudis was awarded a patent by the Greek authorities, no. 22 453 entitled 'A method for making a pharmaceutical preparation for the treatment of ulcers of the stomach and duodenum and of gastritis' (FIGURE 2).

Initially, Lykoudis prepared his 'medication' in the manner of an apothecary, combining the four compounds in powder form, each dose individually wrapped in paper. However, by 1962 the demand far exceeded his capacity to prepare his medication and to keep up with the needs of ever increasing numbers of patients, he purchased a machine for the rapid and efficient preparation of his 'ulcer medication', which was now produced in tablet form from commercial grade compounds. The new antibiotic preparation was named *Elgaco*, from the Greek word for ulcer (= *el*kos), *ga*stritis and *co*litis. Lykoudis claimed that *Elgaco* was very effective against various forms of 'colitis', which was most likely the currently termed 'irritable bowel syndrome'.

Lykoudis treated thousands of patients with his new regimen; based on existing files and the recollections of his physician son, it seems likely that he treated more than 30 000 patients over almost two decades. In a summary of 130 patients that he submitted to the Greek authorities, Lykoudis describes the response to *Elgaco*: by the third day of treatment patients invariably felt much better and by the end of the first week all symptoms of PUD disappeared. Reflecting treatment modalities of that time, Lykoudis makes the point that patients were able to return to a normal diet, abandoning the various restrictive diets that they were following. Recurrences were rare and those that did responded promptly to a repeat course of *Elgaco*.

The success of *Elgaco* cannot be quantified from extant notes on thousands of patients, because the outcome of each patient is not recorded. We have concluded, however, that his treatment was successful, based on the following considerations. First, our current understanding of the etiology and treatment of PUD makes it plausible that his treatment was effective. Second, there is the written testimony (some of it sworn, as explained later) of many of the

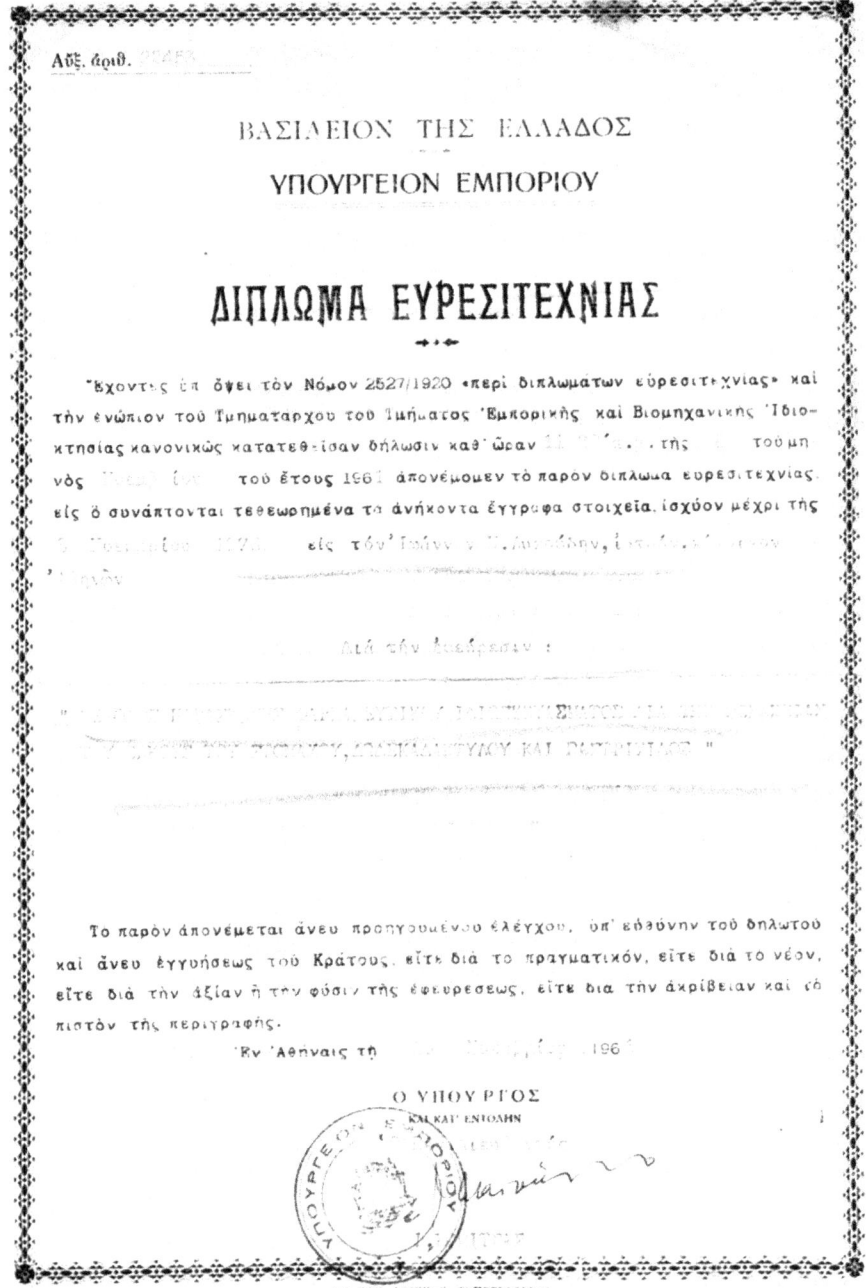

FIGURE 2 Lykoudis' patent for *Elgaco*. The Greek text reads, in part: 'Kingdom of Greece, Ministry of Commerce. Patent Diploma . . . this patent is granted to John Lykoudis, physician, residing in Athens, for his invention: "A method for making a pharmaceutical preparation for the treatment of ulcers of the stomach and duodenum and of gastritis" . . . Athens, 16 November, 1961 . . .'

patients who were treated by Lykoudis. All report prompt responses to his therapy. In some cases, patients even detail that radiographically proven ulcers were cured following treatment with *Elgaco* and that such cure was confirmed by repeat radiological series. Third, Lykoudis had a large following and despite fierce opposition from the establishment, patients flocked to him from all over Greece. It is apparent from thank you notes and other extant correspondence that grateful, cured patients were the main source of referrals to Lykoudis. That he resorted to a commercial level of production of *Elgaco* supports the idea that he treated a large number of patients and constitutes an eloquent indirect testament to the effectiveness of his treatment. Finally, some patients of that period who received *Elgaco* have been interviewed recently and confirmed Lykoudis' descriptions.

Lykoudis ignored

As is apparent, Lykoudis had no difficulty convincing patients of the superiority of his approach to PUD compared with the then standard treatment. He did, however, encounter formidable obstacles in convincing the medical establishment, the Greek regulatory authorities and the pharmaceutical industry. In fact, Lykoudis spent the remaining years of his life engaged in incessant activity to propagate his treatment of PUD and gastritis. His archives, some made recently available by his family, make it clear that he was fully aware of the importance of his discoveries. They also convey vividly an almost suffocating sense of frustration. One is reminded of the proverbial one-armed fisherman who is unable to demonstrate how big was the fish he had caught.

Lykoudis sought to educate his fellow physicians on the merits of his method through presentations at local medical meetings; for example, at the 4 May 1964 meeting of the Medico-Surgical Society. Lykoudis was, however, completely shunned by the medical academic establishment of his time or, at best, considered an eccentric provincial physician. Frequently, the opinion leaders of his day simply derided him.

In 1966, Lykoudis attempted to publish his observations in the *Journal of the American Medical Association*, but his manuscript entitled 'Ulcer of the Stomach and Duodenum' was rejected on 1 September 1966, because '[it] does not seem appropriate for our journal' (FIGURE 3). Unfortunately, no copy of this manuscript survives for re-evaluation in the light of current knowledge. Undeterred, Lykoudis published privately a booklet entitled, 'The Truth About Gastric and Duodenal Ulcer', summarizing his thoughts on PUD and gastritis.[8] On page 32 he writes,

There is no doubt that gastritis and duodenitis, which have gastric and duodenal ulcer as their complication, are inflammations due to an infectious agent ... Hyperchlorhydria, hypersecretion and gastric spasms are due neither to acid nor to neurogenic spasm, rather they are consequences of the inflammation ... Hyperchlorhydria, the so-called gastric neurosis and aerophagia are not diseases but symptoms of gastroduodenitis with or without ulcer and they abate rapidly with our combination of antimicrobial agents ... Ulcer is a local disease and not the manifestation of a generalized illness.

This unambiguous statement conveys an unparalleled iconoclastic insight into PUD, which becomes even more impressive when one considers his limited formal training, the era in which it was made, and Lykoudis' lack of access to non-Greek literature. Lykoudis knew some German and French, but it is almost certain that he had no knowledge of or access to any of the (limited) literature on the bacterial hypothesis of PUD.

A second substantial difficulty for Lykoudis was the Greek regulatory authorities, which rejected his repeated applications to approve *Elgaco*, ostensibly because it lacked the support of appropriate clinical trials. On 12 August 1961, Lykoudis submitted a closely reasoned, but rather subdued, request for the Drug and Pharmacies Administration to reconsider its position on *Elgaco*. He tried to make the case that *Elgaco* owed its success (vouched for by Lykoudis) to its antimicrobial properties, claiming that his treatment of PUD was similar to the treatment of infectious colitis with antibiotics. He contrasted *Elgaco*'s success to the dismal failure of antacid agents and spasmolytics, and claimed that the gastritis accompanying every case of PUD was further evidence of a microbial etiology, which he considered responsible for almost all of the PUD symptoms. He then stated,

> The good results with *Elgaco* on every [type of] gastritis force us to accept its microbial nature and not the chemical, neuronal, etc. However, no medicinal preparation is available to date to treat the infectious etiology of gastritis and the clinical manifestations of ulcer.

He claimed that *Elgaco* was totally free of side-effects and that no ulcer had been resistant to the thousands of *Elgaco* courses already administered to patients. He then concluded,

> *Elgaco* opens up a new therapeutic avenue, and will become a strong therapeutic weapon in the hands of physicians and patients to conquer gastric ulcer, gastritis and colitides, the true scourge of society in 1961.

Lykoudis was rejected again.

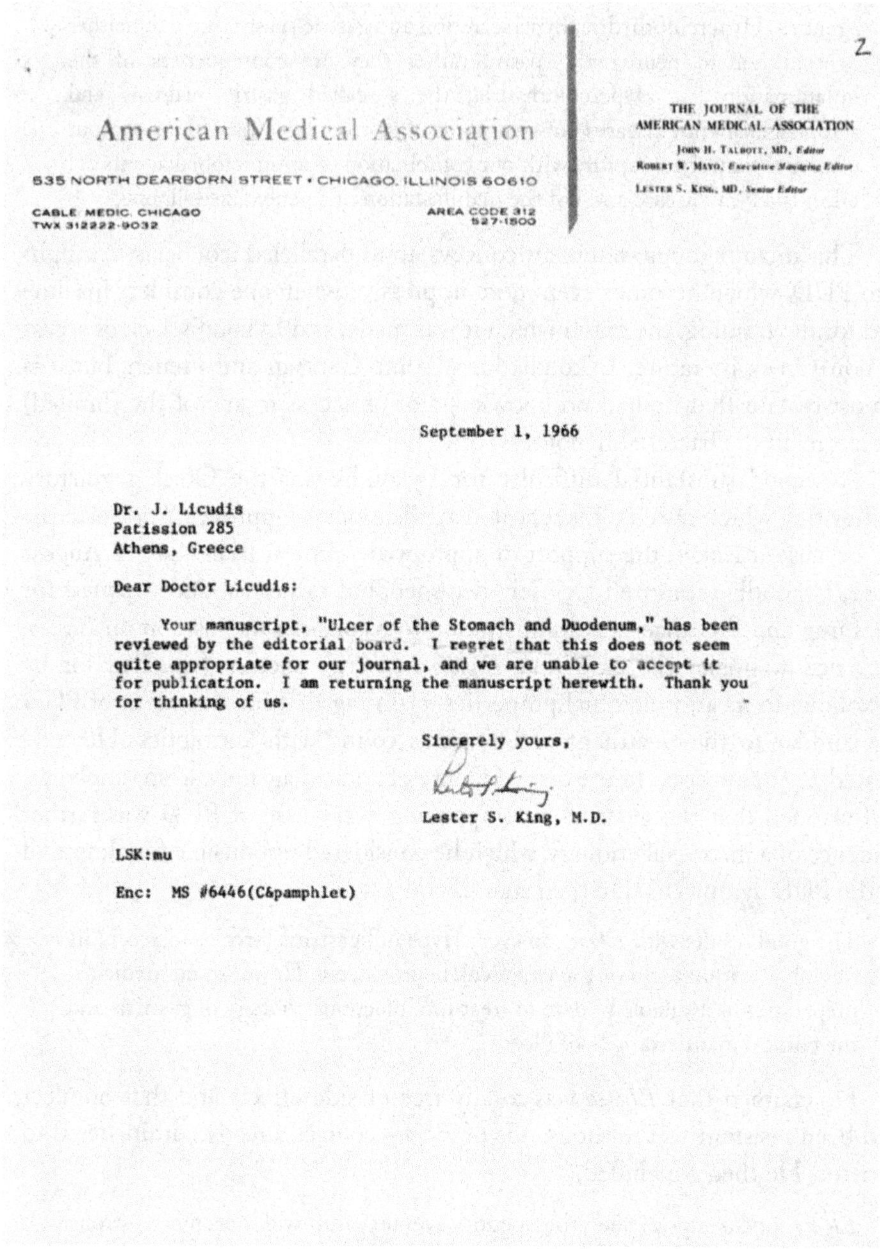

American Medical Association

THE JOURNAL OF THE
AMERICAN MEDICAL ASSOCIATION

JOHN H. TALBOTT, MD, *Editor*
ROBERT W. MAYO, *Executive Managing Editor*
LESTER S. KING, MD, *Senior Editor*

535 NORTH DEARBORN STREET · CHICAGO, ILLINOIS 60610

CABLE MEDIC CHICAGO
TWX 312222-9032

AREA CODE 312
527-1500

September 1, 1966

Dr. J. Licudis
Patission 285
Athens, Greece

Dear Doctor Licudis:

Your manuscript, "Ulcer of the Stomach and Duodenum," has been reviewed by the editorial board. I regret that this does not seem quite appropriate for our journal, and we are unable to accept it for publication. I am returning the manuscript herewith. Thank you for thinking of us.

Sincerely yours,

Lester S. King, M.D.

LSK:mu

Enc: MS #6446(C&pamphlet)

FIGURE 3 Letter of rejection from the *Journal of the American Medical Association* for Lykoudis' manuscript on peptic ulcer disease. This is the only surviving evidence that Lykoudis submitted his observations on peptic ulcer disease to a medical journal.

He protested these rejections strenuously. Surviving correspondence makes it clear that the Greek authorities were annoyed with Lykoudis, to say the least, and his requests were now rejected on trivial technicalities. The director of Drug and Pharmacies Administration, for example, rejected one of his petitions because 'it was not written in the manner appropriate for the correspondence of a private citizen with a Civil Authority'. He probably expected a reverential tone, but the opening salvo of an angry Lykoudis on 16 October 1961 was 'I fail to comprehend why the Supreme Health Council vetoes the approval of *Elgaco*.'

He submitted two lists of cured patients, one with the names, addresses and a brief clinical summary of 130 patients and another one with 12 500 (!) names; we have a copy of the former, and submission of the latter is referred to by Lykoudis in one of his rebuttals to the Greek authorities.

Convinced that his direct approach was failing, Lykoudis resorted to his political connections and in 1965 enlisted the help of the Vice-Premier who, conveniently, was being elected in his district. The Vice-Premier requested careful consideration of Lykoudis' claims, starting from the Minister of Health down to all the decision-making bodies. The matter was referred to the various chairs of Medicine at Athens University, but all, including the respected and powerful Professor B. Malamos, who was also the President of the Supreme Health Council, were negative and apparently paid only token attention to his claims, refusing to test *Elgaco*'s presumed efficacy. *Elgaco* was rejected again, but this time in polite terms. In 1967, Lykoudis succeeded in getting the attention of the Prime Minister's office. His correspondence with the Minister of Health on 21 August 1967, a sad document indeed, is revealing. He registers his frustration that medications with apparently no effect on PUD were approved, whereas *Elgaco* was repeatedly rejected. He proposes, in essence, a phase III trial: 100 PUD patients to be treated at a State hospital by the eminent professors, 50 with conventional treatment and 50 with *Elgaco*. 'Their refusal to approve it is understandable, but their refusal to test it is not!' he writes.

> If the study proves them correct, they will be vindicated and I will become a laughing stock . . . It is dramatically urgent to clarify this issue . . . Too much, endless talking, which leads nowhere, while it is so simple to resolve this in a practical way. Only the facts constitute the truth.

Needless to add, the Supreme Health Council made another negative decision.

Undeterred, Lykoudis approached, in parallel, almost every pharmaceutical company he could reach, including J. R. Geigy SA, Farbwerke Hoechst AG,

Schering AG, Bayer, Leo Pharmaceutical and Specia of Rhone Poulenc, but the negotiations were not successful. In their responses, written in English, but also in German, French and Greek, these companies cited either different research and development objectives (Schering) or, more often, the lack of formal studies. On 13 January 1964, Hoechst mentioned the need for 'a clinical study with statistical evaluation', but also expressed the reservation that the dose of streptomycin was too low. A crucial obstacle, however, seemed to be that Lykoudis was using already approved medications and, at least according to Bayer (10 March 1962), his preparation would require sublicensing from the other companies prior to its marketing. We also suspect that, for similar reasons, they thought it easy for competitors to circumvent Lykoudis' intellectual property protection. The available correspondence also suggests that Lykoudis might have been too careful in disclosing the details of his preparation.

Lykoudis persecuted

> He who ascends to mountain-tops, shall find
> The loftiest peaks most wrapt in clouds and snow;
> He who surpasses or subdues mankind,
> Must look down on the hate of those below.
> Lord Byron, *Childe Harold's Pilgrimage*.[9]

Lykoudis attracted the envy, and perhaps the hate, of lesser minds, as Byron might have predicted. As a result, he was referred for disciplinary action to the Athens Medical Association, of which he was a member, 'because (a) he prepared and distributed an unapproved medicinal preparation ... and (b) he made his method publicly known to attract patients and also treated patients with methods and medications that are not approved ... and also sold through his doorman these medications to patients coming to his office'. On 6 November 1968, Lykoudis' explanations were considered inadequate and the Disciplinary Committee, presided over by a neurology professor, fined him 4000 drachmas, a substantial but not inordinately large amount of money at that time.

A more serious problem for Lykoudis was his indictment in the Greek Courts (FIGURE 4). His son is uncharacteristically laconic about this matter, but we obtained copies of the sworn depositions of two grateful patients who supported Lykoudis, one of whom was the retired Director General of the venerable Red Cross Hospital in Athens. On 17 June 1967 he testified that,

> having become aware from articles in the daily press of the persecution of Dr Lykoudis ... he volunteered his testimony out of gratitude for him who cured his ulcer without receiving a fee; several famous physicians had failed to treat successfully his disease.

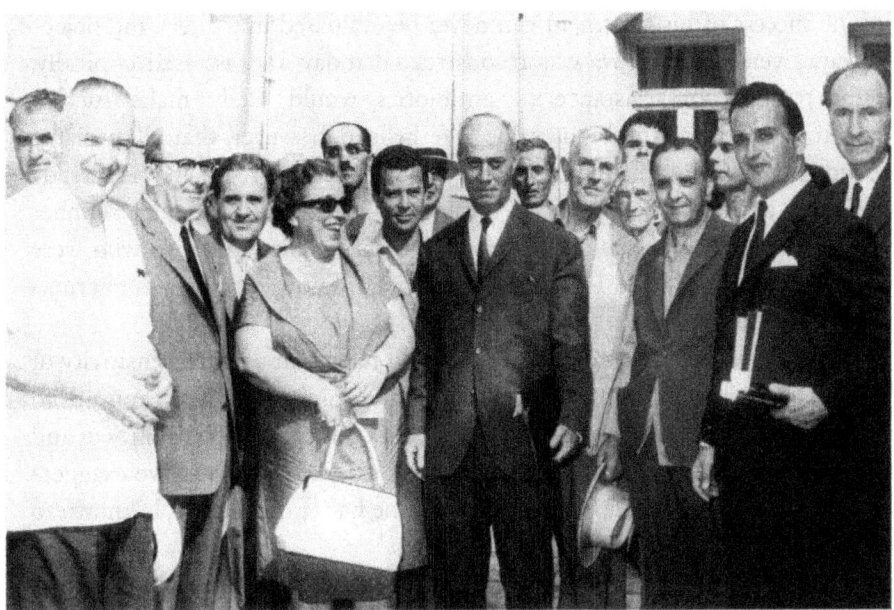

FIGURE 4 Lykoudis (center) outside a Greek courthouse surrounded by his former patients who were showing their support for him.

He also stated that Lykoudis 'treated also many poor ulcer patients free of charge'. We do not know precisely what happened with this persecution of Lykoudis and, unfortunately, the deadline for this chapter precluded a thorough investigation.

An appraisal

Lykoudis' impressive insight into the pathogenesis of gastritis and PUD was based on an astute clinical observation and his indefatigable efforts to assess it clinically. Equally remarkable is his ingenious development of an apparently effective treatment.

All the documents that we have read and the other evidence that we have been able to gather make it clear that Lykoudis had firmly concluded that an infectious agent or agents were responsible for gastritis, PUD and some forms of colitis. Unfortunately, when he was compelled to identify these elusive organisms, particularly when dealing with regulatory agencies, he meandered around known pathogens, unable to build a strong case for any of them. His main argument, and the strongest one that he could marshal in all his writings in favor of the infectious etiology of these clinical entities, was the response to treatment that he had witnessed.

The success of his treatment can never be evaluated in a direct and objective way. Even if his *Elgaco* was reconstructed today and assessed clinically, current patterns of resistance to antibiotics would likely make such a metachronous study of dubious value. We believe, however, that all available evidence makes a compelling case for a highly effective regimen. As already mentioned, our conclusion is based on patient testimonies, the huge number of patients treated by Lykoudis, interviews with patients still alive who were treated by Lykoudis in the 1960s and on posterior knowledge (i.e. its pharmacological plausibility).

The claimed 100% success of *Elgaco* could reflect an unusual sensitivity of *H. pylori* to antibiotics in a population that had minimal, if any, exposure to antibiotics; postwar Greece was, after all, a poor country and availability of and access to medications was limited. Alternatively, Lykoudis may have exaggerated somewhat to achieve approval (Mendel, the father of genetics, is known to have succumbed to such temptation).

In addition to his clinical acumen, Lykoudis displayed unusual tenacity in the pursuit of acceptance. It was evident from talking to his wife and son that not for a moment did he waver in his convictions about PUD and its treatment. Given his level of training and exposure to academic medicine, his relentless efforts betray the passion of a visionary, if not a missionary.

As we have argued elsewhere recently,[10] a question to be pondered in this case is why Lykoudis failed, despite his heroic effort. We still believe that his lack of academic credentials contributed, to some extent, to this failure, but the dominant reason is that his thesis was contrary to established, albeit unsubstantiated, dogma. Unconventional ideas are sometimes discarded without proper evaluation. Such was the reaction of the Greek medical establishment during Lykoudis' time. Unfortunately, his case is not unique in this respect. Staying within the confines of contemporary ideas is intellectually painless, if not comforting. The history of medicine records several examples of ideas, which have been rejected by so-called opinion leaders, making a quantum leap over background thought. K. S. McCully and his homocysteine theory of atherosclerosis are but one, and a sadly recent, example.[11] A similar attitude seems to have influenced the response of the pharmaceutical companies, although financial considerations might also have been at play. In retrospect, it is astonishing that, given the enormous market for the treatment of PUD and gastritis and the simplicity of Lykoudis' *Elgaco*, none of the companies undertook a simple preliminary study. The dogma of the day obviously reigned supreme in everybody's minds.

Lykoudis died a disappointed man who, nevertheless, believed to the end that gastritis and PUD had an infectious etiology and could be permanently cured with antibiotics. He repeatedly asked his wife to bring to his grave the proof of his theory, which he believed was inevitable. The discovery of *H. pylori* and the now firmly established treatment of PUD with antibiotics represent a form of vindication for Lykoudis.

We therefore offer this chapter to the memory of Dr John Lykoudis in the hope that it will provide posthumous solace to the spirit of this unjustly tormented man.

References

1   Kidd M, Modlin IM. A century of *Helicobacter pylori*: paradigms lost–paradigms regained. *Digestion* 1998; **59**: 1–15.
2   Spiro HM. Peptic ulcer: Moynihan's or Marshall's disease? *Lancet* 1998; **352**: 645–6.
3   Moynihan B. Duodenal ulcer. *Practitioner* 1907; **76**: 249.
4   Marshall BJ, Warren JR. Unidentified curved bacilli in the stomach of patients with gastritis and peptic ulceration. *Lancet* 1984; **1**: 1311–15.
5   McNulty CA. The discovery of Campylobacter-like organisms. *Curr Top Microbiol Immunol* 1999; **241**: 1–9.
6   Buckley MJ, O'Morain CA. Helicobacter biology: discovery. *Br Med Bull* 1998; **54**: 7–16.
7   Fremont-Smith P. The new germ theory (Letter). *Atlantic Monthly* May 1999; **283**: 10.
8   Lykoudis J. 'The Truth About Gastric and Duodenal Ulcer'. Athens: 1966 (in Greek; published privately).
9   Lord Byron. *Childe Harold's Pilgrimage*. In: McConnell FD (ed.) *Byron's Poetry*. New York: W. W. Norton Co., 1978.
10 Rigas B, Feretis C, Papavassiliou ED. J. Lykoudis: An unappreciated discoverer of the infectious etiology and treatment of peptic ulcer disease. *Lancet* 1999; **354**: 1634–5.
11 Larkin M. Kilmer McCully: pioneer of the homocysteine theory. *Lancet* 1998; **352**: 1364.

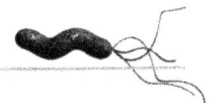

CHAPTER 8

How I discovered helicobacters in Boston in 1967

Susumu Ito

Introduction

I first encountered gastric helicobacters in the early 1960s, when I knew them as gastric spirilla. However, I did not publish any of my observations until in 1967 I saw some incidental micrographs of these bacteria included in a general paper on the fine structure of the gastric mucosa. Paradoxically, although I have made numerous observations on these fascinating *Helicobacter* species, I have to this day not published an entire article solely of these organisms. In my limited search of the literature, I thought that there was only one species of the gastric bacteria that I had called a gastric spirillum, but which was referred to by several other less generic designations. When I was invited by Barry Marshall to contribute some recollections of my encounter with the *Helicobacter* genus, I was delighted to accept.

Background

Although I retired from my academic position in 1990, I have continued to work daily in the laboratory doing electron microscopy of the stomach, as well as other projects. My entry into the field of digestive tract structure and function studies was fortuitous. As a new member of the Anatomy Department at Cornell Medical School in New York City in 1956, I was asked to teach digestive tract histology because no-one else in the new department was particularly knowledgeable of the gut. To prepare my lectures, I searched the literature and was dismayed to find only limited, poor quality electron micrographs of the stomach cell types. Although the stomach was then not an area of special interest to me, I became fascinated by its unusual cells and the mysteries of its unique secretory functions. Thus, I started fixing and examining stomachs of various animal species whenever they became available in the department. These were the early days of biological electron microscopy when almost everything we examined resulted in new, exciting and sometimes perplexing observations. The stomach was no exception. There were numerous areas of the unknown. For example, at that time the actual source of gastric HCl at concentrations of pH 1 or lower was yet to be determined!

After moving to Boston in 1960, my work on the stomach started to take more time from my interests in the testes, mitosis, rickettsiae, and cell surface coats. At this time I was using cat intestine on a regular basis to define the structure and characteristics of the fuzzy surface coat or glycocalyx.[1] On occasion I would fix stomach samples for further observations of the gastric cell types. The ubiquity of helicobacters in many stomachs made an encounter with them inevitable. Initially, these bacteria were passed off as curiosities of little significance. However, their presence in the stomachs of most older cats aroused my curiosity (FIGURES 1–3). I started making fresh mounts of mucosal scrapings and by phase contrast microscopy I was able to see numerous, spectacular spiral bacteria, often more than 10 μm long, swimming rapidly (FIGURE 4). Their corkscrew movement appeared to be produced by terminal flagella at either end, which were clearly visible when their normal speed was reduced in moribund organisms. Because they divided by binary fission, I sometimes saw short forms with a polar flagellar tuft at only one end and these swam in either direction as rapidly as the longer bipolar bacteria by using the tuft as a push or pull propeller.

The bacteria remained motile for hours when mounted *in vitro*. Pathology textbooks of the early 1960s indicated that the stomach did not harbor living bacteria, but older publications described microorganisms in mammalian stomachs even before 1900.[2,3] Few attempts had been made to culture them using modern techniques. Their remarkable swimming ability and behavior was so interesting that I spent many hours observing their antics. I became so fascinated that I made a 16-mm movie film and presented it at a meeting of the American Society for Cell Biology, as well as including a number of electron micrographs. I labeled the bacteria as gastric spirilla, but later thought they must have been *H. felis*, because they were found in cat stomachs. I was surprised when I tried to confirm their identity by comparing them with more recently published electron micrographs of *H. felis* (FIGURES 5–7): they were very different! What I had always thought to be *H. felis* closely resembled micrographs of *Gastrospirillum hominis*. At this point I contacted Barry Marshall to avoid an embarrassing misidentification and though they are still

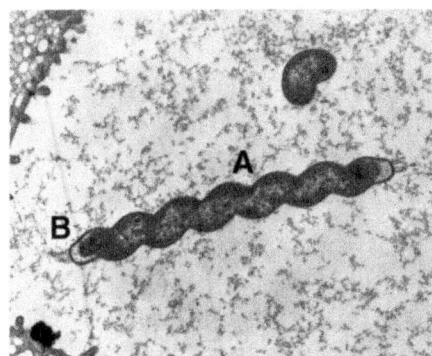

FIGURE 1 *Helicobacter heilmannii* in longitudinal section. The organism has 7–12 wavelengths (A) and multiple flagella at each end (B) (cat stomach, ×40 000).

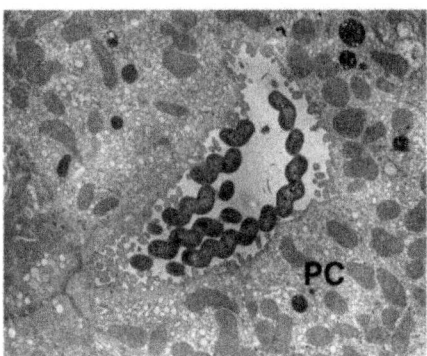

FIGURE 2 Five *H. heilmannii* organisms in a gastric gland, surrounded by parietal cells (PC) (cat stomach, ×20 000).

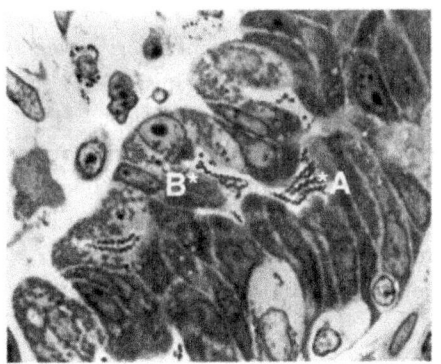

FIGURE 3 Light micrograph showing *H. heilmannii* in (A) gastric glands and (B) parietal cell canaliculi. (Cat stomach, semi-thin 0.5 μm plastic section, ×2500.)

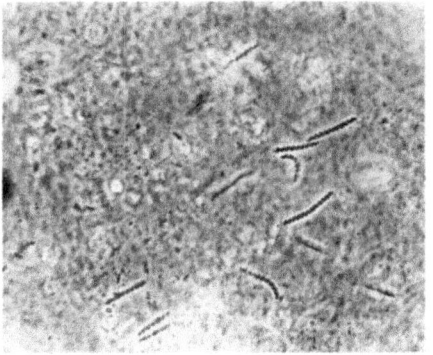

FIGURE 4 Mucosal scrapings viewed by phase contrast microscopy showing numerous *H. heilmannii* in longitudinal section; most of the organisms are straight. In these preparations, graceful motility can be seen in fresh specimens (cat stomach, ×500).

not yet definitively identified, he suggested that they were most likely *H. heilmannii*. Further communication with Jani O'Rourke concerning the identification of the *Helicobacter* species that I was studying resulted in a further evaluation of definitive species identification and we agreed that I probably had *H. heilmannii*-like bacteria. It now seems obvious that the gastric spirillum, which I thought was simply one, or only a few, species that colonized different mammals, is not quite so simple.

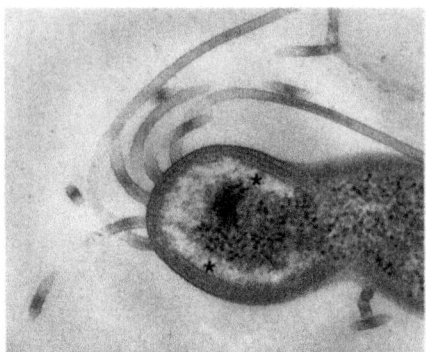

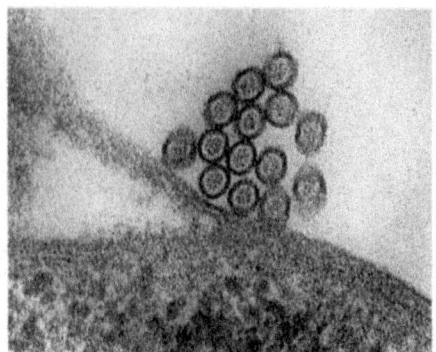

FIGURE 5 *Helicobacter heilmannii* showing terminal plate (*) and flagella (cat stomach, ×40 000).

FIGURE 6 Flagella of *H. heilmannii* in cross-section, showing the flagellin filaments as dots within the outer limiting structures (cat stomach ×220 000).

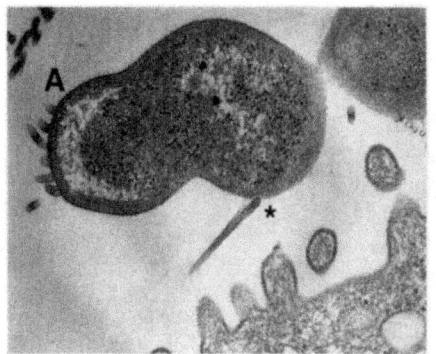

FIGURE 7 Detailed view of *H. heilmannii* flagella and the end of organism. Note the pale area (A) under the flagella insertion points. Nearby, the terminus of a flagellum is shown (*), and there does not appear to be a 'swelling' present as is often seen in *H. pylori* flagella (cat stomach, ×40 000).

The gastric spirilla that I collected were from a number of different cat stomachs. All the samples had *H. heilmannii*-like bacteria, with the exception of a few that had mixed infections with other organisms that were clearly *H. felis* by their distinctive morphology.

Electron microscopy of *Helicobacter*

The structure of helicobacters interested me because I was concurrently studying the ultrastructure of several rickettsial species. I noted that, as with other Gram-negative microorganisms, they had two limiting membranes. Both species are trilaminar. The outer membrane or cell wall was readily preserved by the usual glutaraldehyde or osmium tetroxide fixation procedure, but the inner or plasma membrane was either poorly retained or absent; it was much better preserved when uranyl acetate fixation was carried out prior to osmication and embedding. The reason for this is not known, but the uranium treatment also prevents the core clumping or aggregation of the bacterial DNA, which is fine and filamentous. These observations indicate that the plasma membrane and DNA of microorganisms share similar special needs for their detailed ultrastructural preservation.

A question that intrigued me was, what is the structural basis for the amazing flagellar activity of this organism? Electron microscopy revealed that each flagellar tuft comprised a few, but sometimes more than 15, individual sheathed bacterial flagella (FIGURES 5–7). Each is about 30 nm thick and 2–3 μm long. The size is limited by a single linear density flagellar sheath, which is 4–5 nm thick and contiguous with the outer leaflet of the cell wall. The inner leaflet of the cell wall does not extend into the flagella. Immediately beneath the flagellar sheath there is a clear space of about 4 nm, which must be the structure enclosing the central 10 nm area containing the thin flagellin filaments. Thin cross-sections of the sheathed flagella at very high magnification reveal some 10–14 transverse naked flagellin filaments, which appear as tiny dots of 1–2 nm (FIGURE 6). The filaments can also be seen in favorable longitudinal sections (FIGURE 5).

The lucent polar cytoplasm at the flagellar insertion site does not have the prominent flagellar basal complex found in some other bacteria. Alternative preparation methods may be needed to visualize that, if indeed it is present. However, there are some features that may be relevant for the rotation of the flagella. At the base of each flagellum, the flagellin filaments appear to traverse the inner leaflet of the cell wall and also the plasma membrane. This bundle of filaments, together with the interfibrillar material, is about 35 nm in diameter and extends some 20 nm into the terminal lucent cytoplasm (FIGURE 7).

Another structure consistently present in the terminal cytoplasm of *H. heilmannii*-like spirilla is the 'polar membrane', described very clearly by Lee and O'Rourke.[4,5] This structure is an electron-dense band, starting just lateral to the area of the flagellar insertion site and about 20 nm below the plasma membrane, that extends about 0.25 μm from the polar end.

The core of the lucent cytoplasm has a cone of dense cytoplasm containing numerous ribosome-like particles in a moderately dense ground substance (FIGURE 5). How the flagella generate their rapid and powerful propulsive activity is not obvious from their structure, but by studying the biochemistry of flagellar motility, more light has been shed on the mechanisms involved.

As on all cell surfaces, the helicobacter cell wall has an outer coat of fuzzy material, the equivalent of the glycocalyx of eukaryotic cells. The preservation and prominence of this material is dependent on the cell type and the preservation method employed. Because this coat is the interface between the microorganism and its environment, it is of obvious importance in adaptation and survival. The coat is probably a glycoprotein and studies have suggested that it binds to antigens on the surface of stomach cells and thus facilitates the bacterium's attachment to the epithelium. A better understanding of the surface coat would reveal much about helicobacter biology.

The cytoplasm of *H. heilmannii*-like organisms appears to be similar to that of other bacteria; that is, in a rather homogeneous cytoplasm there are regions that contain the filamentous DNA, small dense inclusions, larger dense bodies, low-density aggregates and clear vacuoles (FIGURE 7).

While working on the electron microscopy of the cat and other mammalian stomachs, I was able to obtain biopsies of human gastric mucosa, including samples from my own stomach. Some of these were used to study the *in vitro* incorporation of radioactive sugars in cells by electron microscope autoradiography, and also to further define gastric cell morphology. It was in one of these samples that a few *H. pylori* were observed. These differed distinctly from the helicobacters that I had been examining: they were not tightly coiled and were only rarely found in the corpus glands, being more commonly found in the pyloric glands (FIGURES 8,9).

Quite recently, while writing this chapter, I looked for the embedded blocks of human stomach in my residual collection. Fortunately, I had saved some of the specimens after moving out of my laboratory when I retired in 1990 and again after the Anatomy and Physiology Departments were combined to form the new Cell Biology Department. Since my retirement 11 years ago, I have been allowed to have a small laboratory and free access to

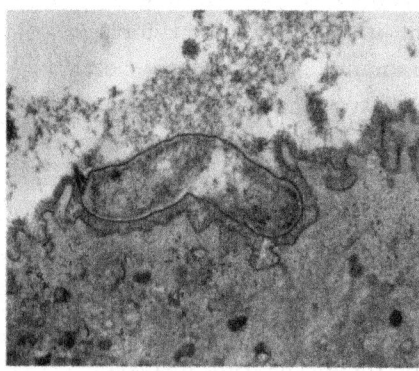

FIGURE 8 *Helicobacter pylori* on the surface of a mucus cell from the author's own stomach (human stomach, ×40 000).[1]

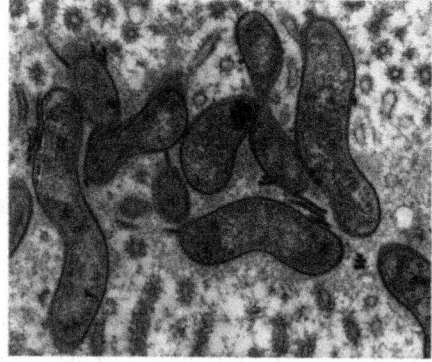

FIGURE 9 Family of *H. pylori* adjacent to a surface mucus cell in the human stomach (×20 000).

the electron microscopes and equipment to continue my collaborative research, which I pursue during the early morning hours. I still enjoy doing all of the embedding, thin- and thick-sectioning and the electron microscopy myself. The blocks I sought had been prepared in 1965 and even earlier, but they still thin-sectioned well and much of the ultrastructural features were still quite good. It thus seems that our specimens will retain their fine structure long after we are gone!

Helicobacter localization within the gastric mucosa

Each *Helicobacter* species seems to have preferential sites in specific glandular regions of the gastric mucosa. *Helicobacter heilmannii-like* organisms are abundant in the corpus area in the superficial mucus layer, in the stomach lumen, throughout the gland lumen and even in the intracellular canaliculi of the parietal cells (FIGURES 2,3,10). Habitation in parietal cells where gastric acid is secreted at high concentrations would seem hazardous, but they manage to flourish, suggesting that there must be some ecological or physiological advantage.

The localization of *Helicobacter* in parietal cells presents an unusual opportunity to use the bacteria as a marker of the cell's structural changes when it reverts from the active secreting to the resting stage. It is generally agreed that during HCl secretion the extensive intracellular canalicular network with numerous microvilli is open to the gland lumen. The prevailing hypothesis is that the resting (nonsecreting) cell depletes its abundant tubulovesicular membranes to produce canalicular microvilli, which are abundant during the secretory configuration. However, when active acid secretion ceases, the tubulovesicular membranes increase concomitantly with a corresponding decrease in microvilli and surface membrane. What is the fate of the unfortunate helicobacters trapped in the canaliculi of acid-secreting parietal cells that are reverting to the resting configuration? Some, no doubt, escape back into the gland lumen, but others are confined in the canaliculi as the microvilli are somehow transferred or

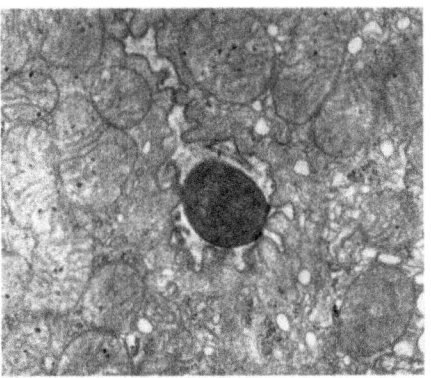

FIGURE 10 Cross-section of a parietal cell canaliculus containing *H. heilmannii*. Normal-looking flagella and cell wall confirm that this organism is comfortable in this environment, although the short microvilli nearby show that the cell is not actively secreting acid (cat stomach, ×40 000).

transposed to become tubulovesicular membranes (FIGURE 11). In the fully resting parietal cell the canaliculus is no longer open to the lumen and almost completely disappears. Thus, the canaliculi are truly intracellular in the resting parietal cell.

Although these cellular changes, I believe, are reasonable interpretations based upon the morphological evidence, they have not yet been demonstrated experimentally because appropriate tracer methods do not exist. Thus it is fortunate that helicobacters in the parietal cell canaliculi appear to afford an unusual and fortuitous marker of the cells' cyclical, secretory morphological changes (FIGURES 2,10,11).

An indication that a particular parietal cell may undergo several cyclic secretory changes during its normal lifespan of several weeks is evident in electron micrographs of helicobacter-infected parietal cells. Bacteria with flagella are clearly in the process of being degraded in parietal cell vacuoles or remnants of the intracellular canaliculi (FIGURE 12). The very dense inclusions in the same or neighboring parietal cells are most likely the unidentifiable remains of helicobacters that were trapped during some earlier secretory cycle.

I have been trying for years to relate the parietal cell's morphological changes to its physiological activity. To this end, I have tried to force electron-dense tracers, such as horseradish peroxidase, iron dextran or ferritin, into the intracellular canaliculi of living parietal cells, starting as early as 1965, but my efforts have never been successful. The objective was to determine whether the canalicular lumen was contiguous with the lumen of the tubulovesicular membrane system. To this day, I believe that convincing

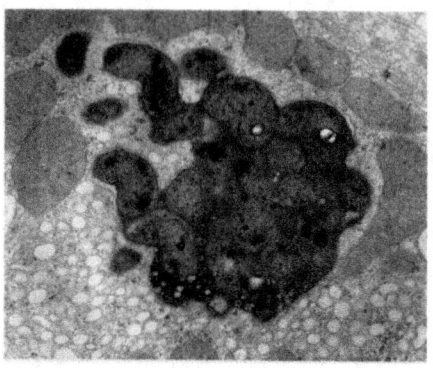

FIGURE 11 Parietal cell, resting stage. Several *H. heilmannii* organisms have been caught within a vacuole (cat stomach, ×40 000).

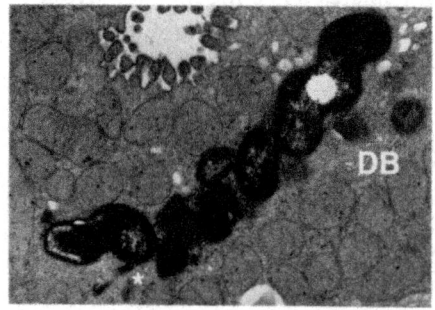

FIGURE 12 *Helicobacter heilmanii* organism apparently undergoing degradation within a lysosome. Although the cell wall is indistinct in some areas and fuzzy dense bodies (DB) are seen nearby, the flagella remain largely intact (*) (cat stomach, ×40 000).

evidence of tracer continuity between these compartments has not been demonstrated, but some recent morphological evidence of probable connections have been shown by high-resolution scanning electron microscopy.[6]

It should be noted that there is a possible alternative process that would account for some of the internalized helicobacters in parietal cells. Almost all cells have the capacity to phagocytose large amounts of extracellular material when appropriate receptors are present on the cell surface. Although apparent phagocytosis of helicobacters is seen in all the cell types in the epithelium, and in some connective tissue cells, these occurrences are rather infrequent. Therefore, some of the intracellular bacteria in the parietal cells are likely to have been phagocytosed from the intracellular canaliculus, but the evidence is strong that some, if not most, have been internalized when the cell goes into the resting stage.

Most of my observations have been made in cat gastric mucosa, but there were several monkey stomachs that I examined that had similar bacteria in the gastric glands. In some samples the incidence of internalized helicobacters in the parietal cells was striking, with numerous bacteria in varying stages of degradation while trapped in canaliculi that were much reduced in size.

Other observations were made of stomach specimens from Japanese monastery monkeys supposedly infected with *H. heilmannii*, provided by Professor Shinichi Takahashi of Kyorin University, Tokyo, Japan, in which the organisms were so numerous in the oxyntic glands, and in particular the parietal cells, that they illustrated and reinforced the observations of *H. heilmannii*-like spirilla in the cat (FIGURE 13).[7] In retrospect, I was puzzled by the similarity of what I believed were two different species: *H. heilmannii* and *H. felis*. Since then I have decided that many *Helicobacter* species have a very similar fine structure, but the species vary according to their host.

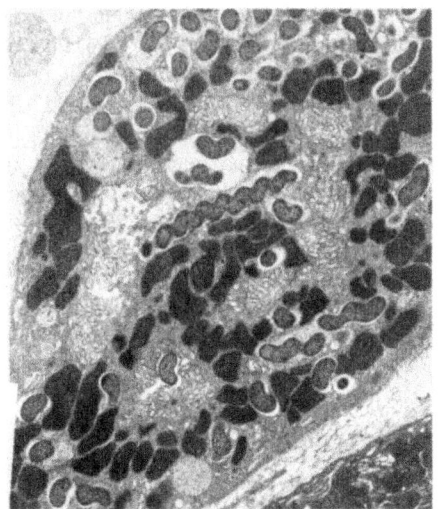

FIGURE 13 In this section from a Japanese monkey, apparent *H. heilmannii* can be seen. In cross-section the organisms appear to be the same diameter as mitochondria, but stain slightly more densely. In this image, all the helicobacters appear to be within vacuoles or in the canaliculi. (Specimen from Dr Shinichi Takahashi, ×14 000.)

To sum up my encounter with the *Helicobacter* genus, it has been a fun experience and, as it turned out, I was only looking at them because they were interesting bacteria! In this rather superficial compilation of some of my numerous observations, I have learned much more about these spirilla than I ever expected, and I am grateful to have had this opportunity. If it were not for this attempt to gather up the many loose ends of my long affair with *Helicobacter*, all of my material and observations would, I am certain, have ended up in the trash can. It has been most rewarding and a pleasure to partake in this endeavor.

References

[1] Ito S. Anatomic structure of the gastric mucosa. In: Heidel US, Code CF (eds). *Handbook of Physiology.* Section 6: *Alimentary Canal,* Vol. 2: *Secretion.* Washington DC: American Physiological Society, 1967; 705–41.

[2] Bizzozero G. Ueber die Schlauchformigen Drusen des Magendarmkanals und die Bezienhungen ihres Epithels zu dem Oberflachenepithel der Schleimhaut. *Arch Mikr Anat* 1893; **42**: 82.

[3] Salomon H. Ueber das Spirillum des Saugetiermagens und sien Verhalten zu den Belegzellen. *Zentralbl Bakteriol* 1896; **19**: 433–42.

[4] Lee ASL, Hazell SL, O'Rourke J, Kouprach S. Isolation of a spiral-shaped bacterium from the cat stomach. *Infect Immun* 1988; **56**: 2843–50.

[5] O'Rourke JL, Neilan BA, Lee A. Phylogenic relationship of *Helicobacter heilmannii*-like organisms originating from humans and animals (Abstract HE4). In: Mobley H (ed.) Proceedings of the 10th International Workshop on Campylobacter, Helicobacter and Related Organisms. Baltimore, 1999.

[6] Ogata M, Araki K, Ogata T. An electron microscopic study of *Helicobacter pylori* in the surface mucous gel layer. *Histol Histopathol* 1998; **13**: 347–58.

[7] Takahashi S, Igarashi H, Ishiyama N *et al.* Serial change of gastric mucosa after challenging with *Helicobacter pylori* in the cynomolgus monkey. *Int J Med Microbiol Virol Parasitol Infect Dis* 1993; **280**: 51.

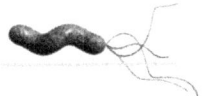

CHAPTER 9

How we discovered in China in 1972 that antibiotics cure peptic ulcer

Shu-Dong Xiao, Yao Shi and Wen-Zhong Liu

W HEN WARREN AND MARSHALL published 'Unidentified curved bacilli on gastric epithelium in active chronic gastritis' in *The Lancet* in 1983,[1] only a few gastroenterologists in the Chinese medical community believed that the curved bacillus, called *Campylobacter pyloridis* and later named *Helicobacter pylori*, which had been cultivated from biopsied gastric mucosa, was the most important etiological factor of active chronic gastritis. Now it is well known that *H. pylori* is the pathogen for this disease and for peptic ulcer, and in 1994 the International Agency for Research on Cancer of the World Health Organization declared *H. pylori* a Group I (or definite) carcinogen of gastric cancer in humans.[2] Hence, the eradication of *H. pylori* has become crucial in the treatment of *H. pylori*-positive peptic ulcer disease, and triple therapies based on bismuth and proton pump inhibitors (PPI) are currently the main regimens. After eradication therapy, the recurrence rates of duodenal ulcer and gastric ulcer drop from 70% to 3% or less, and this is generally regarded as one of the greatest advances in medicine in the 20th century. Unbelievably, in China, before any knowledge of *H. pylori*, many doctors were using an antimicrobial agent, furazolidone, to treat active chronic gastritis and peptic ulcer,[3] and curved bacilli had been found on the gastric mucosa, but were not recognized as pathogenic for gastroduodenal disease.[4]

In 1960, a colleague reported informally that oral antibiotics, such as penicillin V, gentamycin and kanamycin, were effective in relieving symptoms in patients with active chronic gastritis. At that time, neither medical textbooks nor medical journals had any evidence that gastritis was caused by bacterial infection, and so there was no clinical reason for antimicrobial treatment. However, patients' symptoms, such as upper abdominal pain, could be relieved by this empirical therapy, and so before 1980, when Tagamet® became available in China, many doctors in outpatient clinics and small hospitals were using furazolidone, with good effect, for patients with refractory peptic ulcer.[5]

Furazolidone was used in the late 1940s as an oral antibacterial and antiprotozoal agent, effective against many Gram-negative organisms, in the treatment of diarrhea and enteritis. Its use in peptic ulcer was first reported in China in 1972[6] and was widely used all over the country; it is estimated that in nearly 15 years, thousands of patients were treated. To confirm its efficacy, Professor Zhi-Tian Zheng, from Beijing Medical College Affiliated No. 3 Hospital, conducted a double-blind, randomized and placebo-controlled clinical trial from November 1982 to May 1983 using a 2-week regimen of furazolidone (200 mg t.i.d.).[5] The ulcer healing rate was 72.9% in the furazolidone group versus 24.2% in the placebo group, a statistically significant difference between the two groups ($P < 0.001$).

After the report of the association between *H. pylori* and chronic gastritis by Drs Warren and Marshall in 1983,[1] we re-investigated the anti-*H. pylori* effect of furazolidone in a randomized double-blind placebo-controlled clinical trial.[7] Seventy-two patients with *H. pylori*-associated chronic gastritis were randomized to a 3-week oral regimen with furazolidone 100 mg t.i.d., metronidazole 200 mg t.i.d. or placebo. Endoscopy was performed before and after treatment, and biopsy specimens were taken from the gastric antrum for histological examination and bacterial culture. The clearance rates of *H. pylori* in the furazolidone, metronidazole and control groups were 80%, 33.3% and 14.3%, respectively. There was a significant difference between the furazolidone group and the metronidazole and placebo groups ($P < 0.01$), but not between the metronidazole and placebo groups ($P > 0.05$). In the patients receiving furazolidone, the eradication of *H. pylori* was accompanied by marked improvement in both inflammatory infiltration in the gastric mucosa and clinical symptoms.

From 1995, our group conducted the 5-year 'Dutchigas Project' with Professor Guido Tytgat of the Department of Gastroenterology and Hepatology, Academic Medical Center, Amsterdam, the Netherlands, supported by the Ministry of Education and Science of the Dutch Government and the Ministry of Public Health of the People's Republic of China. We did a series of collaborative research projects on the eradication of *H. pylori* using bismuth/furazolidone-based and PPI furazolidone-based triple or quadruple therapies (TABLE I).[8–11] Among the short-term PPI-based triple therapy regimens, most of which included metronidazole, the eradication rate was at least 90%. However, the resistance of *H. pylori* strains to metronidazole, and to a lesser extent to clarithromycin, has increased rapidly in recent years and will

TABLE 1 One-week regimens containing furazolidone for eradication of *Helicobacter pylori*

Regimen	Drug combination	Dosage	H. pylori eradication rate	95% CI
FCB	Furazolidone	100 mg b.i.d.	91%	82–99%
	Clarithromycin	250 mg b.i.d.		
	TDB	240 mg b.i.d.		
FCL	Furazolidone	100 mg b.i.d.	91%	82–99%
	Clarithromycin	250 mg b.i.d.		
	Lansoprazole	30 mg q.i.d.		
FCO	Furazolidone	100 mg b.i.d.	86%	74–95%
	Clarithromycin	250 mg b.i.d		
	Omeprazole	20 mg q.i.d.		
FJB	Furazolidone	100 mg b.i.d.	77%	66–87%
	Josamycin	1000 mg b.i.d.		
	TDB	240 mg b.i.d.		
FBJFa	Furazolidone	100 mg b.i.d.	94.7%	88.9–99.6%
	TDB	240 mg b.i.d.		
	Josamycin	1000 mg b.i.d.		
	Famotidine	20 mg b.i.d.		
FAO	Furazolidone	100 mg b.i.d.	87%	82–91%
	Amoxicillin	1000 mg b.i.d.		
	Omeprazole	20 mg b.i.d.		

TDB, tripotassium dicitrato bismuthate.

eventually affect eradication rates. In Shanghai, for example, the resistance rate of *H. pylori* strains to metronidazole has increased from 42% in 1995 to nearly 70% in 1999, and to clarithromycin from 0% in 1995 to 10% in 1999.[12] Our studies indicate that furazolidone may replace metronidazole in PPI-based or bismuth-based triple therapies in developing countries where the resistance of *H. pylori* strains to metronidazole is high.

From 1978 to 1981, Dr Yao Shi, one of the present authors, was a graduate student majoring in gastroenterology at Shanghai Second Medical University. His thesis, entitled 'Scanning Electron Microscopic Observation in Chronic Gastritis', was defended in 1981 and published in 1983.[4] Dr Shi studied the gastric mucosa using electron microscopy (both transmission and scanning electron microscopes) in 26 cases of chronic gastritis, investigating the structural changes of the stomach, particularly of its microstructure. He found that in the progression from superficial to atrophic gastritis in the corpus of the stomach, the opening of the foveolae changed from a round to a slit-like shape, thus changing the original honeycomb-like microstructure to one resembling the antral mucosa (FIGURE 1). In the antrum, the mucosa with severe intestinal metaplasia had a similar appearance to the villi of the small intestine (FIGURE 2).

Surprisingly, on scanning electron microscopy, Dr Shi found curved bacilli on the surface of the gastric mucosa (FIGURE 3), sometimes so small that it was difficult to differentiate them from residual mucus flakes, but as the morphology and size of the organisms were similar, they were considered to be bacteria. At that time it was considered that these were 'passenger' bacteria and not the pathogen for gastroduodenal diseases, because in gastric biopsy specimens the bacteria were seldom seen, a result of the mucus on the mucosal surface having been washed out in the preparation process. Although it was well known that gastric acid and enzymes were capable of killing bacteria, the presence of a few 'passengers' in the stomach was not uncommon.

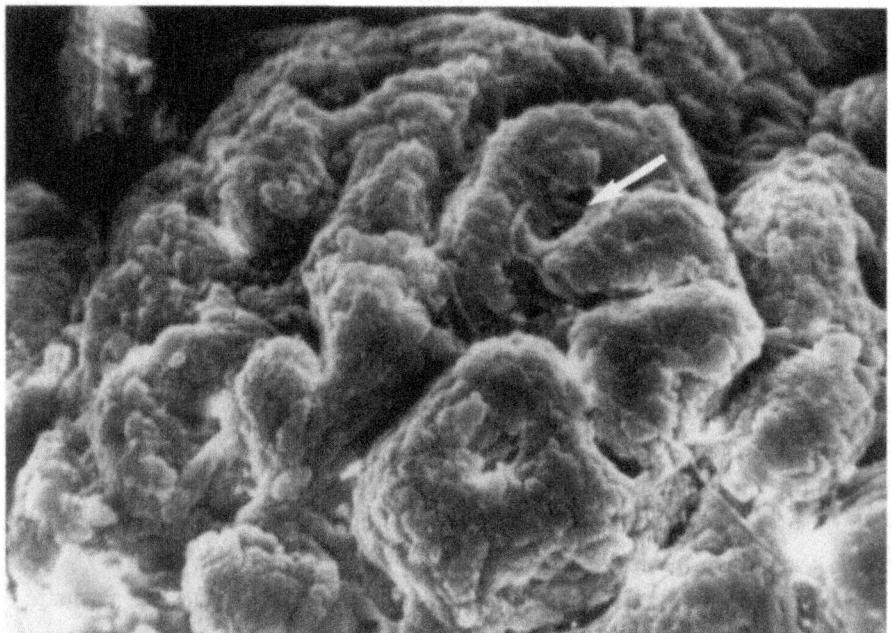

FIGURE 1 In the progression from superficial to atrophic gastritis of the mucosa of the corpus, the opening of the foveolae changes from a round to a slit-like shape, causing the mucosa to resemble that of the antrum. The white arrow indicates a bridge-like connection in a slit-like foveola.

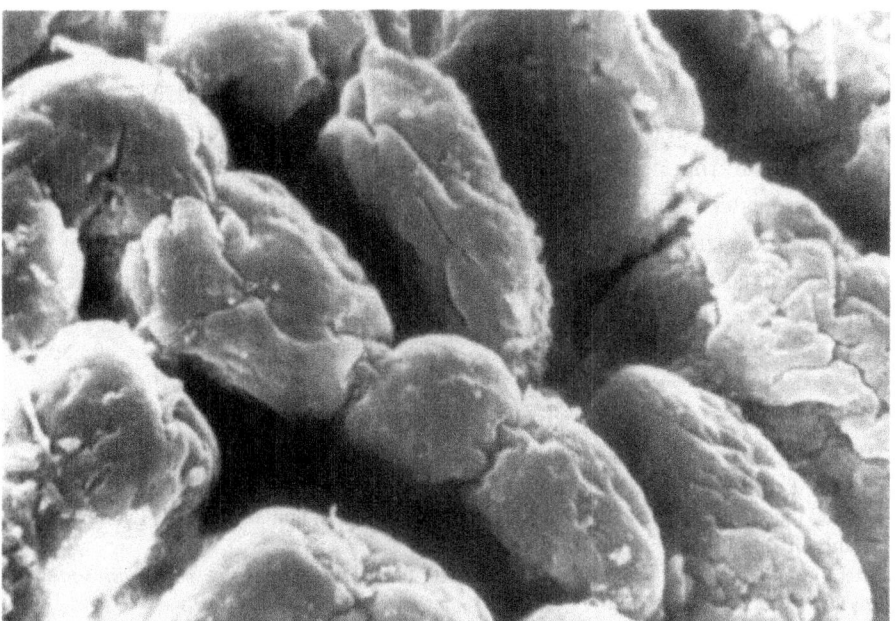

FIGURE 2 The gastric mucosa with severe intestinal metaplasia has a similar appearance to the villi of the small intestine.

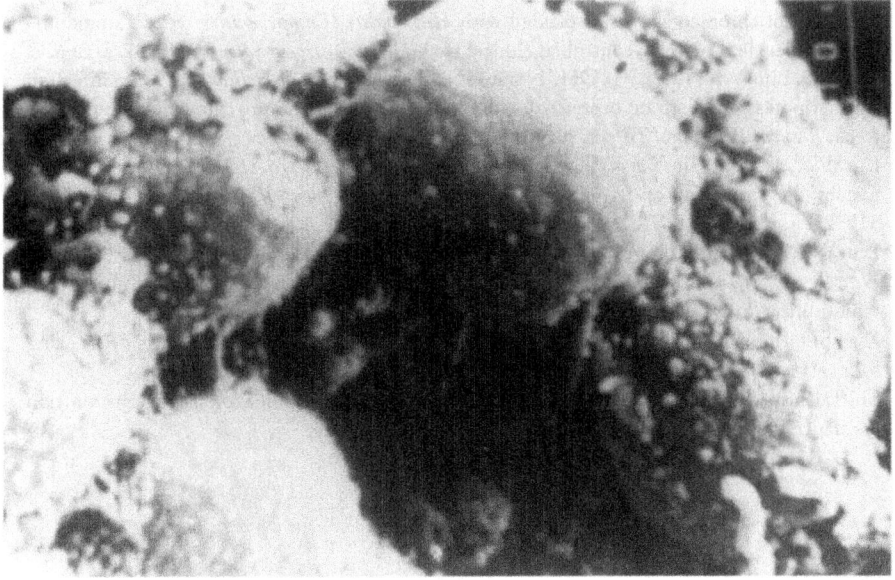

FIGURE 3 A few curved bacilli can be seen on the surface of a gastric epithelial cell (lower righthand corner).

Sometimes, we can find a new, peculiar thing in our daily work, but those who decipher the meaning and function of it are outstanding. Two decades have elapsed since the report of *H. pylori* by Drs Warren and Marshall in Perth, Western Australia and we now understand a lot about this organism and its role in the pathogenesis of active chronic gastritis, peptic ulcer, mucosa-associated lymphoid tissue lymphoma and gastric cancer, as well as how to diagnose and cure *H. pylori* infection. However, there are still a lot of questions related to this bacterium and the gastroduodenal diseases associated with it.

References

[1] Warren JR, Marshall B. Unidentified curved bacilli on gastric epithelium in active chronic gastritis. *Lancet* 1983; **1**: 1273–5.

[2] IARC Monographs on the evaluation of carcinogenic risks to humans, Vol. 61. Lyon: World Health Organization, 1994; 177–240.

[3] Zheng ZT, Wang YB. Treatment of peptic ulcer disease with furazolidone. *J Gastroenterol Hepatol* 1992; **7**: 533–7.

[4] Shi Y, Xiao SD, Jiang SJ, Han YS, Zhu JG. Scanning electron microscopic observation in chronic gastritis. *Chin J Digest* 1983; **3**: 23–5 (in Chinese).

[5] Zheng ZT, Wang TY, Zhu YS *et al.* A double-blind short-term clinical trial of the effect of furazolidone on peptic ulcer. *Chin J Intern Med* 1984; **23**: 195–7 (in Chinese).

[6] Anonymous. A report of 12 cases of duodenal ulcer treated with furazolidone. *Shandong Med* 1972; **5**: 68 (in Chinese).

[7] Xiao SD, Liu WZ, Xia DH *et al.* The efficacy of furazolidone and metronidazole in the treatment of chronic gastritis associated with *Helicobacter (Campylobacter) pylori*: a randomized double-blind placebo-controlled clinical trial. *Hepatogastroenterology* 1990; **37**: 503–6.

[8] Xiao SD, Liu WZ, Hu PJ, Xia DH, Tytgat GN. High cure rate of *Helicobacter pylori* infection using tripotassium dicitrato bismuthate, furazolidone and clarithromycin triple therapy for 1 week. *Aliment Pharmacol Ther* 1999; **13**: 311–15.

[9] Liu WZ, Xiao SD, Shi Y *et al.* Furazolidone-containing short-term triple therapies are effective in the treatment of *Helicobacter pylori* infection. *Aliment Pharmacol Ther* 1999; **13**: 317–22.

[10] Liu WZ, Xiao SD, Hu PJ, Lu H, Cui Y, Tytgat GN. A new quadruple therapy for *Helicobacter pylori* using tripotassium dicitrato bismuthate, furazolidone, josamycin and famotidine. *Aliment Pharmacol Ther* 2000; **14**: 1519–22.

[11] Xiao SD, Liu WZ, Hu PJ *et al.* A multicentre study on eradication of *Helicobacter pylori* using four 1-week triple therapies in China. *Aliment Pharmacol Ther* 2001; **15**: 81–6.

[12] Shi T, Liu WZ, Xiao SD, Xu WW. The changing trend of metronidazole and clarithromycin resistance rates. *Chin J Intern Med* 2000; **39**: 576 (in Chinese).

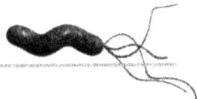

CHAPTER 10

Helicobacter pylori was discovered in Russia in 1974

Igor A. Morozov

L ET ME RECALL the beginning of the 1970s. All the scientific world, including the USSR, had a consensus regarding the etiology and pathogenesis of chronic gastritis and the ulcerative diseases of the stomach. Chronic gastritis was conceptualized as a morphological disruption of the mucosa with evidence of an inflammatory process, but varying in its etiology and pathogenesis. There was no generally recognized and universal classification of chronic gastritis; pathologists classified it by the distribution of inflammation and atrophy. Two main forms of chronic gastritis (superficial and atrophic) were taught by Dr Schindler well in advance of the development of such methods as directed biopsy using fiberoptic gastroscopy. Soviet gastroenterologists proposed a borderline form, namely, chronic gastritis with glandular alteration, but without atrophy.[1] The clinical classification of gastritis was based on the acidity of the gastric juice (i.e. ana-, hypo-, normo- and hyperacidic gastritis) and in the USSR before 1973 the most widespread clinical classification of chronic gastritis was Ryss's,[2] which took into account the 'modern' etiology, the morphological alterations of the mucosa of the stomach, the functional condition of the stomach, and clinical symptoms. Chronic gastritis was further subdivided by etiology into exogenous and endogenous types.

The exogenous causes thought responsible for chronic gastritis were long-term nutritional disruptions, chronic smoking and alcohol intake, and chemical, mechanical, thermal, occupational or other agents. Endogenous gastritis was subdivided further into neuroreflex (signals from other affected organs), neuroendocrine, hematogenic, hypoxemic and allergic gastritis. According to the current trends in science, most of these factors would not be considered as etiological causes.

Beginning in 1973, after the publication of a reappraisal by Strickland and MacKay,[3] chronic gastritis began to be divided into A (autoimmune) and B types, the former being differentiated by its etiology. Infectious agents were not mentioned in this classification.

Nonetheless, it was a time of innovative research. The renowned French gastroenterologists, Moutier and Cornet, had published their concept of a possible infectious origin of chronic gastritis and they recommended treating chronic gastritis with antibiotics as well as with autovaccines prepared from microbes isolated from the oral cavity and gastric juice. The Bulgarian gastroenterologist Dr Tashev believed that microbes (streptococci, staphylococci, enterococci etc.) contaminating the oral cavity, larynx and lung could be responsible for chronic gastritis,[5] but his opinion was not well accepted. Dr Fishson-Ryss from the USSR did not denounce completely the microbial factor in the etiology of chronic gastritis, but nonetheless, wrote in 1974, 'There is no need to go into extremes and to assign a seemingly leading role in the etiology of chronic gastritis for the infectious-toxic damage to the mucosa of the stomach'.[6]

At this time, better defined concepts existed in the USSR for the etiopathogenic mechanisms of peptic ulceration. The simplified corticovisceral theory was discarded and replaced by a neuro-peptic theory in which the ulcer diathesis was put down to a disturbed balance between the aggressive and defensive factors. The leading factors in ulceration were thought to be acidic–peptic and neurotrophic, and among the defense mechanisms were the normal mucus secretion, prostaglandins, self-replacing epithelium and stable blood circulation in the mucosa of the stomach. However, the neuro-peptic theory could not explain the absence of ulcers under some conditions; for example, with very high activity of aggressive juice, as well as after biopsy or polypectomy, when a full thickness lesion of the mucosal layer did not result in an ulcer, but rather complete restoration several days later.

The role of chronic gastritis as an etiological factor of peptic ulcer was denied by most of the leading gastroenterologists in the USSR who believed in the independence of these nosological forms. Chronic gastritis occurring together with peptic ulcer was considered as an independent disease entity. In the USSR, as in the whole scientific world, Dr Konjetzny's 'gastritic theory'[7] was not accepted because of its total disapproval of peptic and other pathogenic factors. At the same time, there were no confirmed cases of either gastric or duodenal ulceration in the absence of the morphological markers of chronic gastritis or duodenitis. This consideration was the main motivating force for the quest of a verification of the hypothesis that chronic gastritis and peptic ulcer have unified etiological origins and pathogenesis, but the first concepts developing this idea were put forward only at the beginning of the 1980s. The idea that chronic gastritis set the stage for peptic ulcer created the basis for acceptance of the theory of the infectious origin of gastritis-associated ulcerative disease.

Let us look further into the history of medicine. In 1936, the First Edition of the Russian *Large Medical Encyclopaedia*[8] indicated infection as one of the etiological causes of peptic ulcer, and during the next decades several papers describing the successful treatment of peptic ulcer with antibiotics were published. Thus, the pathogenic role of infection as an initiating factor for peptic ulcer has a long tradition in Russian gastroenterology.

In 1955, Dr Tarnopolskaya proposed using the so-called 'penicillin probe' (routinely 200 000–300 000 U of benzylpenicillinum-natrium 2 or 3 times per day by injection for 7–10 days) with the aim of providing a differential diagnosis between peptic ulcer and stomach cancer.[9] According to his roentgenological investigations, the infiltrated rolled edge around the ulcer either decreased or dispersed after penicillin treatment, whereas the cancer infiltration was unaffected. In 1958, Dr Gordon and coworkers from the same clinic as Dr Tarnopolskaya published data on the successful treatment of 100 patients with complicated peptic ulcer using a penicillin–streptomycin combination,[10] but unfortunately, the mutual mechanism of the antibiotics' effect on reducing the infiltrated rolled ulcer edge and precipitating ulcer healing was not adequately explained.

Gastroenterologists also made some strides toward healing of ulcerative disease with metronidazole injection.[11] Combined with the standard antiulcer treatment using anticholinergic and antacid preparations, metronidazole led, in 84% of cases, to the rapid disappearance of abdominal pain and ulcer healing within 2 or 3 weeks, which was much quicker than with treatment that did not include metronidazole. These clinical data were confirmed in 1981 by other Russian authors[12] and were referenced by Drs Marshall and Warren.[13] In the 1970s, metronidazole was not considered an antibiotic, but rather as a regenerative process stimulator, and 20 years later, this mistake, as well as the widespread use of metronidazole alone for the treatment of both peptic ulcer and urological infection, has resulted in the creation of a large proportion of *Helicobacter pylori* strains (approx. 50%) that are resistant to this drug.

Having made a retrospective journey into the history of medicine to review the reunification of the infectious and peptic ulcer pathogeneses, let us now look into my own achievements. At the beginning of the 1970s, I worked in Moscow in the Laboratory of Pathology of the Institute of Gastroenterology under the supervision of Professor Leonid Aruin, studying the influence of some normal and artificial conditions (long-term clinical fasting, hyperacidic conditions, vagotomy complications etc.) on the function and ultrastructure of parietal cells, in both humans and laboratory animals. During this time, some other scientists and I began to cast doubt on the statement that the mucosa of the stomach and duodenum could not be contaminated by any residential microbes because of the high acidity of the gastric juice. During light and electron microscopy investigations of the stomach and bowel of Wistar rats and C57Bl/6 mice, we routinely found a large number of spiral-shaped bacteria with flagella either at one end or both (Figure 1a,b). These bacterial colonies were located deep in the crypts adjacent to the Paneth cells, thereby excluding the possibility that they were contaminants from the lumen. Later, these bacteria were isolated and identified as *H. muridarum*.[14]

At last we are coming to the main theme of my narrative; namely, the discovery of the role of *H. pylori* in the pathogenesis of peptic ulcer. In 1974, we carried out electron microscopic analysis of the antral mucosa of the stomach of a patient, 4 years after a vagotomy performed to relieve the symptoms of ulcer disease. When examining a section of mucosa in which the mucus layer was well maintained, we discovered numerous cocci-shaped bacteria located in both the mucus itself and in the valleys between epithelial cells (Figure 2). Unfortunately, the mucus from the fundal sections of the stomach of the same patient had washed off during biopsy preparation. Nonetheless, individual cocci were also found in the clefts of the intracellular secretory canaliculi of the parietal cells (Figure 3), abutting the microvillus membrane, without any apparent deleterious morphological effects.

We were quite surprised to discover an S-shaped bacillus, 2.5 μm in length, 0.4 μm in width and with two short flagella at one end, located inside a parietal cell from the same section (Figure 4). It appeared quite different from the cocci and was located within a vacuole. Initially it was believed that the bacillus had penetrated deep into the parietal cell, followed by cytolysis, but further investigations revealed that it was located within a dilated intracellular canaliculus of which the membrane was partially damaged. This conclusion was confirmed by further sections from other patients after vagotomy in which the same bacilli were revealed within the intracellular secretory canaliculi of parietal cells (Figure 5).

It should be emphasized that these data on the S-shaped bacillus disposition in secretory canaliculi of parietal cells were only obtained from patients after either stem or selective proximal vagotomy. According to clinical observations at this time, successful vagotomy resulted in a significant depletion of hydrochloric acid secretion; namely, basal secretion declined to zero and stimulated secretion was reduced to the range of 8–16 mEq/L per hour. The same pathophysiological mechanisms could have resulted in uncontrolled growth of

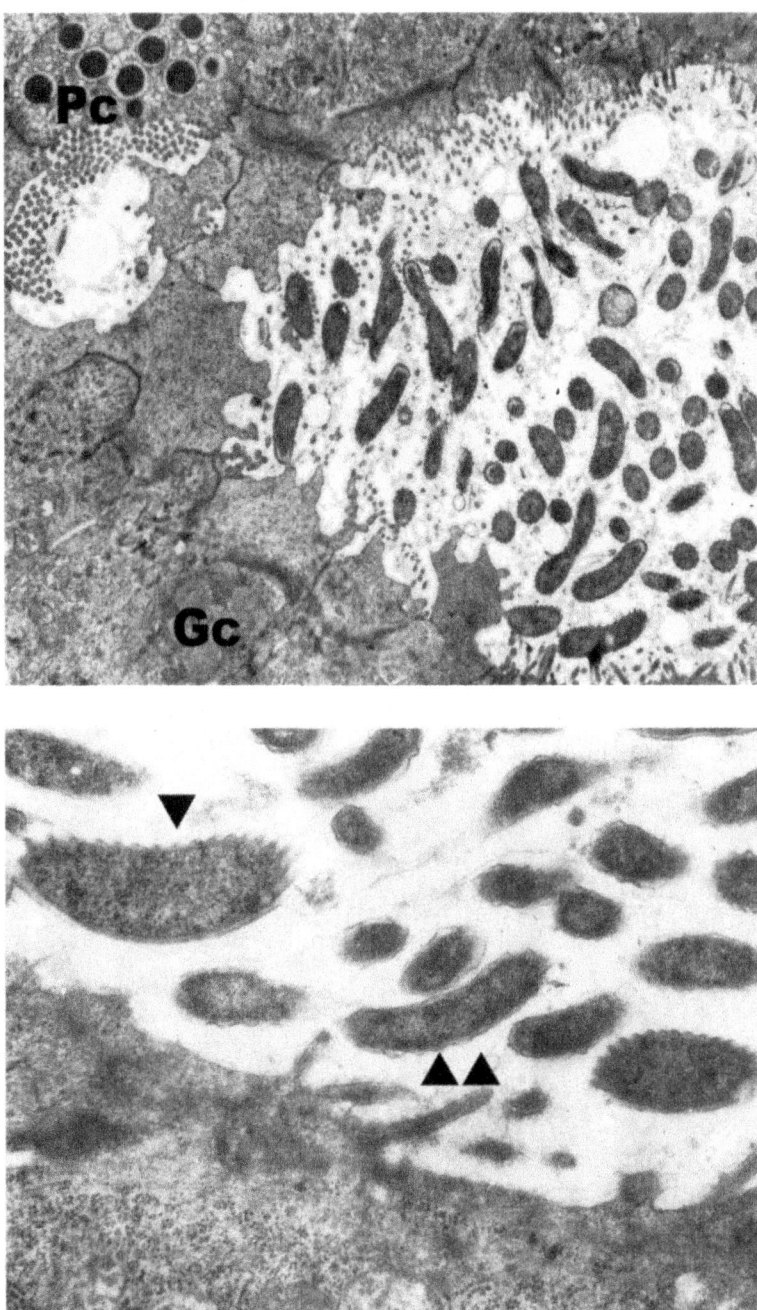

FIGURE 1 Spiral-shaped bacteria (*Helicobacter muridarum*). (Top) Bacterial colonies deep within the crypts of C57Bl/6 mice duodenum, adjacent to the Paneth cells (Pc) and Goblet cells (Gc) (×10 000). (Bottom) The same *H. muridarum* (arrowhead) and another strain of bacteria (*E. coli* ? double arrowheads) are located between the duodenal villi (×20 000).

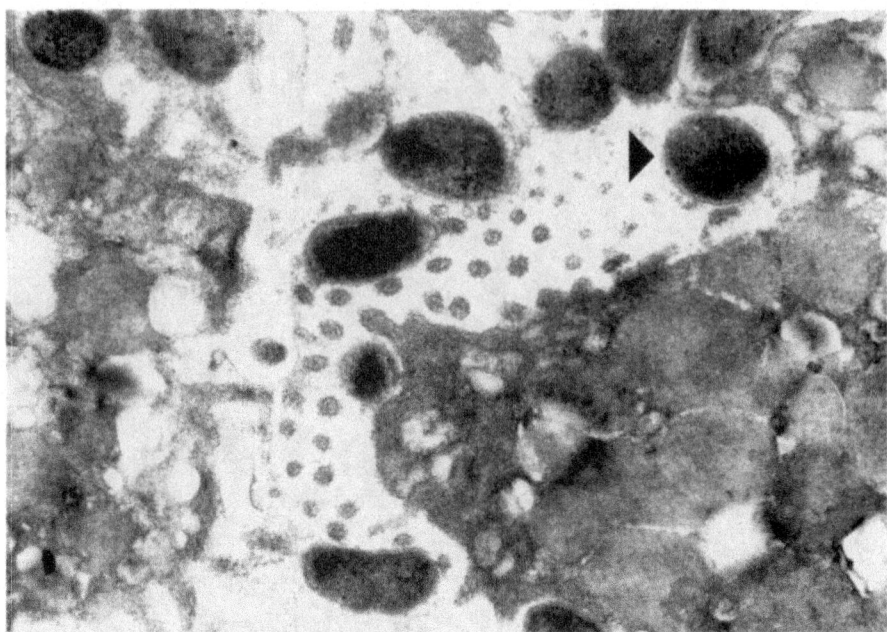

FIGURE 2 Numerous coccoid form of *H. pylori* (arrowhead) in the mucus layer of the antrum of the stomach from a patient with peptic ulcer, 4 years after selective proximal vagotomy (×30 000).

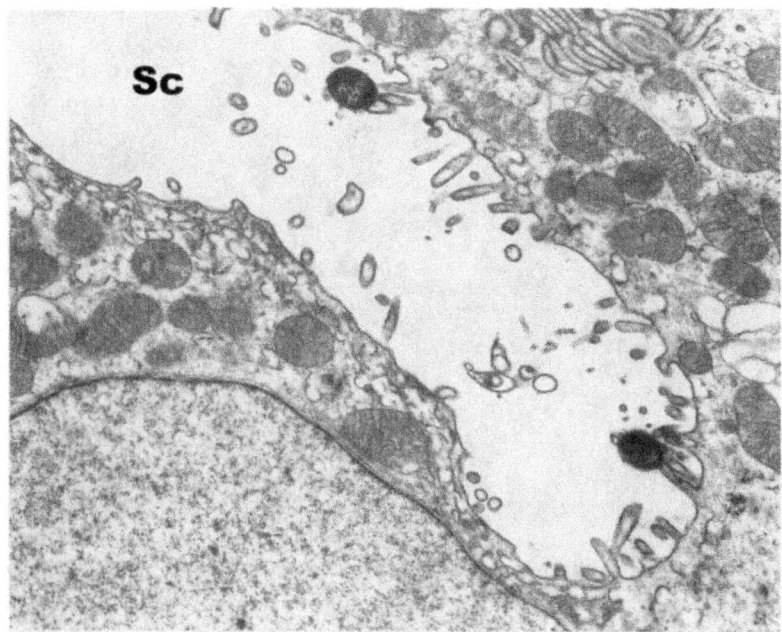

FIGURE 3 Coccoid form of *H. pylori* within the secretory canaliculus (Sc) of a parietal cell (patient in FIGURE 2; ×10 000).

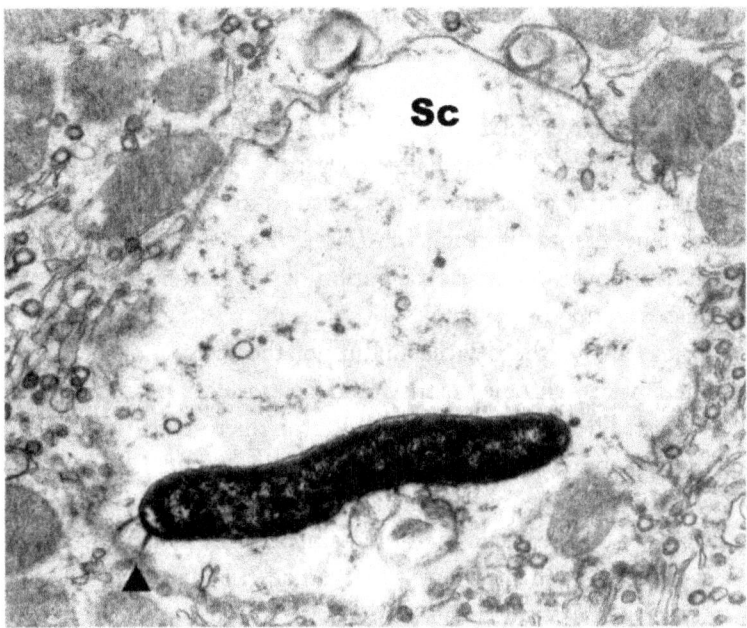

FIGURE 4 S-shaped bacterium (*H. pylori*) with flagella (arrowhead) within the dilated secretory canaliculus (Sc) of a parietal cell (patient in FIGURE 2; ×15 000).

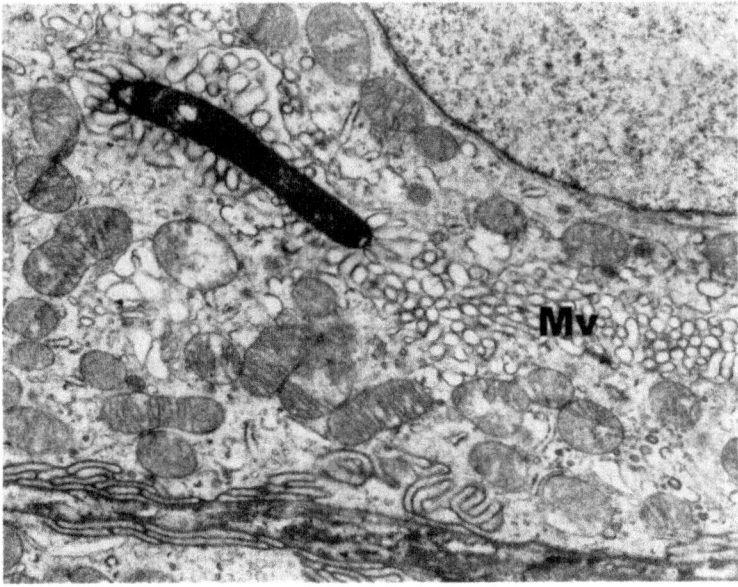

FIGURE 5 S-shaped bacteria (*H. pylori*) between the secretory channel microvilli (Mv) of a parietal cell of a patient with peptic ulcer, 2 years after vagotomy (×10 000).

the cocci and bacilli in the stomach. This was the reason why these observations might not have been interpreted according to current concepts and is the point of view on the origin of the discovered bacilli that I described in my Dissertation for the degree of Doctor of Medical Sciences in 1977.[15]

The publication from Drs Marshall and Warren[13] regarding the infectious nature of chronic gastritis and peptic ulcer forced us to recall our previous data of 1973–1975. The first publication on *H. pylori* in the Russian language included a description of our first observation of the bacteria and was illustrated by our electron micrographs.[16]

The main reasons for the delayed finding of the connection between the bacilli discovered by us, chronic gastritis and peptic ulcer pathogenesis have become clear at last. The first is the specific electron microscope technique. The mucus layer that is considered to be the main ecological niche for *H. pylori* was mostly washed off during the routine fixation method, followed by specific processing of specimens. A few bacilli might remain, but only by being attached to the mucosal surface. It is well known now that our described position of *H. pylori* is limited to special cases and in this connection, to have found any of these organisms during electron microscope analysis was quite an accidental boon.

The second reason is that those years were not a time for understanding such unusual data. In 1974, most pathologists were not ready to search for global changes in ulcer pathogenesis, including a possible bacterial basis of chronic gastritis and peptic ulcer. Similarly, routine light microscopic analysis by hematoxylin–eosin without special staining techniques, made it unlikely that bacilli would be reported in the usual histological sections.

Now it is quite clear why vagotomy, performed without preceding bacterial eradication, resulted in *H. pylori* being found as coccal forms in the antral portion of the stomach. *Helicobacter pylori* may have been sequestered in the secretory canaliculi of parietal cells in a vegetative form and influenced by either impaired hydrochloric acid secretion or its absence during starvation, the bacteria migrated in the direction of the more acid pH to survive. The analog to this phenomenon was shown later in peptic ulcer studies in which *H. pylori* dissemination only in the mucosa of the antral portion of the stomach was noted. Under inadequate therapy using metronidazole, De-Nol and omeprazole (20 mg nocte for 7 days), *H. pylori* from the antral portion of the stomach took on the coccoid form after 3–4 days, and after 5–7 days of the same treatment, *H. pylori* were found in the mucus of the fundal portion of the stomach. Two weeks after the completed treatment, the entire stomach was contaminated by *H. pylori* (FIGURE 6).[17]

Gaining a complete understanding of how the early results formed the basis for further understanding, we should refer to Dr Zufarov's publication of

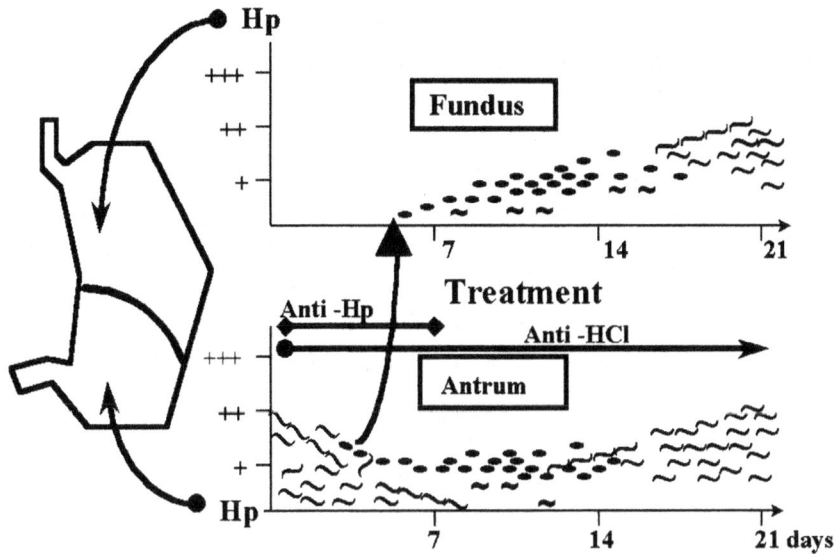

FIGURE 6   The response of a resistant strain of *Helicobacter pylori* to quadrotherapy in a peptic ulcer patient with primary dissemination in the antrum of the stomach only.

1974.[18] He is a scientist from Uzbekistan, which was part of the USSR. He and his coworkers studied electron microscope sections of the mucosa of the stomach from patients with peptic ulcer before and after gastrectomy and discovered contamination of the stomach by some strains of microbes, including streptococci, staphylococci, enterobacteria etc. The concentrations of these microbes were found to be much higher than in healthy people and these pathogenic flora were also found to possess a very aggressive enzyme composition, including catalase, hyaluronidase, fibrinolysin, hemolysin and others. The invasiveness and cytopathogenic capacities of these microbes were increased after gastrectomy that was followed by anacidic conditions. The microbes migrated from breaks in the glands through the intracellular canaliculi of the parietal cells towards the cytoplasm. One of the illustrations in Dr Zufarov's publication clearly showed intracellular canaliculi contaminated by bacilli of the *Helicobacter* family and may be recognized as *H. heilmannii* (*Gastrospirillum hominis*), having 4–5 screw-shaped bends of the bacillus body.[18] Initially, the lysosomes of the parietal cells had been thought to be bacilli in the cytoplasm.

The discovery of *H. pylori* in our laboratory and Dr Zufarov's discovery of *H. heilmannii* in the secretory channels of parietal cells were both made under similar physiological conditions marked by impaired hydrochloric acid secretion.

We kept these investigations going during the years after our initial discovery with the result that we made new observations on the morphological evidence regarding infectious contamination of the mucous membrane of the stomach. However, we could not explain these results at that time. In April 1977, on studying the mucous membrane of the stomach of patients with peptic ulcer, we observed contamination of the lamina propria by individual unusual bacilli, distinct from known bacilli by their form and ultrastructure (FIGURE 7). Such contamination was absolutely unknown before and would have been explained as a pathogenic bacterial invasion of the lamina propria either via intercellular conjunctions or through the broken epithelial layer of the mucosa.

After the recognition of the pathogenic role of *H. pylori* in peptic ulcer, there were publications concerning the possible invasion of *H. pylori* into the lamina propria under special conditions; for example, in acquired immune deficiency syndrome (AIDS).[19,20] Using immunohistochemical methods, we confirmed that in patients with AIDS and chronic gastritis (approx. 25% of cases) the gastric mucosal surface and its intima were both contaminated by *H. pylori*, following epithelial and basal membrane penetration.

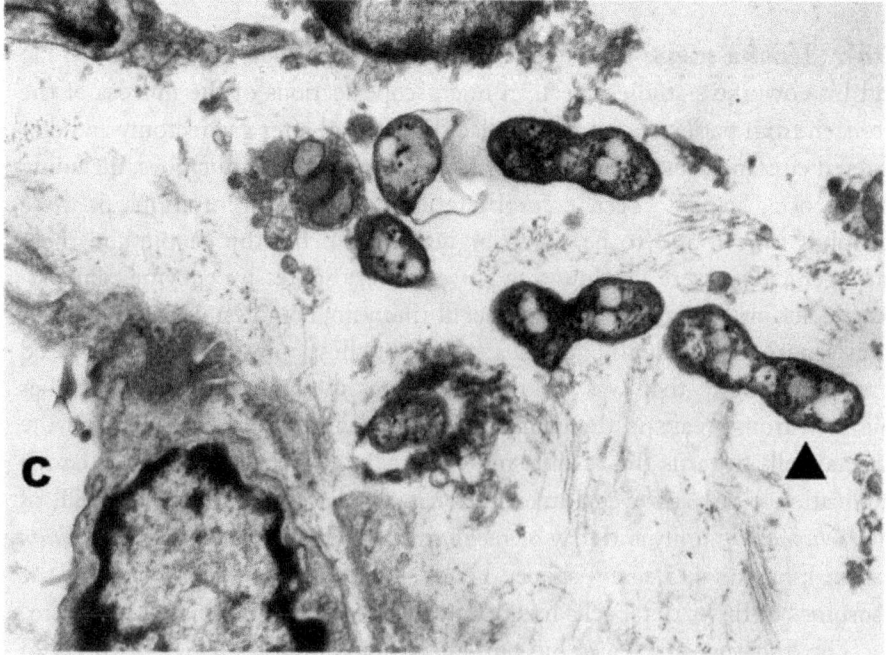

FIGURE 7 Deformed bacteria (arrowhead) in the lamina propria of the mucosa of the antrum of the stomach from a patient with peptic ulcer (×20 000). C, capillary lumen.

It is reasonable to compare the morphological evidence of ulcerative disease with nonulcerative dyspepsia. This clinical form was occurring in patients in their 30s after the Chernobyl reactor accident. Twenty-five such patients had morphological evidence of light antral gastritis and in 60% of cases this clinical condition was associated with the presence of *H. pylori*. Four patients had complicated pangastritis also associated with *H. pylori*. A close examination of the morphological sections revealed *H. pylori* in the gastric pits and mucus as well as in the lamina propria among the glands. Three patients had small colonies in the lamina propria, all of which included from 6 to 10 bacilli. In one case, a very high concentration of *H. pylori* was responsible for bacilli migrating through the intercellular junction (FIGURE 8) into the lamina propria, followed by colony formation (FIGURE 9). Electron microscopic analysis showed great detail. The bacilli that penetrated the intercellular space of the epithelial barrier (FIGURE 10) and located under the epithelial cells (FIGURE 11) appeared to hold their shape, although the cytoplasm in the center of each bacillus was brighter. Much more alteration of the cytoplasm was found in the bacilli located in the depths of the lamina propria among the mononuclear cells infiltrating this layer. Here, most had the markers of degeneration; namely, brighter cytoplasm and cytoplasmic vacuoles, as well as small granules with very high electron density (FIGURE 12).

The described data concerning the persistence of *H. pylori* in the lamina propria were examined in detail, leading to the inference that massive ingress of infection was possible only with a significantly impaired immune response, both mucosal and general. This last circumstance was confirmed in all cases of sharply defined dissemination of *H. pylori*.[21,22]

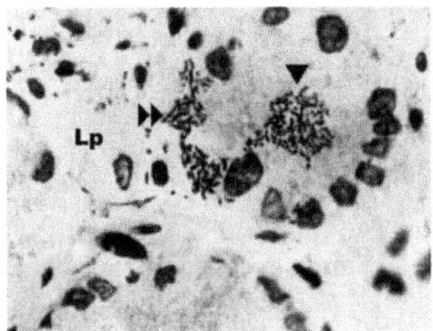

FIGURE 8 *Helicobacter pylori* penetrating from the lumen (arrowheads) of the gland into the lamina propria (Lp) of the mucosa of the antrum of the stomach from a patient with non-ulcerative dyspepsia (×630).

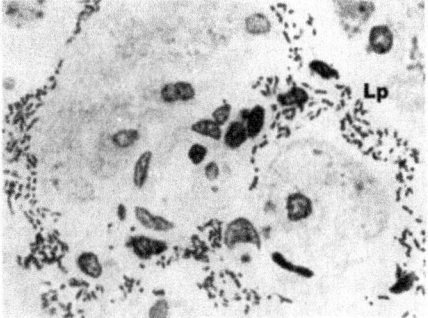

FIGURE 9 Numerous *H. pylori* located in the lamina propria of the mucosa from the patient in FIGURE 8 (× 630).

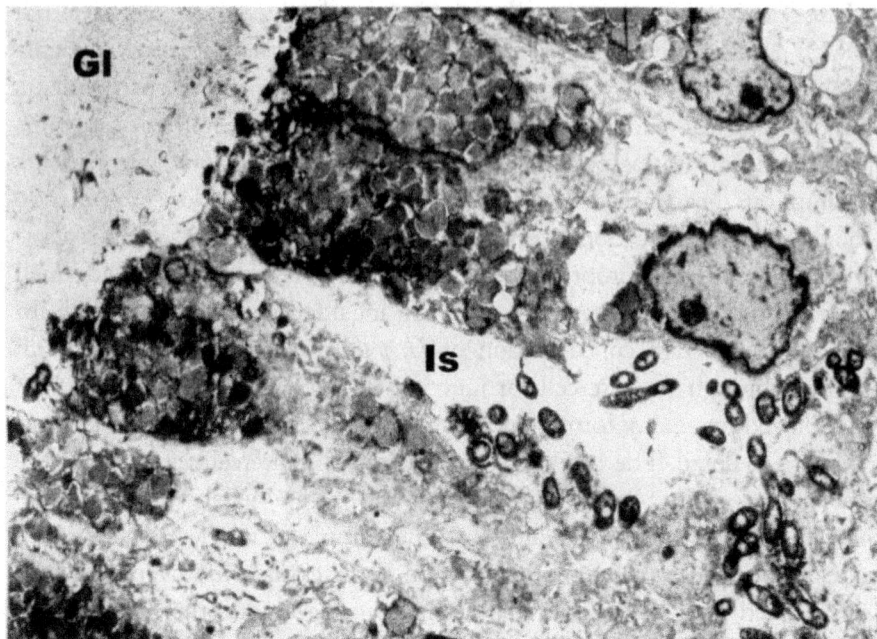

FIGURE 10 *Helicobacter pylori* localized in the intraepithelial space (Is) in the antrum of the stomach from a patient with chronic gastritis (×3000).

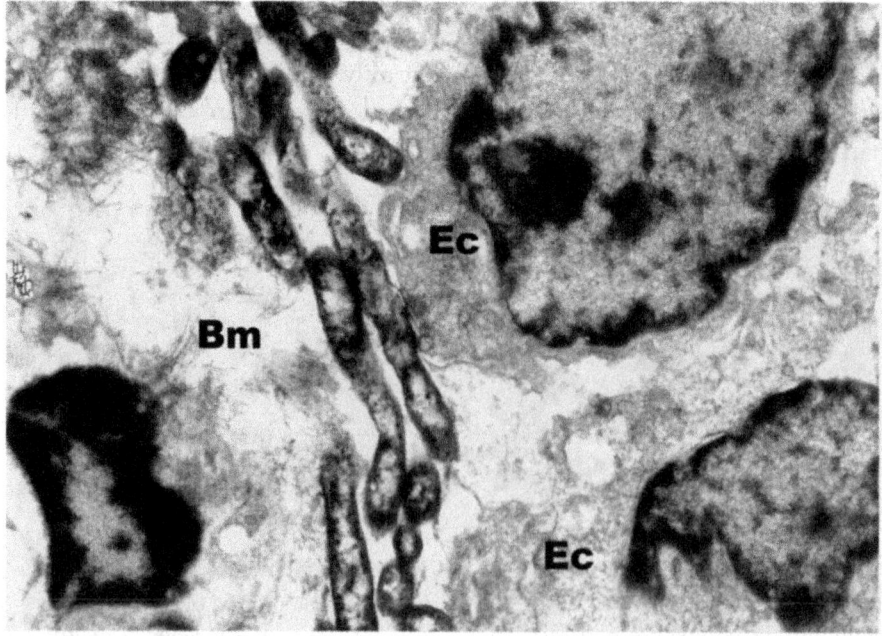

FIGURE 11 *Helicobacter pylori* localized under the epithelial cells (Ec) of the lamina propria of mucosa from the same patient in **FIGURE 11** (×20 000). Bm, basement membrane.

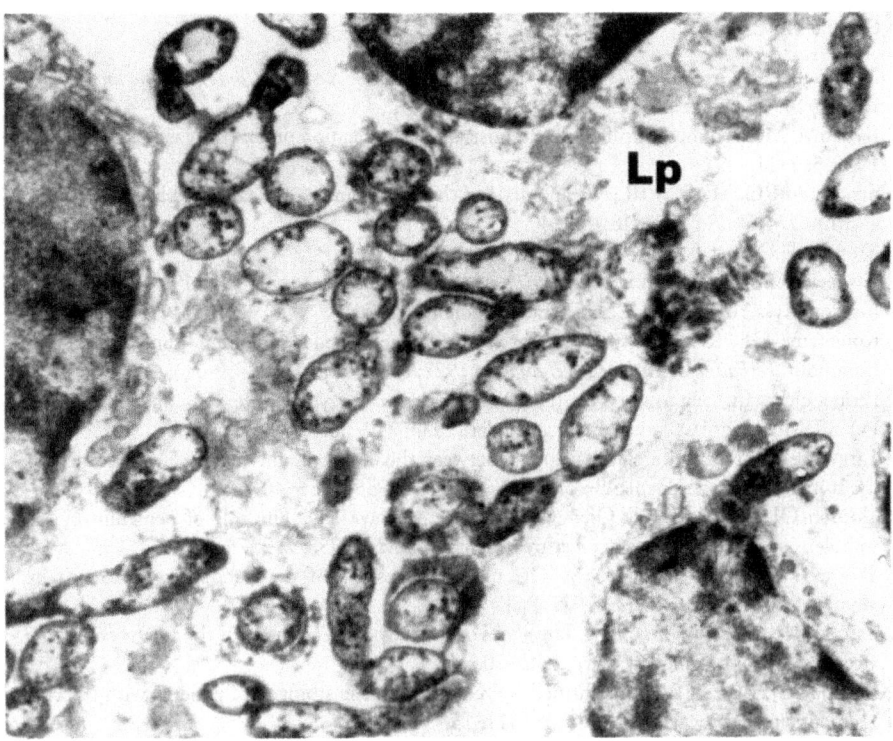

FIGURE 12   Cytoplasmic alterations of *H. pylori* located in the lamina propria (Lp) (see text; ×20 000).

Helicobacter pylori was discovered in Russia in 1974 during electron microscopic observation of sections of the mucosa of stomach from patients after either stem or selective proximal vagotomy in connection with peptic ulcer. The cocci and vegetative forms were found in antral and fundal portions of the stomach, as well as in the gastric mucus layer when it was retained, in gastric pits, and within the intracellular secretory canaliculi of parietal cells. The last location was the most surprising. According to the existing clinical concepts, we explained the microbial contamination of the stomach as a result of impaired hydrochloric acid secretion. Unfortunately, we did not try to identify these bacilli and did not combine the discovered invasion of the mucous membrane of the stomach with successful Russian results of ulcer disease treatment using antimicrobial preparations. Fortunately though, this new concept helped open up a new chapter in gastroenterology.

References

1 Masevich TsG. *Aspirate Biopsy of the Mucous Membrane of the Stomach, Duodenum and Bowel.* Leningrad: 'Medicine', 1967.

2 Ryss SM. Modern methods for the diagnosis and classification of chronic gastritis. *Ther Arch* 1966; **5**: 5–11.

3 Strickland RG, MacKay IR. A reappraisal of the nature and significance of chronic atrophic gastritis. *Dig Dis Sci* 1973; **18**: 426–40.

4 Moutier F, Cornet A. *Les Gastrites.* Paris: Masson, 1955.

5 Tashev T. Gastritis. In: *Stomach, Intestine and Peritoneum Diseases.* Sophia, 1964; 177–88.

6 Fishson-Ryss YuI. *Gastritis.* Leningrad: 'Medicine', 1974.

7 Konjetzny GE. Die Gastritis in ihrer pathogenetischen Beziehung zum Ulcus und Karzinom. *Verhandl Geselschaft F Verdauungs* 1927; 63–78 und 108–24.

8 Peptic ulcer. In: Semashko NA (ed.) *Large Medical Encyclopaedia*, 1st edn, 1928–1936, Vol. 35. Moscow: AO 'Soviet Encyclopaedia', 1936; 719–26.

9 Tarnopolskaya PD. Differential diagnosis between the innocent and malignant cancer ulcer of the stomach using the 'penicillin probe'. *Soviet Med* 1955; **2**: 36–40.

10 Gordon OL, Markova GF, Oleneva VA, Tarnopolskaya PD. The role of penicillin in the complex concept of the peptic ulcer treatment. *Clin Med* 1958; **2**: 22–6.

11 Skornetsky BD, Gavrilenko YaV. The ulcerative disease of the duodenum treatment by metronidazole. *Military Med J* 1977; **8**: 37–40.

12 Shirokova KI, Phillimonov RM, Polyakova LV. Metronidazole used in the treatment of the ulcerative disease. *Clin Med* 1981; **2**: 48–50.

13 Marshall BJ, Warren JR. Unidentified curved bacilli in the stomach of patients with gastritis and peptic ulceration. *Lancet* 1984; **1**: 1311–15.

14 Lee A, O'Rourke J. The *Helicobacter felis* mouse model. In: Lee A, Megraud F (eds). Helicobacter pylori: *Techniques for Clinical Diagnosis and Basic Research*, 2nd edn. Philadelphia: W.B. Saunders Co. Ltd, 1996; 188–205.

15 Morozov IA. Submicroscopic aspects of the hydrochloric acid secretion under normal and pathological conditions (Dissertation for the Degree of the Doctor of Medical Science). 1st Sechenov's Moscow Medical Institute, Moscow, 1977.

16 Aruin LI. *Helicobacter* (*Campylobacter*) pylori in the etiology and pathogenesis of gastritis and gastric ulcer. *Arch Pathol* 1990; **10**: 3–8.

17 Morozov IA, Lukina EV, Lopatina IV, Greenberg AA. The reparation speed of the bleeding ulcerative duodenum dependence of the *Helicobacter pylori* eradication. In: *Diagnosis and treatment of the diseases associated with* Helicobacter pylori. Proceedings of the HP 2nd International Symposium, Moscow; 43–7.

18 Zufarov KA. *Cellular Mechanisms of Adaptive Processes in the Stomach and Intestine of the Patients Suffering From Ulcer Before and After Gastroectomy.* Tashkent: UzSSR Publications House 'Medicine', 1974.

19 Meiselman MS, Miller-Cathpole R, Christ M, Randale E. *Campylobacter pylori* gastritis in Acquired Immune Deficiency Syndrome. *Gastroenterology* 1988; **95**: 209–12.

20 Andersen LP, Holck S. Possible evidence of invasiveness of *Helicobacter pylori*. *Eur J Clin Microbiol Infect Dis* 1990; **9**: 135–9.

21 Morozov IA. *Helicobacter pylori* colonies in lamina propria mucous barrier under non-ulcerative dyspepsia (Abstract): the HP VIIth Workshop of the European Helicobacter Study Group, Houston. *Am J Gastroenterol* 1994; **89**: 1328.

22 Morozov IA. Possibility of *Helicobacter pylori* invasion into lamina propria of the stomach mucous membrane. *Arch Pathol* 1994; **56**: 19–22.

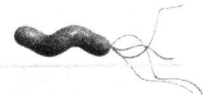

CHAPTER II

The discovery of *Helicobacter pylori* in England in the 1970s

Howard W. Steer

Preface

The *Helicobacter pylori* story goes back a long time, covering several different periods, and investigators in numerous countries have contributed to the present state of our knowledge.

Initial interest in gastric bacteria started in the late 19th century and the scientific results of that early period are historically recorded,[1-4] but any manuscripts giving more detailed accounts of the highs and lows of the research process have been lost in the passage of time. There were no further developments until the 1970s, and an account of this phase in the advancement of knowledge is chronicled here.

The beginning

After completing my preregistration houseman post in surgery at St Thomas's Hospital, London, I moved to Southampton, a university town better known for its docks, with my family on Sunday, 31 January 1971 to begin a preregistration houseman post in medicine at Southampton General Hospital with Dr John Bamforth. This post gave me considerable clinical experience, both in quality and quantity, and it was a happy, if exhausting time. It was here that I met Dr Duncan Colin-Jones (FIGURE I), who was then senior registrar and later became a Professor of Medicine at Southampton University Medical School.

Towards the end of my six-month post, I decided to pursue a career in surgery. It was usual practice at that time to work in an anatomy department

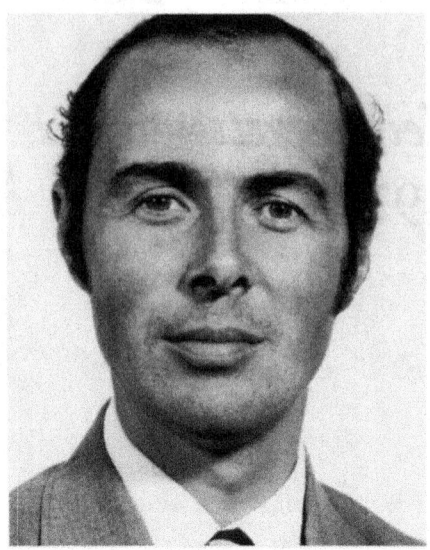

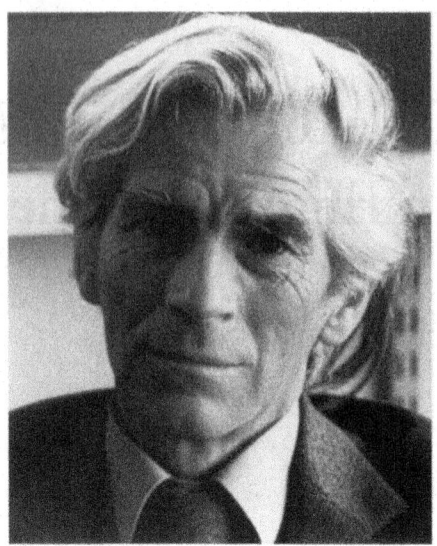

FIGURE 1 Professor Duncan Colin-Jones.   FIGURE 2 Professor David Bulmer.

while studying for the Primary Fellowship examination of the Royal College of Surgeons of England. As it happened, Southampton University was in the process of setting up a new Medical School, with the first intake of students scheduled to start their studies in October 1971, and the School was looking for anatomy demonstrators/temporary lecturers to teach topographical anatomy to these students. I therefore arranged to meet the Foundation Professor of Human Morphology, the late Professor David Bulmer (FIGURE 2). We immediately established a cordial rapport, as not only were we both anatomists and cell biologists by training, but also, as students, our supervisor and mentor had been the late Professor D. V. Davies (FIGURE 3). 'D. V.' had inspired both of us: David Bulmer while at Cambridge and myself at St Thomas's Hospital. Over the years, David Bulmer and I enjoyed many 'one to one' discussions, over cups of coffee, about anatomy and medical education – we were kindred spirits!

I arranged to start the anatomy demonstrator/temporary lecturer post on Monday, 2 August 1971. When Duncan Colin-Jones learned that I was to work in the Human Morphology department, he asked if I would like to carry out some research into the reasons why carbenoxolone sodium was so effective in healing benign peptic ulcers. I agreed readily.

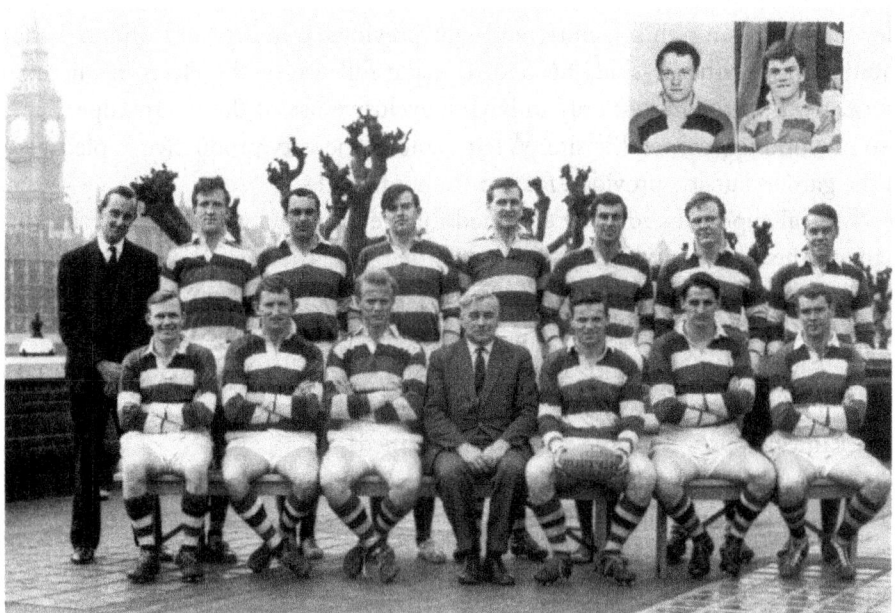

FIGURE 3 St Thomas's Hospital Rugby Football Team on the Embankment beside the Thames outside the hospital, with Big Ben in the background. Standing (L–R): John Ormsby-Gore, Bob Logan, Nicholas Silk (English Rugby International, former captain Oxford University), Alasdair Boyle (Scottish Rugby International, British Universities International), Brian Whitcombe, George Smythe, Tony Twite, David Child. Seated (L–R): John Gosnold, Iorrie Evans, Howard Steer (British Universities International), Professor D. V. Davies (President), Richard Stephenson (Captain), Quentin Livingstone, Michael Cracknell. Inset: Martin Smith, Roger Tapper.

Pleasures and pains

At that time, the Department of Human Morphology was a most interesting unit for many reasons, not least of which was its location! The department was newly established and temporarily existed on two sites while awaiting completion of the new medical school building. One site comprised two adjacent semidetached houses on University Road, which no longer exist. The second site, at Southampton General Hospital, was a converted hospital mortuary that had been licensed for the teaching of topographical anatomy to medical students.

The site of the department's scientific research activities at that time was one of the semidetached houses. Obviously this house had not been purpose-built for research and adaptations for its new function included light-sealing the kitchen before installing an electron microscope in the center of the room. No-one was using this facility, and my previous training in London had equipped me with the skills needed to make full use of the electron microscope. I was fortunate not only in having exclusive use of the microscope, but also in working in an idyllic site. What is more, the very productive apple tree in the garden outside provided for refreshment breaks!

Ethical approval had to be obtained for the proposed research. The chairman of the University's Ethical Committee was the late Professor Ralph Wright, Professor of Medicine at the University and an internationally renowned hepatologist. Duncan Colin-Jones (who had by now become a Senior Lecturer in Medicine at the University) and I had to attend a meeting of the Ethical Committee in Professor Ralph Wright's unit to present our case. Ethical approval for the study was obtained.

After starting my demonstrator/temporary lectureship post on 2 August 1971, I collected my first gastric biopsy specimens on Thursday, 5 August at Southampton General Hospital. They were from a 61-year-old woman who had had a right nephrectomy for hydronephrosis and pyelonephritis resulting from renal calculus disease in 1966. Later, she developed a duodenal ulcer for which she underwent a truncal vagotomy and pyloroplasty on 30 March 1967. The surgery was complicated by a subphrenic abscess. She recovered well, but it was not recorded whether she had been investigated for parathyroid disease. In December 1970 she began to have further abdominal pain, diarrhea and weight loss. The gastroduodenoscopy was normal and biopsies were taken from the body and fundus of the stomach to be examined with the electron microscope. They were not colonized with any bacteria.

Biopsies were obtained from further patients, none of whose mucosae were ultrastructurally colonized by bacteria, until the 11th patient to be studied. The 51-year-old man had previously been diagnosed as having a benign gastric ulcer, which was treated with carbenoxolone sodium. His follow-up gastroduodenoscopy was performed on 26 August 1971 and revealed multiple superficial gastric ulcers. Biopsies were taken from the superficial ulceration at the incisura angularis and high on the lesser curve of the stomach. Histologically, the biopsies showed benign acute-on-chronic gastritis and ultrastructurally there were numerous mucosa-related bacteria (FIGURE 4). This was the first time I had seen bacteria and my initial thought was that they were contaminants from the preparation process, but this was discounted for various reasons, particularly their distribution and ultrastructural location.

Further mucosa-related bacteria were found in the 18th and 21st patients (9 September 1971) and subsequently the number of patients with mucosa-related bacteria simply increased.

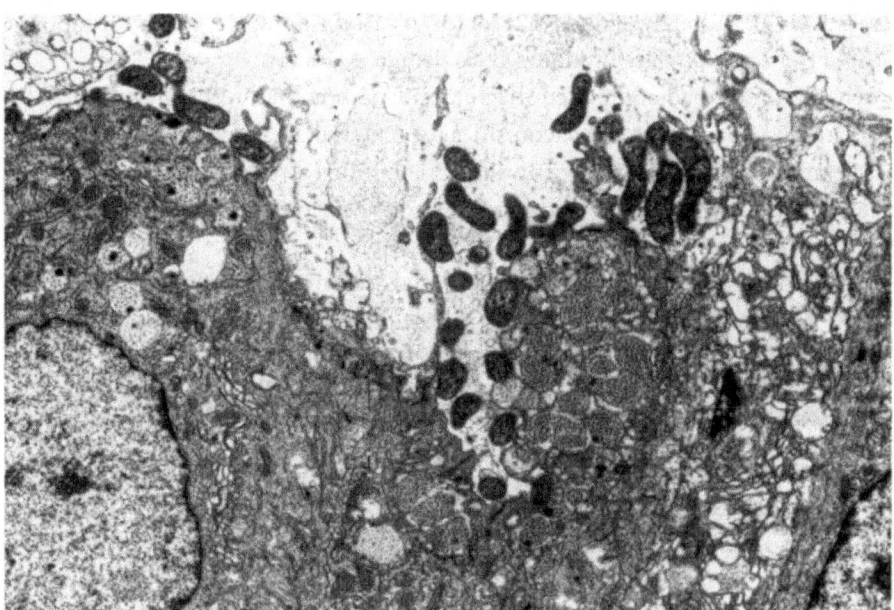

FIGURE 4 Transmission electron micrograph of the epithelial surface of an antral biopsy from a patient with a chronic duodenal ulcer. Numerous *H. pylori* abut the luminal surface of the epithelial cells (×5962).

The bacteria were found to (i) be related to the epithelial surface, (ii) have a patchy distribution, (iii) be deep to the gastric mucus, (iv) be unrelated to intestinal metaplasia, and (v) be related to the presence of polymorphonuclear leukocyte migration and even occasionally to be phagocytosed by these leukocytes. The bacteria were not found in the normal stomach.

Identification of these bacteria proved difficult. Bacteriological help was sought, but was not forthcoming, so it became a 'do it yourself' effort using incubators that had become 'surplus to requirements' at the Royal South Hants Hospital, Southampton. Aerobic cultures were established as the technology for anaerobic culturing was unavailable and not surprisingly the only bacterium I was able to culture was *Pseudomonas aeruginosa*, an endoscope contaminant.

The number of patients studied significantly increased while I was an anatomy demonstrator. I took and passed the primary Fellowship examination at the first attempt on 1 November 1971, but rather than following the usual practice of resigning from the demonstrator post and returning to clinical duties, I decided to continue as a demonstrator for one further year so that I could continue the research that I was enjoying and finding so scientifically satisfying. I was not concerned about using the research for a postgraduate thesis as I had already gained a Doctor of Philosophy degree in London (1968) after my first class Honours B.Sc degree in anatomy.

By the time I had completed the anatomy demonstrator post in June 1972 I had studied 84 patients. The acquisition of material and the evaluation of the data continued while pursuing my surgical training. Professor David Bulmer generously permitted me to continue to use the facilities in his department, which enabled me to carry out two further studies.

(1) The relationship between bacterial colonization and gastric acid secretion using the pentagastrin test. The last pentagastrin test of this study was performed on 7 March 1974.

(2) The effect of vagotomy on bacterial colonization of the stomach using mucosal biopsies taken before and after ulcer curative surgery for chronic duodenal ulceration. Between April 1973 and May 1974 I studied 10 patients who had had a truncal vagotomy and 7 patients who had had a highly selective vagotomy.

With the accumulation of data, the question of disseminating the results had to be addressed. At the time, accepted medical opinion stressed the importance of gastrin and acid secretion in benign peptic ulceration and considerable human and financial resources were directed to studying their effect. In 1974, a study of the ultrastructure of the mucosa in peptic ulcer disease was published[5] by researchers from one of the foremost surgical institutes in the United Kingdom run by Professor Sir A.P.M. Forrest, Regius Professor of Surgery at Edinburgh. They did not mention any bacteria or bacterial colonization. In fact, on examining their illustrations it was difficult to believe that they were examining the same pathological processes that I had been studying.

However, two papers were written and published without significant delay in 1975,[6,7] following which Duncan Colin-Jones attended a meeting in Mexico City. While traveling on a coach he was joined by Dr Morton Grossman, the then doyen of gastroenterology in the USA, who in the course of conversation asked Duncan, 'Do you believe what you wrote about infection in ulcer disease?' Obviously, he had read our papers, but medical opinion exclusively favored gastrin and acid secretion in the etiology of peptic ulceration. Dr Grossman was also chairman of the Editorial Board of *Gastroenterology* from 1973 to 1978 (the leading gastrointestinal journal in the world) and this phenomenon of the medical establishment ignoring or not believing there was bacterial involvement in ulcer disease continued throughout the 1970s[8,9] and the general medical scepticism continued into the 1980s and 1990s. My initial paper[6] had shown an ultrastructural association between *H. pylori* and the acute inflammatory response. Later, this association was evaluated with light microscopy and a quantitative calculation of the numbers of bacteria and polymorphonuclear leukocytes was made. Although this was time consuming it resulted in the first quantitative correlation between these two parameters for *H. pylori* and was published in 1985.[10] There have not been other publications detailing bacterial numbers, presumably because it is such time-consuming work.

To the pre- and postoperative cases studied in 1973–1974, a further eight patients were added in the early 1980s when I returned to Southampton from Oxford and the results were published in 1989.[11] Surgery (vagotomy) and healing of chronic duodenal ulceration was found to be accompanied by a significant decrease in the number of *H. pylori*, independent of whether or not there was a pyloroplasty. It was therefore concluded that the decrease in acid secretion, resulting from the vagotomy, had altered the gastric microenvironment and thus decreased the gastric bacterial colonization. The persistence of infection may have accounted for the small, but recognized ulcer relapse rate after curative surgery; persistence of bacterial colonization and (hence the risk of relapse) had been noted after medical treatment with carbenoxolone sodium in 1975.[7]

The investigation correlating bacterial colonization, vagotomy and its effect on acid secretion is one that is unlikely ever to be repeated because of the current success in eradicating *H. pylori* by pharmacological means. Surgery for benign peptic ulcer disease is now rare, except occasionally in the event of complications.

Concerning my study of bacterial colonization and the pentagastrin acid secretion tests, in spite of numerous prior attempts the findings were not accepted for publication until 1998, but were presented at an international meeting in Bologna, Italy in 1991.[12] Scientific study of gastric acid output in chronic *H. pylori* infection had unequivocally demonstrated an association between bacterial colonization mass and acid secretion, but did not answer the question as to whether this was a direct or indirect effect of the infection. My impression has been that it is indirect, but it has been demonstrated that *H. pylori* infection and acid secretion are interrelated and cannot be considered in isolation. My gastric acid output study was finally published as part of a more extensive study including nonulcerative dyspepsia in 1998.[13]

The frustrations

Having passed the Final Fellowship examination of the Royal College of Surgeons of England at the first attempt on Wednesday, 6 November 1974, I applied for a Hunterian Professorship at that College on the subject of bacterial colonization of the stomach. The application was unsuccessful, which I presumed was because of insufficient publications on the subject, but I was also conscious of the fact that many senior surgeons in England (in both academic and nonacademic posts) had made their reputations on the subject of gastrin and acid secretion, and were actively involved in researching this topic, with funding based on their research. Bacteria were not being considered, or if they were, the assumption was that they were completely irrelevant to the pathology. It seemed that the medical establishment was not ready to accept the concept that bacteria might be involved in association with gastrin and acid secretion.

Towards the end of my surgical registrar rotation in Southampton I was fortunate enough to be appointed to a clinical lecturer post in the Nuffield Department of Surgery headed by Professor Sir Peter Morris at the University of Oxford, starting on 1 September 1975. This was an exciting opportunity and an invigorating experience, working in a progressive department in which the clinical and research interests were principally directed towards transplantation, vascular surgery and immunology. From a research point of view I acquired a considerable knowledge of immunology, which would prove a useful tool in my subsequent work. I believed it was inappropriate to pursue gastric research while I was in the Department of Surgery as I considered the way forward would be through bacteriological studies.

In 1976 I discussed the gastric bacterial colonization with the Head of the Bacteriology Unit at the Radcliffe Infirmary, Oxford, but was unable to raise any enthusiasm from the bacteriologists for further work on the subject. I decided to write to the Director of the Pasteur Institute in Paris about the research, but did not receive a reply, which in retrospect was not really surprising, because my poor grasp of the French language meant that I had written in English, which I fear was discourteous.

While working in Oxford I was fortunate to spend a sabbatical year working in the Sir William Dunn School of Pathology, in the Cellular Immunology Unit run by Professor Sir James Gowans and the late Professor Alan Williams. I started research work there on 31 January 1977 and it was a truly invaluable experience. Soon after starting to work there, I decided to make one more attempt at generating bacteriological interest in the gastric mucosa-related bacteria and contacted the Wellcome Research Laboratories at Langley Court, Beckenham, Kent. I spoke to Dr Jarmila Miler and Dr J. F. Spilsbury and arranged to visit their unit on Friday 22 April 1977. The unit was happy to collaborate and the meeting was productive in that regard; however, the specimens had to be collected in Oxford and then sent to Beckenham, a distance of at least 87 miles, so it was not surprising that the work was unsuccessful in view of the specific bacteriological requirements of *H. pylori*.

The gastric research could not be taken any further forward during my stay in Oxford, which continued until April 1981.

The ultrastructure studies were not completed until my return to Southampton in April 1981. The Southampton General Hospital Electron Microscopy Unit had acquired a scanning electron microscope in 1976 and after discussions with Mr Chris Inman, the Head of the unit, I arranged to carry out research using this equipment. The first biopsies for this project were taken on 9 August 1982 from a patient who was being treated with cimetidine for a chronic duodenal ulceration and were followed by biopsies from further patients. With the great technical assistance of Chris Inman, I was able to evaluate the association of *H. pylori* with the gastric epithelial surface (FIGURE 5). This research was completed and the resulting paper submitted for publication in the medical journal *Gut* in May 1983. Difficulties were experienced in persuading the journal to publish this research, with the manuscript being referred back to me for minor alterations that were irrelevant to the scientific content. Fourteen months elapsed and I then read two letters in *The Lancet*, one of which included a scanning electron micrograph of *H. pylori*[14] and the other referring to that scanning electron micrograph.[15] Naturally, I became concerned with the delay in publication of my paper. It was eventually published in November 1984 after a telephone call to my friend and former

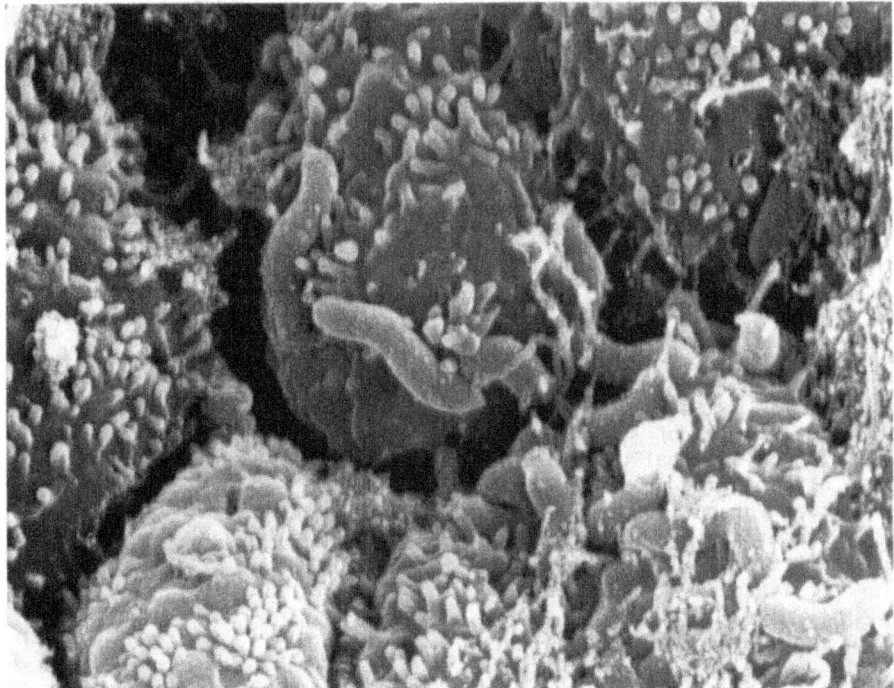

FIGURE 5 Scanning electron micrograph of the epithelial surface of an antral biopsy from a patient with a chronic duodenal ulcer. Numerous bacteria are attached to the surface of the epithelial cells (×13 998).

colleague in Oxford, the late Mr Emanoel Lee on Thursday 20 July 1984. Emanoel was an outstanding gastrointestinal surgeon of international repute, and a gifted artist. He also happened to be on the Editorial Board of the journal (*Gut*) and while I am sure he had no part in the delay, he must have conveyed my anxieties to the Editor because within days the Editor telephoned me to ask if I would accept publication. The paper duly appeared in print,[16] over 18 months after the original submission. This experience highlighted for me the deficiencies of the peer review process and contributed to my scepticism of it in principle and in practice.

The finale – or is it?

Completing the evaluation of the material accumulated in the early 1970s proved time consuming. The findings were presented at international meetings, but proved difficult to publish in conventional medical journals, as exemplified by a letter from the Editor of *The Lancet* in 1984 (FIGURE 6).

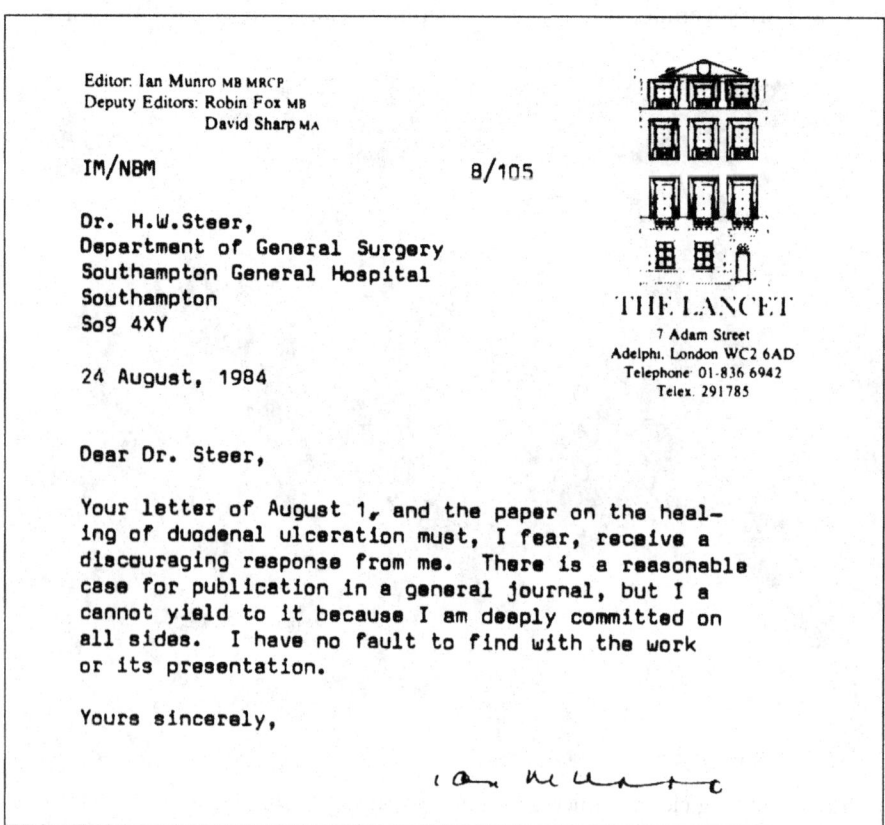

FIGURE 6 Letter from the Editor of *The Lancet*.

I believe that the medical establishment is quite fixed in its views and has great difficulty in considering the merits of any challenge to the accepted view. I think this is an indictment of the establishment. It can be most frustrating and I feel great sympathy with the Hungarian obstetrician, Ignaz Philipp Semmelweis (1818–1865) whose effective antiseptic method of significantly reducing the mortality of puerperal fever in Vienna in 1846 was not immediately recognized by the medical establishment and he shortly afterwards became insane.

References

1   Bottcher. *Dopater Med Z* 1874; **5**: 148.
2   Rosenow EC, Sandford AH. The bacteriology of ulcer of the stomach and duodenum of man. *J Infect Dis* 1915; **17**: 210–26.
3   Appelmans R, Vassiliadis P. Etude sur la flore microbienne des ulcers gastro-duodeneaux et des cancers gastriques. *Rev Belg Sci Med* 1932; **4**: 198–203.
4   Seley GP, Colp R. The bacteriology of peptic ulcers and gastric malignancies: possible bearing on complications following gastric surgery. *Surgery* 1941; **10**: 369–80.
5   Patrick WJA, Denham D, Forrest APM. Mucous change in the human duodenum: A light and electron microscope study and correlation with disease and gastric acid secretion. *Gut* 1974; **15**: 767–76.
6   Steer HW. Ultrastructure of cell migration through the gastric epithelium and its relationship to bacteria. *J Clin Pathol* 1975; **28**: 639–46.
7   Steer HW, Colin-Jones D. Mucosal changes in gastric ulceration and their response to carbenoxolone sodium. *Gut* 1975; **16**: 590–7.
8   Grossman MI. A new look at peptic ulcer (UCLA Conference). *Ann Intern Med* 1976; **84**: 57–67.
9   Grossman MI. Peptic ulcer: the pathophysiological background. *Scand J Gastroenterol* 1980; **15**(Suppl. 58): 7–16.
10 Steer HW. The gastroduodenal epithelium in peptic ulceration. *J Pathol* 1985; **146**: 355–62.
11 Steer HWJ, Hawtin PJ, Newell DG. The effect of surgical treatment of chronic duodenal ulceration on *Campylobacter pylori* colonisation of the stomach. In: Megraud F, Lamouliatte H (eds). *Gastroduodenal Pathology and* Campylobacter pylori. Amsterdam: Exerpta Medica, 1989; 525–7.
12 Steer HW. Gastric acid output studies and *Helicobacter pylori* colonisation in patients with chronic duodenal ulceration. *Ital J Gastroenterol* 1991; **23**(Suppl. 2): 177.
13 Mullins P, Steer H. *Helicobacter pylori* colonisation density and gastric acid output in non-ulcer dyspepsia and duodenal ulcer disease. *Helicobacter* 1998; **3**: 86–92.
14 Phillips AD, Hine KR, Holmes GKT, Woodings DF. Gastric spiral bacteria. *Lancet* 1984; **2**: 100–1.
15 Meyrick-Thomas J, Poynter D, Gooding C *et al.* Gastric spiral bacteria. *Lancet* 1984; **2**: 100.
16 Steer HW. Surface morphology of the gastroduodenal mucosa in peptic ulceration. *Gut* 1984; **25**: 1203–10.

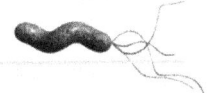

CHAPTER 12

We grew the first *Helicobacter* species and didn't even know it!

Adrian Lee, Michael Phillips and Jani O'Rourke

THIS STORY BEGAN in 1968, well before the momentous discoveries of Barry Marshall and Robin Warren in the early 1980s.[1,2] At the Rockefeller University in New York, two great microbiologists, Russell Schaedler and Rene Dubos considered that an unexplored, but very important, field of human medicine was the composition of the bacterial flora of the intestinal tract.[3-5] This normal flora was likely to play an important role in health and disease, and yet there had been virtually no systematic studies on the composition of the gut bacteria of any animal species. Therefore, they selected the mouse as their model and determined to try and culture and understand the organisms that inhabit the normal rodent intestinal tract. Viewed under the microscope it was clear that the dominant bacteria in the large intestinal contents, the cecal contents and the stools were fusiform (i.e. bacteria with pointed ends), present in very large numbers, but had never ever been cultured.

As a young, fresh-faced postdoctoral fellow, Adrian Lee traveled to Rockefeller University from Australia, and was given the task of trying to grow these fusiforms. The Rockefeller team reasoned, based on the work of Aranki and Freter's team,[6] that these bacteria were likely to be extremely sensitive to oxygen, which was why normal culture techniques had failed. So Lee created one of the first anaerobic culture cabinets: a large, rigid, plastic glove box from which the oxygen was removed by continually inflating and deflating a large atmospheric research balloon and replaced by nitrogen that had been passed through a column of heated copper filings. The remaining oxygen was then removed by placing mung beans in the chamber and allowing them to germinate! This bizarre methodology worked, although the smell on opening the cabinet was horrid. Adrian Lee remembers vividly that moment when he looked at the culture plates and saw beautiful purple-speckled colonies that no one had ever seen before. The fusiform bacteria had been cultured! The work was considered of sufficient moment to be published in *Nature* and FIGURE 1 is the illustration from that paper showing the pointed fusiform bacteria.[7] But have a look at FIGURE 1D! What can be seen clearly are spiral-shaped bacteria. Lee, however, had very little interest in these organisms, but as he had grown them, he felt he had better report on this culture:

> It should be stated here that large numbers of colonies of spiral-shaped organisms were recovered from most of the animals studied. These organisms produced discrete, tiny, pale, convex colonies with a zone of green homolysis on plates inoculated inside the chamber but they spread over the plates when inoculation was carried out in the open air. No detailed study of these spiral shaped organisms as yet has been carried out but it seems worthwhile to note that they appear to be extremely numerous in all animals tested.

If only he had known that the first *Helicobacter* species had been born! This was Lee's first lost opportunity for fame and fortune.

Work on the fusiforms continued. The Rockefeller researchers wanted to know when these organisms colonized the mouse intestinal tract, so they cultured the feces of mice at varying ages and clearly determined when the fusiform bacteria first colonized the murine intestine. The spiral organism, which they now called the 'spirochete-like organism', was still there and, indeed, they reported that both these organisms appeared in the mouse intestine between days 12 and 14 of age. That paper, which was published in the *Journal of Experimental Medicine*,[8] contained an observation that became the focus of the work of the Lee group during the next 35 years.[9]

> There may be significance in the fact that the anaerobic tapered rods and spirochetes characteristically inhabit the mucous layer of the large intestine and caecum where they seemed to constitute a barrier between the outside world and the intestinal mucosa.

At the end of 1969, Lee, now a still very young lecturer in medical microbiology, had moved to The University of New South Wales in Sydney, Australia. Interest in the spiral bacteria had become a focus of his work and, indeed, with Bill Leach, a Master's student, he published a paper in *Infection and Immunity* in 1973, which mapped the localization of these spiral bacteria in the gastrointestinal tract and even proposed them as a possible explanation for the disease condition of animals called intestinal spirochetosis.[10] The spiral bacteria were seen to inhabit only the mucous lining and the mucous crypts of the intestinal tract and

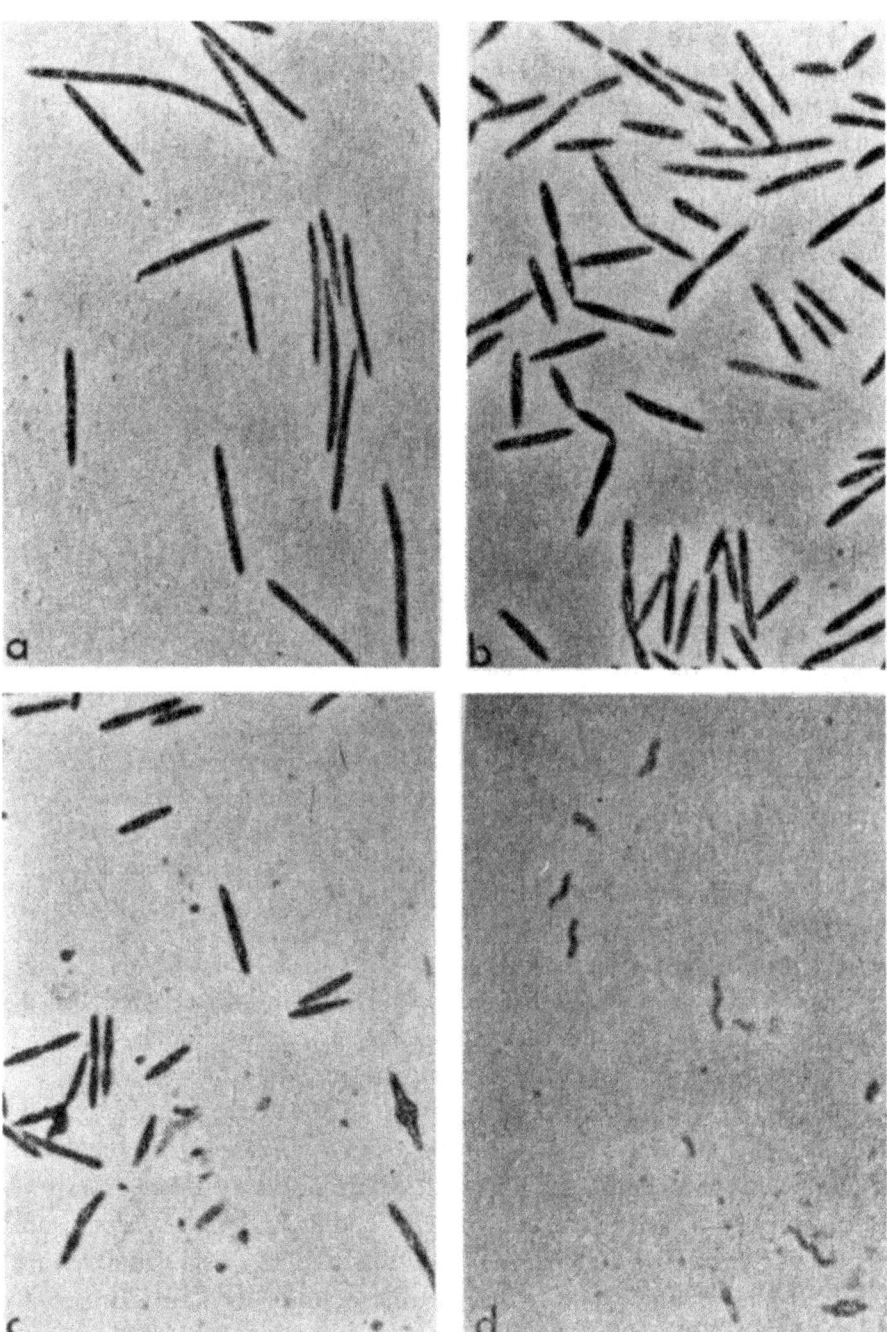

FIGURE 1 Anaerobic bacteria from the ceca of specific-pathogen-free mice (phase contrast, ×3000). (a–c) Fusiform rods; (d) spiral-shaped organisms. (Reproduced with permission from *Nature (Lond)* 1968; **220**: 1137–9.)

in fact very few spiral bacteria could normally be seen in the intestinal lumen or the stools of mice. However, if diarrhea was induced in these animals with Epsom salts (i.e. magnesium sulfate), extremely high numbers of diverse spiral-shaped bacteria were flushed out and seen in the stools (Figure 2). Remember this organism.

In 1977, Michael Phillips, a bearded Australian, began his path towards not only a doctorate, but what we now know was the very first culture of the first proven *Helicobacter* species. He joined Adrian Lee's group as an honors student studying microbiology and his project was to try and grow those spiral bacteria that Leach had shown were flushed out of the diarrheal rodents. Phillips' first paper showed clearly that there were at least six different morphologies of the spiral bacteria in the rodent intestinal tract and he mapped their location (Figure 3).[11] Using anaerobic techniques, Phillips cultured many of these lower bowel spi-

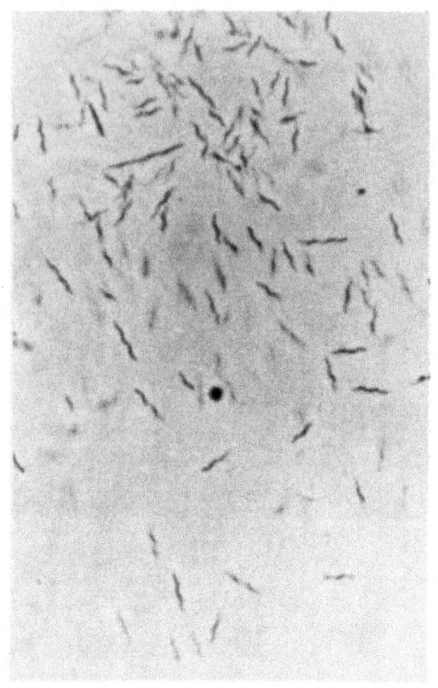

FIGURE 2 Fluid stool from a rat with induced diarrhea showing numerous spiral-shaped organisms (phase contrast, ×4340). (Reproduced with permission from *Infect Immun* 1973; 7: 961–72.)

rals, but the favorite organism of the research group, affectionately called 'Stubby' because of its characteristic shape, was not cultured. FIGURE 4 shows 'Stubby' in an ileal crypt of a mouse; note the very unusual surface structure.

Phillips recalls a Research Meeting with Adrian Lee who had just read about the newly discovered spiral gut pathogen *Campylobacter jejuni*, published by Jean Paul Butzler and Martin Skirrow.[12] 'Why not use the Butzler/Skirrow selective media and microaerophilic growth conditions?' This was done and 'Stubby' was grown for the first time in 1981. In 1982 Michael traveled to Hobart to present this work at the meeting of the Australian Society of Microbiology in May. Here the plot thickens. An observer of Phillips' presentation was a Perth microbiologist, Dr Doug Annear, who reported the finding to a young internist, Dr Barry Marshall, who was trying to grow the spiral bacteria that a pathologist, Dr Robin Warren, had seen in gastric biopsies.

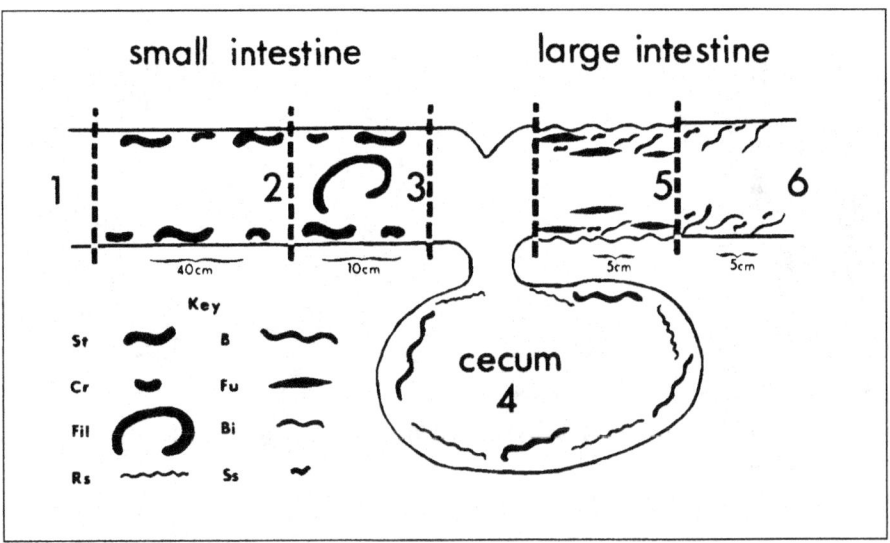

FIGURE 3 Diagram of the intestine of the rat, showing the location of mucosa-associated microorganisms. (Reproduced with permission from *Aust J Exp Biol Med Sci* 1978; **56**: 649–62.)

Annear had clearly thought that 'Stubby' looked like the Warren/Marshall bacteria (FIGURE 5). Marshall immediately sent his first letter to Michael Phillips on 4 June 1982. He coyly refers to his work, giving nothing away, and asking for some pictures of the Phillips bacterium.

> I was shown an abstract of your paper 'Isolation and Characterization of Spiral Shaped Bacteria from the Intestinal Mucosa of Rodents', and would be very interested to receive a copy. I am a Medical Registrar undertaking research into human campylobacters and on occasions we have isolated an apparently similar organism from human biopsy material. We have also seen them on electron microscopy and I would be delighted if you could send a copy of your electron microphotographs, especially any showing these organisms inhabiting the mucosa and intestinal crypts.

The pictures of 'Stubby' were sent to Perth and clearly further impressed Marshall because he soon replied from Port Hedland Hospital where he was now working, reading the gastric literature and forming his first major hypotheses about *Helicobacter pylori* as a pathogen.[13] This was an important letter as it contained one of the first pictures of *H. pylori*, a hand-drawn

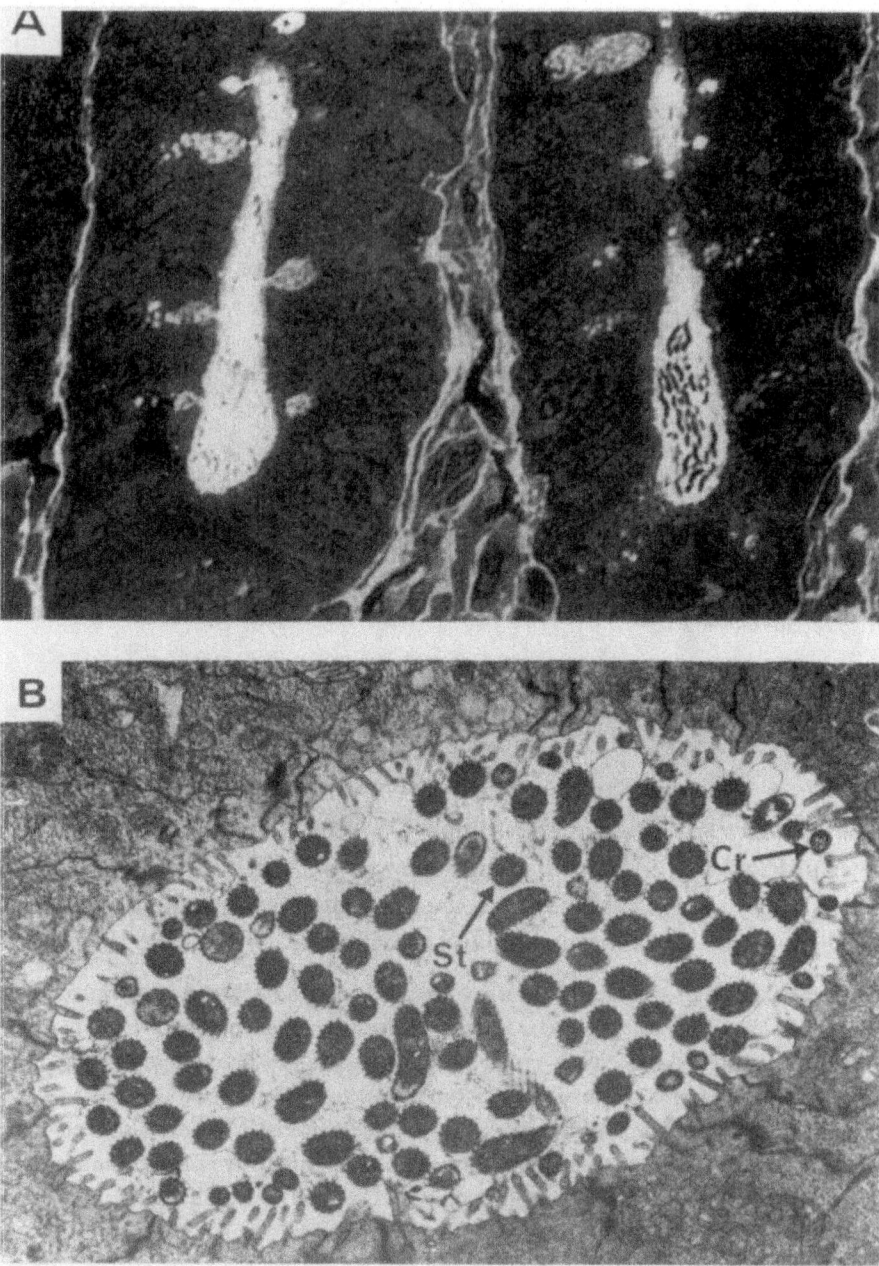

FIGURE 4 Section of the rat ileum showing mucosa-associated microorganisms. (a) Light micrograph showing localization of spiral-shaped bacteria at the base of a crypt (×1100). (b) Electron micrograph of a section through the base of a crypt showing (St) organisms in the lumen and (Cr) bacteria associated with the tissue surface (×7400). (Reproduced with permission from *Aust J Exp Biol Med Sci* 1978; **56**: 649–62.)

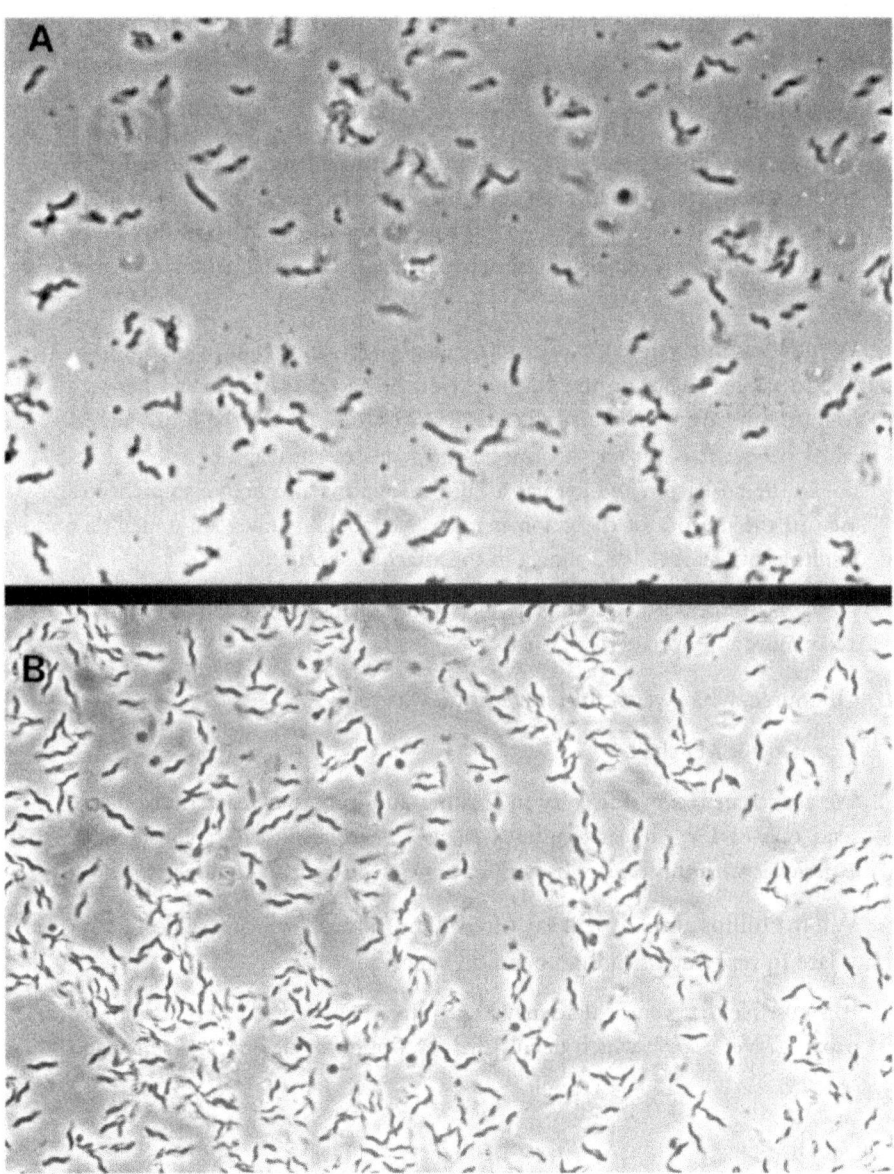

FIGURE 5 Comparison of (a) *H. pylori* and (b) *H. muridarum*, viewed by phase contrast microscopy, showing their similar S-shaped morphology (×1000).

cartoon by Marshall, shown in FIGURE 6. In his second letter in October 1982 Marshall said,

> Dear Michael,
>
> We have been finding spiral bacteria in the gastric antrum of man since 1979 and believe it is associated with gastritis. The bacteria can be seen on gram stains, silver stains of biopsies, and has been cultured regularly at Royal Perth Hospital. Dr Doug Annear has viable freeze-dried specimens for further study.
>
> While I was in Perth in October Dr Annear suggested I contact Prof Adrian Lee to ask his advice on the Taxonomy of the bacteria. I have read Bergey's Manual 8th Ed and of course all the references to yours and the Prof's papers and I believe it is yet another species or genus of spirilla. The organism is unlike the rat bacteria which has axial fibrils and is also unlike spirochaetes seen in the mucosa of the colon in man. Metabolic studies are under way, results as of October 1982 shown in the attached sheet.
>
> Please ask Professor Lee for his opinion and perhaps guide me on the path to a few more appropriate references.

Of course, what we should have done was reply:

> Dear Doctor Marshall,
>
> We are fascinated by this very interesting and important bacterium. Please send one of Dr Annear's cultures to us so we can use our considerable experience with this type of bacterium to help you identify it quickly!

What Phillips actually did say on 17 December 1982, after apologizing for being late in replying as he had been on vacation, was:

> It is possible that your isolate may belong to a new genus. I have included a paper (Davis *et al.*[14]) which details the description of such a new genus and

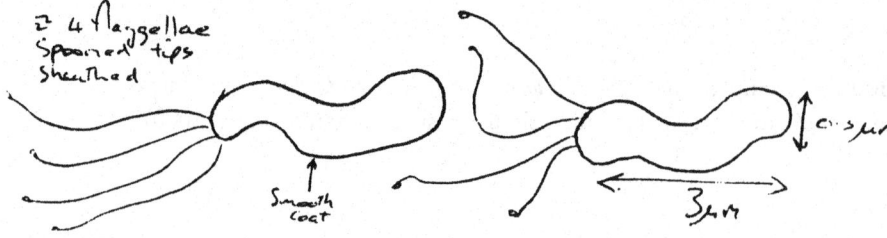

FIGURE 6 Hand-drawn cartoon of an organism, now known to be *H. pylori*, grown in the microbiology laboratories of Royal Perth Hospital, in the letter written by Dr Barry Marshall to Michael Phillips in October, 1982.

hope this will serve as useful guide. I am sorry we cannot be of more help, however, the taxonomy of the spiral organisms associated with the gastrointestinal mucosa is, as you will be aware, very poorly understood.

And so our second chance for fame and fortune passed us by! We knew nothing about stomachs. In 1982, what microbiologist did?

Meanwhile, back in the lab, Jani O'Rourke, who had joined Adrian Lee's group one year after Phillips in 1978, was happily obeying the instructions of her boss to keep growing the mouse spirals and she collected a remarkable collection of intestinal spirals from many animals. She too was interested in 'Stubby' and all of us were convinced it was a member of a new genus. Indeed, we proposed the name *'Mucospirillum ileocryptum'* in a manuscript entitled *'Mucospirillum ileocryptum* General nov., sp. nov., a microaerophilic bacterium with a novel ultrastructure isolated from the intestinal mucosa of the rat'. The bacterium was lodged as the type culture 'Stubby 1' (St1) with the American type culture collection (Reference Number: ATCC 49282). By now Barry Marshall's discovery was well known and the Lee group had become very interested in *H. pylori*; in 1984, Stuart Hazell, later a major researcher in the *Helicobacter* field, started his doctorate, possibly the first on *H. pylori*.

'Stubby' was forgotten in our excitement about the stomach. Then one day when looking at a culture of our now neglected bacterium, someone asked, 'Is it urease positive?' Lee replied, 'I don't know' and taking the Hazell urease solution used for testing *H. pylori*, he did the test. Lo and behold, it was extremely urease positive.[15,16] Could 'Stubby' be a *Helicobacter* species? By now O'Rourke was a *Helicobacter* expert, having grown *H. felis* and *H. heilmannii*.[17–20] She did a wide range of biochemical tests on a culture of St1 and all the results pointed to 'Stubby' being a *Helicobacter*. By now links had been established with Professor James Fox at Massachusetts Institute of Technology and in collaboration with Bruce Paster and Floyd Dewhirst, the 16S rRNA sequence was done and yes, 'Stubby' became *H. muridarum*.[21] This was not only historically the first *Helicobacter* species grown, but also the first non-gastric *Helicobacter* to be officially named. We were actually quite disappointed about 'Stubby' being a *Helicobacter* because of our attempt in 1982 to give it the genus name *Mucospirillum*. If the *International Journal of Systematic Bacteriology* had accepted this name, this book would now be the history of *Mucospirillum pylori*!

To complete this saga, it needs to be said that the many intestinal spirals that Jani O'Rourke had cultured were later shown to be *Helicobacter* species, including *H. bilis*, *H. trogontum*, *H. ganmani* and *H. rodentium*.

Without doubt, the bacterium first grown at Rockefeller University in 1968 was a *Helicobacter*, but Lee did not know it. Phillips grew the first *Helicobacter* in 1981, a year before Marshall, but Phillips did not know it. If

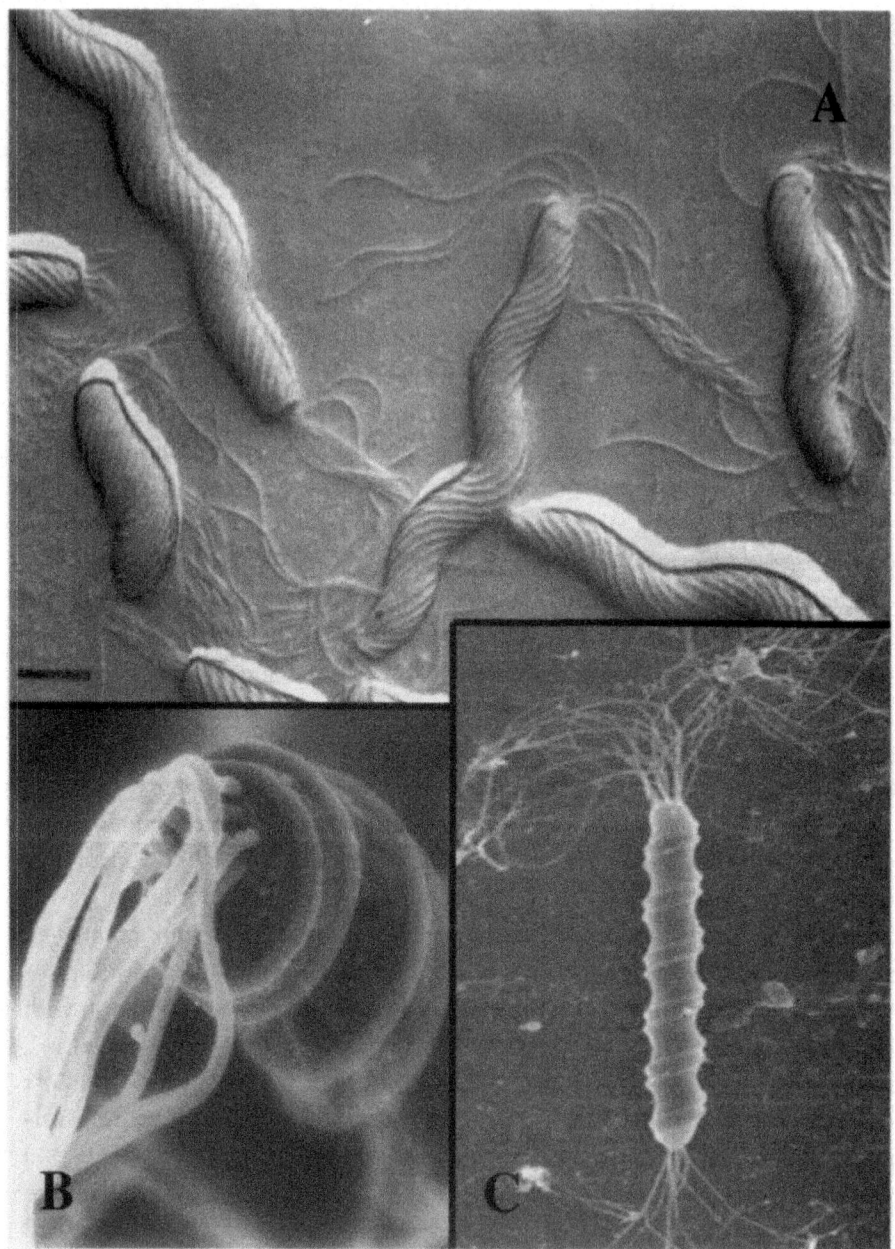

FIGURE 7 (a) *Heliocobacter muridarum* (freeze-dried image viewed by transmission electron microscopy, ×20 000). (Reproduced with permission from *Int J Syst Bacteriol* 1992; **42**: 27–36.) (b, c) *Helicobacter felis* (critical point dried images viewed by field emission scanning electron microscopy, ×16 000 and ×70 000, respectively).

O'Rourke had cultured more isolates of 'Stubby', we would have had the genus name, but O'Rourke did not.

What a story it might have been! We really could have been famous!

We conclude by acknowledging the generosity of Barry Marshall in allowing us to write our side of the story. Many others saw spiral bacteria in the stomach before Robin Warren; many may feel they got there first. But the reality is that Marshall and Warren were the only ones to realize the significance of this bacterium. Barry's inspirational predictions as he sat and wrote at Port Headland in late 1982 revolutionized gastroenterology and caused a paradigm shift in the management of gastroduodenal disease. Thank you Barry and Robin for your discovery! It has been fun, allowing us to travel and make many good friends. Adrian has revelled in the title of 'Felis Leader' of one of the most superb research teams. We did produce the *H. felis* and the *H. pylori* Sydney strain (SSI) mouse models, but that's another story.[19,22,23] We also believe that we have grown the most beautiful *Helicobacters*. Have a look at Figure 7.

References

1   Warren JR, Marshall B. Unidentified curved bacillus on gastric epithelium in active chronic gastritis. *Lancet* 1983; **1**: 1273–5.

2   Marshall BJ, Warren JR. Unidentified curved bacilli in the stomach of patients with gastritis and peptic ulceration. *Lancet* 1984; **1**: 1311–15.

3   Schaedler RW, Dubos R, Costello R. The development of the bacterial flora in the gastrointestinal tract of mice. *J Exp Med* 1965; **122**: 59–66.

4   Dubos R, Schaedler RW, Costello R, Hoet P. Indigenous, normal, and autochthonous flora of the gastrointestinal tract. *J Exp Med* 1965; **122**: 67–76.

5   Savage DC, Dubos R, Schaedler RW. The gastrointestinal epithelium and its autochthonous bacterial flora. *J Exp Med* 1968; **127**: 67–76.

6   Aranki A, Syed SA, Kenney EB, Freter R. Isolation of anaerobic bacteria from human gingiva and mouse cecum by means of a simplified glove box procedure. *Appl Microbiol* 1969; **17**: 568–76.

7   Lee A, Gordon J, Dubos R. Enumeration of the oxygen sensitive bacteria usually present in the intestine of healthy mice. *Nature (Lond)* 1968; **220**: 1137–9.

8   Lee A, Gordon J, Dubos R. The mouse intestinal flora with emphasis on the strict anaerobes. *J Exp Med* 1971; **133**: 339–52.

9   Lee A. Neglected niches: the microbial ecology of the gastrointestinal tract. In: Marshall KC (ed.) *Advances in Microbial Ecology*, Vol. 8. New York: Plenum Press, 1985; 115–62.

10 Leach WD, Lee A, Stubbs RP. Localization of bacteria in the gastrointestinal tract: a possible explanation of intestinal spirochaetosis. *Infect Immun* 1973; **7**: 961–72.

11 Phillips M, Lee A, Leach WD. The mucosa-associated microflora of the rat intestine: a study of normal distribution and magnesium sulphate induced diarrhoea. *Aust J Exp Biol Med Sci* 1978; **56**: 649–62.

12 Butzler JP, Skirrow MB. Campylobacter enteritis. *Clin Gastroenterol* 1979; **8**: 737–65.

13 Marshall BJ, McGechie DB, Rogers PA, Glancy RJ. Pyloric *Campylobacter* infection and gastroduodenal disease. *Med J Aust* 1985; **142**: 439–44.

14 Davis CP, Cleven D, Brown J, Balish E. *Anaerobiospirillum*, a new genus of spiral-shaped bacteria. *Int J Syst Bacteriol* 1976; **26**: 498–504.

15 Hazell SL, Borody TJ, Gal A, Lee A. *Campylobacter pyloridis* gastritis. I. Detection of urease as a marker of bacterial colonization and gastritis. *Am J Gastroenterol* 1987; **82**: 292–6.

16 Ferrero RL, Hazell SL, Lee A. The urease enzymes of *Campylobacter pylori* and a related bacterium. *J Med Microbiol* 1988; **27**: 33–40.

17 Lee A, Hazell SL, O'Rourke J, Kouprach S. Isolation of a spiral-shaped bacterium from the cat stomach. *Infect Immun* 1988; **56**: 2843–50.

18 Dick E, Lee A, Watson G, O'Rourke J. Use of the mouse for the isolation and investigation of stomach-associated, spiral-helical shaped bacteria from man and other animals. *J Med Microbiol* 1989; **29**: 55–62.

19 Paster BJ, Lee A, Fox JG *et al.* Phylogeny of *Helicobacter felis* sp. nov., *Helicobacter mustelae*, and related bacteria. *Int J Syst Bacteriol* 1991; **41**: 31–8.

20 O'Rourke JL, de Groote D, Solnick JV *et al.* 'Heilmannii' at last: *Canditatus Helicobacter heilmannii* as the official name for the major group of non-*H. pylori* gastric bacteria. *Gut* 2001; **49**: A52.

21 Lee A, Phillips MW, O'Rourke JL *et al. Helicobacter muridarum* sp. nov., a microaerophilic helical bacterium with a novel ultrastructure isolated from the intestinal mucosa of rodents. *Int J Syst Bacteriol* 1992; **42**: 27–36.

22 Lee A, Fox JG, Otto G, Murphy J. A small animal model of human *Helicobacter pylori* active chronic gastritis. *Gastroenterology* 1990; **99**: 1315–23.

23 Lee A, O'Rourke J, De Ungria MC, Robertson B, Daskalopoulos G, Dixon MF. A standardized mouse model of *Helicobacter pylori* infection: introducing the Sydney strain. *Gastroenterology* 1997; **112**: 1386–97.

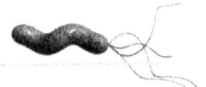

The Dallas experience with acute *Helicobacter pylori* infection

Walter L. Peterson, William Harford and
Barry J. Marshall

Prologue: Gastroenterology, 1978

At the 1978 meeting of the American Gastroenterology Association held in
Las Vegas, the Tuesday morning Plenary Session for upper gastrointestinal
disorders contained two presentations that were to become intimately connected with the discovery of *Helicobacter pylori*. The first of these was
'Duodenal Ulcer Relapse after Withdrawal of Cimetidine', in which Ippoliti
and coworkers at the Center for Ulcer Research and Education (CURE) in
Los Angeles noticed that patients with chronic duodenal ulcer experienced
relapse soon after cimetidine therapy was withdrawn.[1] That paper pre-empted
many hundreds that confirmed that the H2 blockers could not cure the peptic
ulcer diathysis; that is, the underlying defect must have been something else
besides acid excess.

The second paper of interest was by Edward ('Jerry') Ramsey and
colleagues, from John Fordtran's group in Dallas, Texas, who described an
epidemic of acute gastritis, possibly caused by a bacterial (*Helicobacter pylori*)
infection transmitted in their gastric secretion laboratory.[2] Jerry Ramsey, now a
gastroenterologist in Richmond, Virginia, recalls the day he presented the
Dallas epidemic paper at the 10:30 am AGA Plenary session. After the presentation, John Fordtran had lengthy discussions with Basil Hirschowitz (one
of the inventors of fiberoptic endoscopy) and Dr G. Makhlouf of Richmond.
Both these investigators had their own experience with achlorhydria and
gastritis; Hirschowitz had observed similar cases while studying the gastric
effects of corticosteroids in the 1950s[3] and Makhlouf had taken part in many

self-intubations to study his own gastric acid secretion, and had published on episodes of hypochlorhydria.[4] Later that year, Jerry Ramsey attended an interview in Richmond for the gastroenterologist position, which he subsequently gained, but his visit was also memorable for the large hematemesis that occurred during the night and which led to Jerry being admitted to the intensive care unit for observation. Apparently, he was quite blasé about his known duodenal ulcer disease (recently diagnosed at endoscopy in Dallas), and refused further endoscopy, traveling onwards for further interviews a day or so later.

Background

In the mid-1970s, the Dallas laboratory of John Fordtran, MD was actively involved in studying the physiology of gastric acid secretion and its reduction with new pharmacologic agents. Healthy volunteers (including seminary students, medical students and others) were being studied at Parkland Memorial Hospital and the Dallas Veterans Affairs Medical Center (VAMC). Many of the studies measured meal-stimulated acid secretion using the technique of *in vivo* titration in which a standardized meal adjusted to pH 5.0 was infused into the volunteer's stomach. Periodic aliquots of gastric contents would be removed, the pH measured by a pH electrode, and the contents then returned to the stomach. The volume of sodium bicarbonate needed to keep the pH of the gastric contents at 5.0 reflected the amount of gastric acid secreted in response to the meal. This was a common technique of determining the effect of new pharmacologic agents (e.g. histamine-2 receptor antagonists, prostaglandin analogs) on gastric acid secretion.

One day in the fall of 1976, it was noted that the baseline gastric juice of one of the volunteers was particularly thick and viscous with a high pH level. The response to the test meal in that case was particularly weak. Over time, 17 of 37 healthy volunteers and one patient with Zollinger–Ellison syndrome (ZES) became abruptly hypochlorhydric, defined as a reduction in peak acid output to pentagastrin of at least 75% in two consecutive studies. After the first few of these occurrences, a protocol was implemented to study these and future subjects who developed hypochlorhydria and the results of these studies were published in 1979.[2]

Clinical features

Of the 17 subjects who became profoundly hypochlorhydric, 9 described a premonitory illness, characterized by mild to moderate epigastric pain in all, nausea in 4, and vomiting in 2 subjects.

Mucosal biopsies

Gastric fundic mucosal biopsies were obtained using a peroral hydraulic suction instrument under fluoroscopic control in 12 subjects and 8 controls, and these biopsies were coded and read by Jerry Trier, one of the foremost gastrointestinal histopathologists of the time, and Kevin Carey, one of his fellows, at the Peter Bent Brigham Hospital in Boston. Severe fundal gastritis was noted in each of the 12 subjects (FIGURE I), with abundant parietal cells and chief cells that were normal in appearance. Severe fundal gastritis was noted in only one of the eight controls. Antral biopsies were available in only five hypochlorhydric subjects, and in four there was moderate-to-severe gastritis. Serial biopsies were performed in 10 subjects, which showed a gradual decrease in the severity of gastritis and a concomitant increase in gastric acid secretion.

Gastric acid secretion

Gastric acid secretion returned to near-baseline levels in 14 of the 17 subjects, but three subjects remained hypochlorhydric for a further 12 months after detection. The duration of hypochlorhydria in the 14 subjects whose acid secretion had recovered ranged from 53 to 235 days, with a mean of 125 days (FIGURES 2,3).

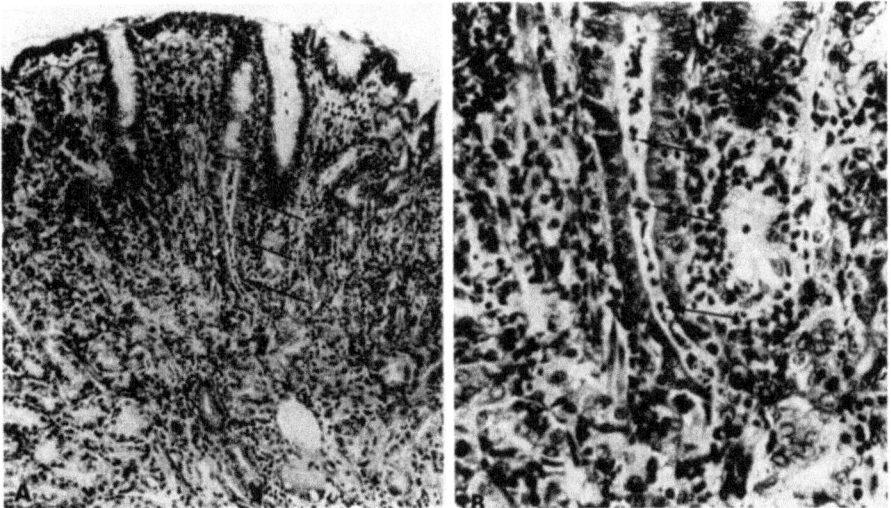

FIGURE I (Left) Arrows show pit abscess containing polymorphonuclear leukocytes in Grade 3 gastritis (×100). (Right) Higher magnification. Arrows again show pit abscess containing polymorphonuclear leukocytes (×250). (Reproduced with permission from Ramsey EJ, Carey KV, Peterson WL *et al. Gastroenterology* 1979; **76**: 1449–57.)

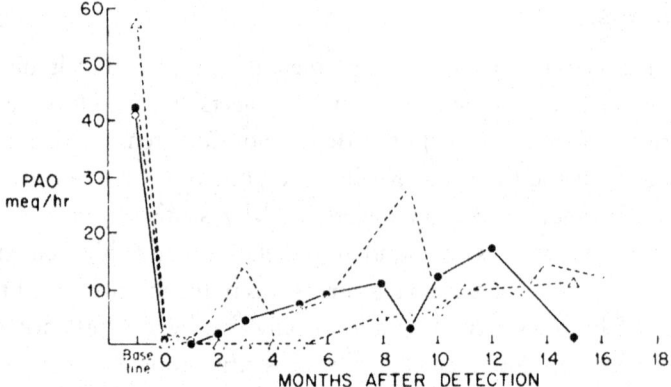

FIGURE 2 Serial peak acid outputs (PAO) for the three persistently hypochlorhydric subjects. (○) Case no. 13; (△) case no. 14; (●) case no. 15. (Reproduced with permission from Ramsey EJ, Carey KV, Peterson WL *et al. Gastroenterology* 1979; **76**: 1449–57.)

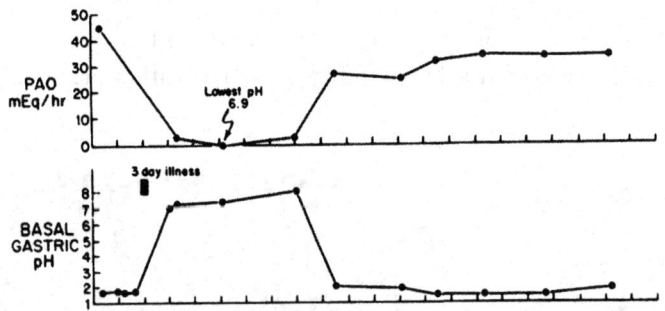

FIGURE 3 Illustrative case. Peak acid output (PAO) and basal gastric pH of case no. 4 before, during and after recovery from hypochlorhydria. (Reproduced with permission from Ramsey EJ, Carey KV, Peterson WL *et al. Gastroenterology* 1979; **76**: 1449–57.)

Gastric permeability

Gastric absorption studies with H^+, ^{22}Na and L_i did not show a significant increase in gastric mucosal permeability in the hypochlorhydric subjects. Thus, the isotopic studies did not provide an explanation of the hypochlorhydria because there was no increase in the back-diffusion of these compounds through the mucosa, and it therefore was related to parietal cell failure, rather than back-diffusion of gastric acid. Apparently, the healthy parietal cells had in some way been switched off.

Serologic studies

The serum levels of pepsinogens, the precursor molecules of pepsin, are generally related to the mass of functional gastric corpus mucosa, and the levels rise when gastric mucosal inflammation is present. Thus it was observed that serum pepsinogen concentrations were abnormally high in hypochlorhydric subjects early in the clinical course, but returned to normal in parallel with improvement of secretory capacity and healing of the gastritis. Parietal cell antibodies were negative in all 14 subjects in whom they were measured. Neither mean fasting serum gastrin nor gastrin in response to a meal was significantly different during hypochlorhydria or after recovery, although two subjects had very high levels during the hypochlorhydria compared with recovery.

Search for an etiologic agent

An infectious agent was strongly suspected, and it was postulated that perhaps this agent was transmitted from subject to subject via the shared pH electrode used during the studies of meal-stimulated acid secretion. This practice was stopped soon after recognition of the syndrome, but cases continued to be identified. More mucosal biopsies were sent to Jerry Trier and Kevin Carey in Boston, but they reported that they had not seen any suspected pathogens. Additionally, cultures of the mucosal biopsies did not disclose an infectious agent and serologic tests for known pathogens were negative.

Our description of acute gastritis with hypochlorhydria (AGH) was not the first,[5-7] but clearly involved the most subjects. Neither the etiology nor the means by which subjects developed the gastritis was known at the time. The occurrence of this phenomenon in a patient with ZES, and the assumption that the etiology was infectious in nature, offered the possibility of treating other patients with ZES. At the time, there was no effective medical therapy to control the gastric acid hypersecretion that is characteristic of ZES. Therapy was surgical, in which either the tumor was found and resected, or total gastrectomy was performed. We thought that administering the gastric juice from the ZES patient with AGH to other ZES patients to induce 'parietal cell failure' might be a nonsurgical treatment. After many months of discussion, the Dallas VAMC Ethics Committee granted permission to use the gastric juice in another patient with ZES, but at the last moment, the patient in question declined to take part in the experiment.

The pathophysiology of spontaneous hypochlorhydria was closely associated with inflammation of the fundic mucosa, although the means by which gastritis led to decreased acid secretion was poorly understood. The parietal cells appeared normal in number and histology and there was no evidence of increased back-diffusion of hydrogen ions. A mechanism whereby inflamma-tion might elicit some compound that inhibited acid secretion was speculated, but no such agent was known at the time.

Long-term follow-up

Upon the suggestion from Barry Marshall that the outbreak we described in 1979 might have been related to *Helicobacter pylori*, we in Dallas decided to review the original clinical material collected from the AGH subjects and then conduct a follow-up study with two goals in mind: (1) to determine the rela-tionship between AGH and *H. pylori* infection and (2) to investigate the long-term outcome of AGH. Since the original report, 17 additional cases had been reported between July 1977 and December 1987, bringing to 35 the total number of AGH cases recognized in the Dallas laboratory and the full report of this investigation has been recently published.[8]

The serum samples we had obtained before the onset of AGH, at the time AGH was first noted and at various intervals after the onset were retrieved from the archive, and the laboratory of Martin Blaser examined these samples for IgA and IgG antibodies to *H. pylori*, as well as for antibodies to CagA pro-tein. In Dallas, Dr Edward Lee examined the archived gastric mucosal biopsies for the presence of *H. pylori* and the presence, degree and type of gastritis.

We were able to locate 28 of the 33 surviving AGH subjects who agreed to participate in some or all of a panel of follow-up studies. Two of the AGH subjects had died of causes unrelated to AGH and the other five could not be located. Each AGH subject participating in the follow-up studies was paired with a control subject matched for the age of the AGH subject at the time of follow-up, as well as for sex, race and profession. The follow-up studies included a questionnaire related to gastrointestinal symptoms, esophagogas-troduodenoscopy with biopsies of the antrum and fundus, basal and stimulated gastric secretory studies, and measurement of serum antibodies to *H. pylori*.

This review of the archived material that had been collected from the AGH subjects provided strong evidence of new *H. pylori* acquisition in a total of 14 subjects within 2 months of recognition of AGH, in 18 within 4 months, and in 22 of 35 within 12 months. The evidence included the development of IgG or IgM *H. pylori* antibodies and/or the presence of *H. pylori* in biopsies taken after recognition of AGH. However, the nature of the archived material was an obsta-cle to determining the exact temporal relationship between AGH and *H. pylori* acquisition. During the time of the epidemic, subjects were not visiting the labo-ratory at regular intervals and this, combined with the fact that the onset of AGH was asymptomatic or minimally symptomatic in the majority of subjects, made it difficult to determine the precise onset. The initial gastric biopsy samples were collected with a hydraulic suction tube, and in some cases the biopsy material available for review was limited. Thus it is likely that the recognition of AGH was often delayed and the evidence of *H. pylori* colonization was also likely missed or delayed in a number of cases. Data collected during the follow-up provided additional evidence of an association between AGH and *H. pylori*: the prevalence of *H. pylori* colonization at the time of follow-up was 82% in AGH subjects, compared with 29% of the matched controls.

The follow-up study also provided information regarding the long-term outcome of AGH and *H. pylori* infection. The AGH subjects were studied for a mean of 12 years after initial recognition of the disease and the development of significant upper gastrointestinal disease was uncommon in them during follow-up. One gave a history of a duodenal ulcer and another had duodenal erosions at follow-up endoscopy. *Helicobacter pylori* infection, once acquired, persisted in all but two of the AGH subjects. Gastritis tended to improve, but also persisted and was associated with *H. pylori* colonization. Despite the persistence of gastritis, the basal and peak acid outputs returned to pre-AGH levels in all but two subjects who remained persistently achlorhydric.

Conclusion

Overall, the follow-up study did not prove that acute *H. pylori* colonization causes AGH, but the data were most compatible with that hypothesis. The study did not provide any additional information regarding the means by which the epidemic was propagated, with one exception: CagA antibodies were present in 23 AGH subjects and absent in 14, suggesting that the epidemic was not caused by a single source of *H. pylori*.

References

[1] Ippoliti A, Elashoff J, Valenzuela J *et al.* Recurrent ulcer after successful treatment with cimetidine or antacid. *Gastroenterology* 1983; **85**: 875–80.

[2] Ramsey EJ, Carey KV, Peterson WL *et al.* Epidemic gastritis with hypochlorhydria. *Gastroenterology* 1979; **76**: 1449–57.

[3] Hirschowitz BI, Streeten DHP, London JA, Pollard HM. A steroid induced gastric ulcer. *Lancet* 1956; **2**: 1081–3.

[4] Makhlouf GM, McManus JPA, Card WI. A comparative study of the effects of gastrin, histamine, histalog, and mecothane on the secretory capacity of the human stomach in two normal subjects over 20 months. *Gut* 1965; **6**: 525–34.

[5] Spiro HM, Schwartz RD. Superficial gastritis: A cause of temporary achlorhydria and hyperpepsinemia. *N Engl J Med* 1958; **259**: 682–4.

[6] Waterfall W. Spontaneous decrease in gastric secretory response to humoral stimuli. *BMJ* 1969; **4**: 459–61.

[7] Gledhill T, Leicester RJ, Addis B *et al.* Epidemic hypochlorhydria. *BMJ* 1985; **290**: 1383–6.

[8] Harford WV, Barnett C, Lee E, Perez-Perez G, Blaser MJ, Peterson WL. Acute gastritis with hypochlorhydria: report of 35 cases and long-term follow up. *Gut* 2000; **47**: 467–72.

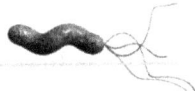

CHAPTER 14

The discovery of *Helicobacter pylori* in Perth, Western Australia

J. Robin Warren

For me, the story of *Helicobacter* started on my birthday, 11 June 1979. I was getting on with my routine reporting, and on examining a gastric biopsy that showed active chronic gastritis, I noticed an unusual blue line on the surface of the gastric mucosa. With higher magnification, I thought I could see numerous small bacilli, closely adherent to the epithelium, and with oil immersion, I saw the bacteria quite clearly. Excited, I showed them to Dr Len Matz, one of the best pathologists in Perth, who worked in the same department – but to my great disappointment, he could not see them. I sat down and turned the problem over and over in my mind. I have always enjoyed such problems.

I was born in Adelaide, South Australia. Most of my mother's relatives were doctors, so that was my future, although dad was a winemaker, from a farming family. I was educated at St Peter's College and attended the Adelaide University medical school (as did Lord Florey). At school, I enjoyed mathematics and the logic related to this has always appealed to me. After graduation, I became a pathology trainee in Melbourne, under Dr Doug Hicks, who was a wonderful teacher and mentor. One day in 1967, after I had passed my College membership, I noticed an unusually large man talking to Dr Hicks, and the next thing he whirled into my room and said, 'Doug tells me you need a job. Well, I will see you in Perth next year.' That was my introduction to Professor Rolf ten Seldam and, as I found out, nobody argued with him! So from 1968, I worked as a consultant pathologist at the Royal Perth Hospital, which is how, 11 years later, I came to be considering the meaning of gastric bacteria.

Basic medical teaching for more than 100 years stated that bacteria do not grow in a normal stomach, probably because of the acid environment. Bacteria or fungi, often *Candida*, do grow in atrophic stomachs or in the necrotic debris in an ulcer. In those cases, the infection appears to be secondary to the underlying lesion and of little significance. Other factors contributed to this widespread belief. Before endoscopy became commonplace in the 1970s, it was unusual to see well-fixed gastric biopsies. Most stomachs coming to a pathology department were surgical (gastrectomy) specimens, and although theatre staff would quickly place the specimens in formalin fixative, the stomachs were usually unopened and the mucosa showed moderate autolysis. Other specimens came from postmortem examinations and by the time these reached the pathologist, the enzyme and acid digestion of the tissues was well under way. Any bacteria were long gone and the fine detail of the gastric mucosa was rarely seen. If medical textbooks showed pictures of well-fixed gastric mucosa, they were often animal tissues that could be fixed immediately.

Because pathologists rarely saw the mucosal detail adequately, chronic gastritis was difficult to diagnose and was thought to be relatively unimportant compared with ulcers and stomach cancer. The system used by many pathologists at the time to describe and classify gastritis made little sense to me, and did not seem to be very useful in practice. It emphasized gross atrophic endoscopically visible gastritis, as seen in pernicious anemia, a classic disease beloved of medical schoolteachers, but uncommonly seen in clinical practice. Most gastric biopsies coming to my laboratory showed some chronic gastritis, with variable degrees of mucosal atrophy, but this was not obviously clinically significant.

In the early 1970s with the appearance of the fiberoptic endoscope, the situation changed from rarely seeing the fine histology of gastric mucosa, to finding that well-fixed fragments of tissue from the gastrointestinal tract were becoming some of the most frequent specimens. In 1972, Richard Whitehead, together with Truelove and Gear, published a new classification of gastritis,[1] which I found logical and easy to use. Although this classification initially appears complicated, it actually uses common features such as the location of the biopsy, the depth, type and severity of the inflammation, the degree of atrophy of the gastric glands and the presence of intestinal metaplasia. Importantly for me, the authors described a specific histological change that they referred to as 'activity' and which is a common feature that had previously been ignored. I could easily see and measure these changes and the results appeared consistent.

I had been experimenting for some time with various stains for bacteria in histological sections. Most bacteria are easily seen in acellular microbiological smears, but most stains for bacteria also stain the tissue structures and it can be very difficult to see microorganisms against this complex background. One exception is the Gram stain. Gram-positive bacteria stain dark blue, in sharp contrast to the totally negative tissue histology. Similarly, acid-fast bacilli stand out, although they are often small and pale, and some fine cellular organelles may also be acid fast. The only other promising stain I found was the Warthin-Starry silver stain, which demonstrates the very small spirochetes of syphilis as dark gray against a yellow-brown cellular background, making them surprisingly easy to see. Donovan bodies (*Calymmatobacterium granulomatis* in granuloma inguinale) also stained well. Another Gram-negative intracellular bacterium that is shown well with the silver stain is *Klebsiella rhinoscleromatis* (in rhinoscleroma). Therefore, I tested the Warthin-Starry stain on numerous Gram-negative bacteria. Some of them stained well; others were negative.

So there I was, on that winter's day in June 1979, with gastric biopsies showing numerous suspicious bacteria on the surface. I had seen the arrival of the endoscope and the subsequent improvement in the quality of gastric biopsies. I had read Whitehead's description of gastric histology and pathology. I was experimenting with the use of the Warthin-Starry silver stain. Therefore, I ordered the stain for this case, and there before my eyes, was a beautiful silver stain, with numerous bacilli clearly visible, even on low-power magnification (FIGURE I).

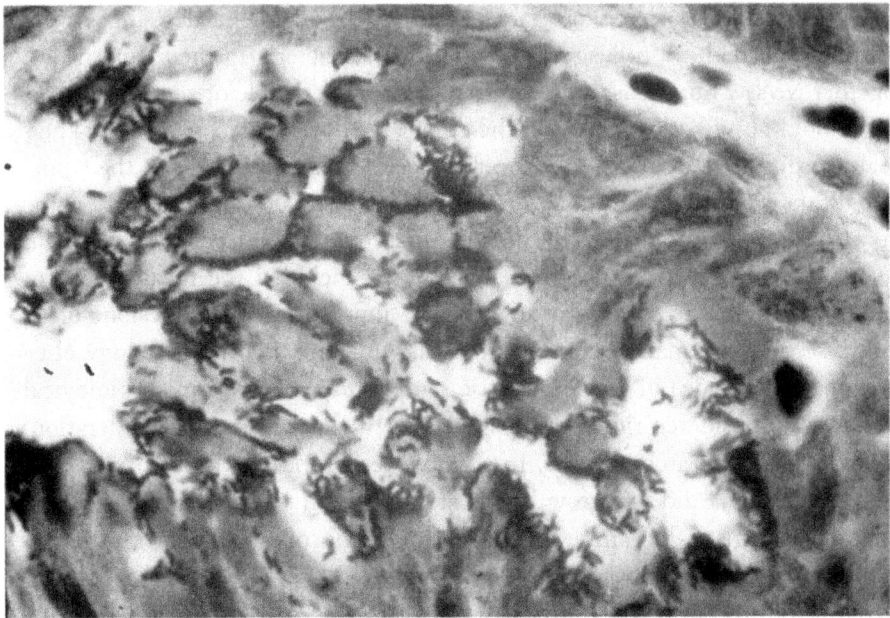

FIGURE I Warthin-Starry silver stained section from my first case of *H. pylori* gastritis.

I am often asked what I thought when I first saw the bacteria and I think the answer is exemplified in my original report (FIGURE 2). The bacteria appeared fixed to the surface of the epithelium of an abnormal mucosa, in a way that looked as if the bacteria were actually causing the damage. They often seemed to be penetrating between the epithelial cells, which were bulging out in the manner of active gastritis. I arranged for thick sections from the tissue wax block to be examined by electron microscopy and those, too, clearly showed the bacteria, closely applied to the epithelial surface (FIGURE 3) and appearing to extend between the bulging cells, but only as deep as the intercellular tight junctions. Finally, my immediate colleagues believed they were there. But what did they mean – if anything? Len Matz said, 'If you really believe they are important, see if you can find some more cases.'

Therefore, I continued to search for the bacteria in more biopsy specimens, not really expecting to find any more. After all, I had never seen them before and it is not uncommon in pathology practice to find one-off cases of an unusual infection. But to my amazement, the bacteria appeared quite often, usually in smaller numbers than in the first case or showing a patchy distribution. It soon became obvious they were closely related to the 'active' form of chronic gastritis, as described by Whitehead, with the specific epithelial distortion and superficial polymorphonuclear cell infiltration. With experience, I found the bacteria in almost half of the biopsies from the gastric antrum, although sometimes they were rare and often the histological changes were mild. I persuaded my colleagues to code for the bacteria in their reports and together we saw hundreds of examples over the next couple of years.[2,3]

I could not get any help from the clinicians, however, at that point. Their goal was different, of course; they took biopsies of abnormalities in the stomach: ulcers or suspected tumors, for example. The tissue samples could come from anywhere in the stomach, which required me to search for the bacteria in a very motley collection of samples that often included the focal lesions of interest to the clinicians. Unfortunately, the mucosa near these lesions often shows secondary inflammation and healing, unrelated to the histology elsewhere. The very idea of sending gastric samples especially for microbiological culture was considered ridiculous. Patient care was the primary consideration, before esoteric research projects. In any case, everyone had known for a century that bacteria did not grow in the stomach. Why would a well-balanced gastroenterologist take samples from apparently normal parts of the stomach in order to look for bacteria?

Whenever I pushed the subject into a discussion, I was often asked two difficult questions. First, 'If the bacteria really are there, why are they not just secondary to the inflammation?' My best answer was that, in my opinion, as

Patient's Classification........PRIVATE....................

Date Received ....08/06/79....................   Date Reported ....12/06/79........................

Specimen: Gastric biopsies

Macroscopic:

(a) Labelled "Antrum" - Six pieces of pale greyish-brown soft tissue,
     each 0.3 cm. in extent.

(b) Labelled "Anterior wall" - Two pieces of brownish tissue, each
     0.3 cm. in extent.

Microscopic:

(a) Fragments of antral mucosa. The pits and surface epithelium are
     somewhat irregular.   The glands show mild evidence of atrophy and
     are mucus-secreting in type. The mucus-secretion on the surface
     of the mucosa appears somewhat more densely staining than normal.
     It contains numerous coiled or curved bacilli up to about 3um in
     length with up to two loose coils. Many of these are in close
     contact with the surface of the epithelium.   Scattered other bacilli
     and cocci are also present. There is one focus of superficial
     erosion with some fibrinous exudate mixed with the mucus and
     containing occasional polymorphs. The lamina propria shows a
     moderate increase in small round cells with scattered plasma cells
     and occasional polymorphs. The glands are mucus-secreting in type,
     with some evidence of atrophy.

(b) One fragment consists of body-type mucosa. The other is a fragment
     of blood clot. The mucosa shows evidence of surface haemorrhage.
     The epithelium and pits are slightly distorted but do not show
     obvious irregularity. The glands are lined by chief and parietal
     cells. The lamina propria is slightly increased in amount with
     a mild increase in small round cells.

Conclusion:

(a) There is chronic gastritis with a small erosion. The quality of
     the surface mucus appears slightly more dense than normal in many
     areas, and it contains numerous bacteria in close contact
     with the surface epithelium. These bacteria have the morphology
     of Campylobacter. They appear to be actively growing and not
     a contaminant. I am not sure of the significance of these
     unusual findings, but further investigation of the patient's
     eating habits, gastro-intestinal function and microbiology may be
     worthwhile.

(b) Mild gastritis.

J.R. Warren
Pathologist

FIGURE 2 The pathology report from my first case, 11 June 1979 (my birthday!)

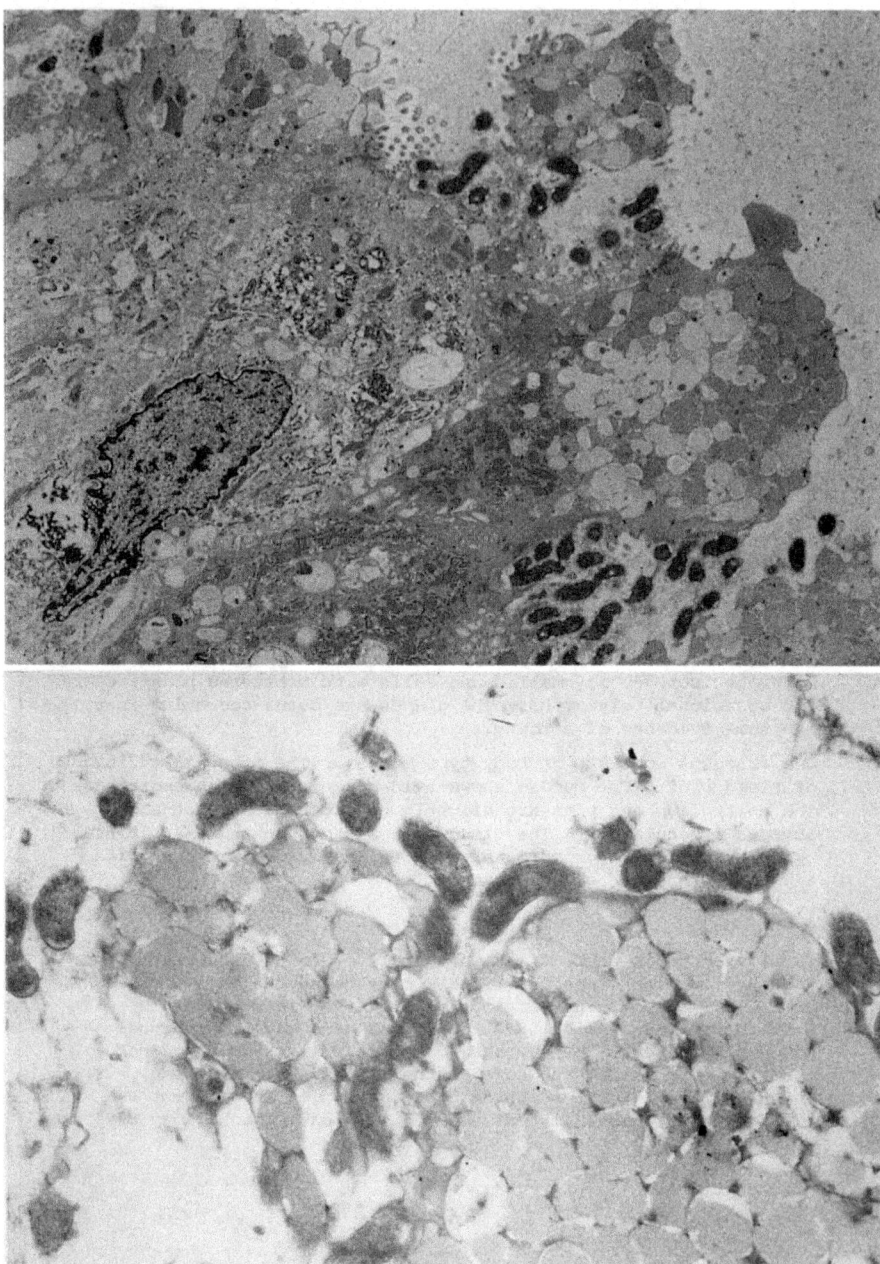

Figure 3 Electron micrographs from two early cases of *H. pylori*. (Top) Prepared especially for electron microscopy, shows abnormal epithelial cells with loss of cytoskeletal structure, absent microvilli, 'pseudopodia' and even intracellular vacuoles. (Bottom) Reprocessed from a paraffin section, but showing the bacterial morphology and their tight attachment to the mucus-secreting epithelial cells.

the consultant pathologist, the features, position and distribution of the bacilli had the appearance of a primary infection, with secondary mucosal damage. However, until I became involved with Dr Barry Marshall and examined the effects of antibacterial therapy on the mucosa,[4] I failed to convince anyone.

The second question people often asked me was, 'Why, if the bacteria really are there, has no-one else reported them?' This was difficult to answer, as I had enough trouble understanding why I had not seen them before. Later, of course, we gradually found numerous reports of them, going back 100 years.[5] Many reports over the previous century had been dismissed as incorrect or of no importance, such was the power of the belief that the stomach was sterile. Freedberg and Barron had published a small article about several cases seen in 1940,[6] but some years later, Palmer 'showed' that no such bacteria existed.[7] I also found a beautiful electron micrograph in a gastroenterology textbook.[8] (Stone Freedberg actually wrote to both Barry and I after we published our work,[9] thanking us for proving he had been right all the time.)

This apparent dearth of reports suddenly changed for me one year later when I decided to report the series. I took my original electron micrographs to the Electron Microsopy Department to try to find some properly fixed sections of gastric mucosa. The technologist was doubtful, but, as we looked at my pictures, his assistant walked past, glanced down, and said, 'Those look like the bacteria that Prof. Papadimitriou was finding a few years ago.' He continued on his way, but he was correct. There was a series of about 100 electron microscopic studies of the stomach, both transmission microscopy and some very impressive surface micrographs. My bacteria were present on many of the images and Papadimitriou had written what I still regard as one of the best short descriptions of them.[10] This was the first previous report I had found. I tried to convince Papadimitriou to review his series and become a co-author of my paper, but he would not, saying, 'It is your work. You write it. I have too many other things to do.'

I thought one useful investigation would be a negative control: how many of the previous gastric biopsies filed as 'normal' also showed the bacteria? This was a harder task than I expected, as most of these so-called 'normal' specimens came from the gastric body and showed mild changes only that were coded as normal. Most accompanying biopsies from the gastric antrum in the same patients showed gastritis and the bacteria were as common as in other cases. There were very few biopsies of normal antrum. Our filing system did not differentiate between different parts of the stomach, so it was difficult to find cases where the antrum was coded as 'normal', but I eventually found 20 such cases. I excluded one of these 'normal' cases because although it actually did show bacteria, there was moderately severe gastritis, which the original

pathologist had reported but incorrectly coded. These new data were supportive, and interesting, but hardly publication material.

By now, I found the bacteria in almost half the biopsies I examined, usually
in biopsies with accompanying chronic gastritis showing active changes. Many
had some degree of atrophy and some had focal intestinal metaplasia. I never
saw the bacteria when the antral histology was normal.

I started to write up my findings, although no-one believed much of what
I was saying. The clinicians gave the project very little attention and most of
them regarded me as a bit eccentric. In fact, there was only one doctor who did
believe in what I was doing; my wife Win, who was a psychiatrist, and who
encouraged me throughout all the long evenings when I was late home from
work, brought more work home with me, and often worked until two o'clock in
the morning (FIGURE 4). With a family of five children, she had every reason to
resent the time and resources I was devoting to this idea. Nevertheless, she
supported me loyally throughout and without her, I do not know how I would
have managed. Looking back now at that time when she was losing her hus-
band to 'nonexistent' bacteria in the stomach, Win had every reason to send
me to her colleagues!

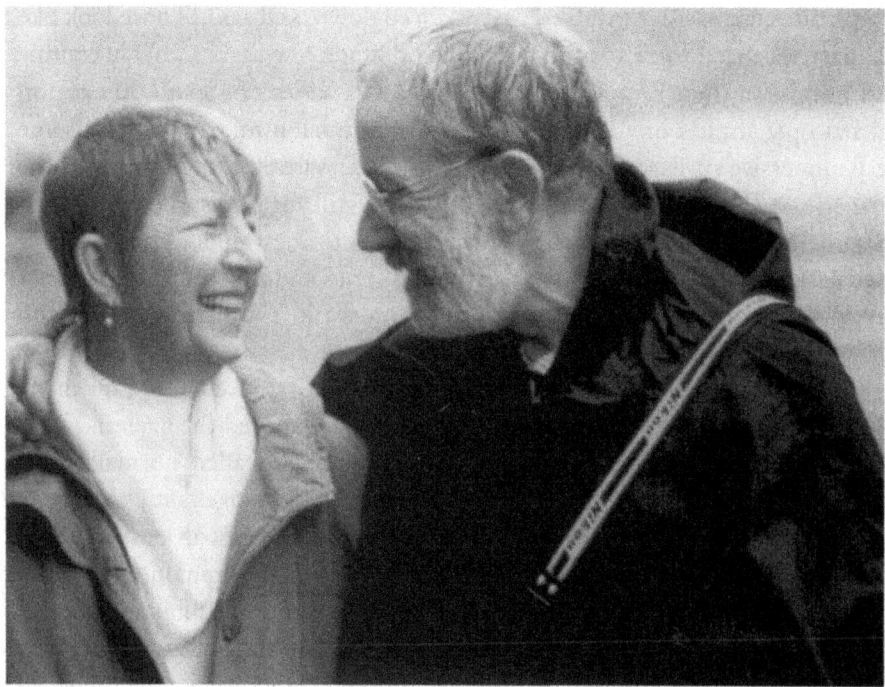

FIGURE 4 Win and I at the first Western Pacific Helicobacter Congress, Guangzhou,
1994.

The paper was almost ready when I first met Barry Marshall in 1981, when he asked to see my work. At the time, Barry was a registrar on the Royal Australasian College of Physicians training program, which expects its trainees to undertake a small research project and write a paper each year. Trainees spend 6–12 months in a series of medical specialties during the three years of their advanced training, and Barry had just arrived in the gastroenterology department. He did not like the project suggested to him by the department, so they suggested he go and see 'that pathologist who is trying to make gastritis into a bacterial infection'. I, on the other hand, had been missing a link in the story: how my histological and bacteriological findings related to patients.

I had been trying for years to get a series of clean biopsies from an area in the antrum not involved by local lesions. Although I initially failed to convince Barry about my work, he did agree to arrange a series of 20 patients, taking samples from areas of the gastric antrum that looked normal to the endoscopic eye. These showed the gastritis histology better than the usual routine biopsies, and the bacteria and accompanying active gastritis were just as common, and easier to see. The changes were not just a consequence of ulcers nearby. At this point, Barry changed his mind and became very enthusiastic about the idea, a position he maintains to this day.

The next stage was to set up a formal study of the next 100 patients referred to the outpatient department for gastroscopy. We used a detailed clinical protocol and took standardized antral biopsies for histology and culture. The results were quite unexpected: the bacteria and gastritis found on histology seemed almost unrelated to most of the clinical symptoms and the endoscopic findings. Only bad breath and burping seemed to be related to the bacteria. Most of the patients had been referred with epigastric pain, regardless of what we found, so we could not test for any relationship to pain. Furthermore, the 'gastritis' seen by the doctor performing the gastroscopy was not related to the histological gastritis as diagnosed by the pathologist on microscopy.

Because I thought the bacteria resembled *Campylobacter*, our colleagues in microbiology at Royal Perth Hospital used the same techniques for culturing *Campylobacter*, but without the antibiotics normally included when trying to culture that organism from fecal samples. However, all the initial cultures were negative. Then chance again took a hand. There was a five-day public holiday for Easter, which included a weekend. The staff was very busy and overlooked the 35th gastric biopsy, which was inadvertently left in the microaerobic culture cabinet. When Helen Royce, one of the microbiology technicians, came in to work after the holiday, she noticed tiny transparent colonies on the culture plate, looking somewhat like diphtheroids. She made a slide, stained it, and thought she saw the bacteria we were looking for. Barry was not convinced, but electron microscopy showed spiral bacilli, similar to *Campylobacter* except with four sheathed flagella showing drumstick-like expansions at the end. This was most unusual, and suggested these bacteria were a new variety. They were eventually placed in a separate genus and named *Helicobacter*.[11]

We obtained several additional positive cultures of the same species, but many cultures were false negatives. Afterwards, it was found that the incubator was leaking and once we repaired it, cultures suddenly became very reliable for diagnosing the presence of this organism. They were almost always positive when I saw the bacteria on biopsy and not otherwise.

Meanwhile, Barry had left the gastroenterology department because his professional training roster moved him to hematology. However, he completed the organization for the trial, persuaded clinicians to have their patients fill in our detailed questionnaires, and collated all clinical findings with my histology report. Later that year, Barry provided medical cover at a remote country hospital in Port Hedland, a somewhat desolate iron ore town, 2000 km north of Perth. At the last moment, he decided to take all the endoscopy reports with him and collate them. He discovered, to our mutual surprise, that I had found the bacterium in all 13 patients with duodenal ulcers, and 24 of 28 gastric ulcer patients.

Thus we could show that the bacteria were related to the 'active' type of chronic gastritis, that they could be cultured and were a new variety of bacterium, and that they were related to peptic ulcer and very strongly to duodenal ulcer. The latter was rather unexpected. We set out to write our definitive report, but Barry wanted an advance letter to *The Lancet* to describe our findings. He left that to me, so I took the opportunity to write a summary of my unpublished paper, written before I met Barry.[3] I was taken aback when Barry read the letter I had prepared and told me there was nothing new in it. He quickly wrote a second letter describing our joint work[12] and after a short discussion the Editor agreed to publish both letters. (My letter represents the only publication of my own findings and conclusions from before I met Barry.) Our findings were also presented by Barry at a Campylobacter conference held in Brussels the same year, which, luckily for us as it happened, Martin Skirrow, a leading UK authority on *Campylobacter*, attended and found our work very interesting.

Soon afterwards, Barry and I completed our definitive paper and sent it to *The Lancet*. I believe the Editor wanted to publish the paper, but the reviewers could not agree and held up publication for months: the findings were too strange and new. Finally, we contacted Martin Skirrow, whose colleagues repeated a short series similar to ours and showed the results were reproducible. They sent their results to *The Lancet* and two weeks later in June 1984, our paper was published,[9] with several letters validating our work in the same issue.

We spent the rest of the early days of *H. pylori* concentrating on diagnosis, treatment and proof. We investigated several methods of diagnosis, most of them suggested by Barry, including pretreatment serology, the C14 urea breath test, the CLOtest and rapid urease test, as well as histology and microbiological smears and cultures.

Treatment went in two main directions: bismuth and antibiotics. Barry had read about the use of bismuth in an old copy of William Osler's *Principles and Practice of Medicine* and thought, correctly, that it might work by killing the bacteria. An alternative assault on the bacteria was antibiotics; in particular, amoxycillin, tetracycline, erythromycin and tinidazole.

For proof of a causative association between *Helicobacter* and gastritis, both Barry and Arthur Morris[13] in New Zealand independently applied Koch's postulates: they drank a suspension of the bacteria and observed the results. Barry rapidly became very sick with acute gastritis, to the disgust of his wife, but then cured himself easily. Dr Morris, on the other hand, developed a chronic gastritis that took years to cure. I still have numerous biopsies he sent me showing the *Helicobacter*-related mucosal inflammation. It improved somewhat after several courses of treatment and, when he finally thought it was clear, I was the one who had to write back and tell him it was still there. Eventually he did succeed in curing it.

Even my wife and I were early patients. Win needed nonsteroidal anti-inflammatory drugs for arthritis and promptly suffered one of the most well-known complications of those drugs: abdominal pain. Whenever she stopped the NSAIDs, the pain went, but the arthritis returned. Therefore, I sent her to Barry for investigation and treatment. The bacteria were there, and once they had been treated, Win could carry on taking the pain-killers without side-effects. Then she noticed that I had bad breath, although like most people with *H. pylori* infection, I did not have any other symptoms. I took a course of treatment too and my bad breath apparently disappeared.

At this stage, Barry left for a year, and I took part in a study of gastric mucosal cultures with Professor C. S. Goodwin. For me, the biopsies were not as uniform as those Barry arranged. They came from many parts of the stomach, but this helped me to see that the histological changes, so obvious in the gastric antrum, were also present in the fundus. Often, there were few bacteria and the inflammation was very mild and superficial or focal. Nevertheless, further careful or high-power examination usually showed the same changes as in the antrum. In addition, with the repaired incubator and improved microbiological expertise, the cultures and biopsies became an almost perfect match. What I, at the time, called campylobacter-like organisms or CLO (hence the name Barry gave to the CLOtest) were present on histology whenever the cultures were positive.

Barry and I next completed a double-blind trial of antibacterial treatment for duodenal ulcer. We designed the trial so that patients with a duodenal ulcer received a course of either antibiotic therapy or placebo. The treatment was arranged blind by the pharmacist, with no communication to the patients or us. The medication packs looked identical. All patients followed an identical protocol, with further endoscopic assessments to demonstrate any recurrent ulceration and to provide biopsies for histological assessment and culture. Barry's ability to retain trial patients was quite amazing. He encouraged them to return again and again and again for what is a relatively uncomfortable investigation – even when they did not have symptoms! In the whole study, only one patient missed one gastroscopy on one occasion.

At the end of the trial, we broke the code to find out which patients had taken which medication. We found that if we eradicated a patient's bacterial infection, there was little risk of recurrent ulceration. If *Helicobacter* remained, the gastritis was unchanged and almost all of these patients showed endoscopic relapse of ulceration within 12 months. For me, this trial provided an ideal chance to study the pathology related to *Helicobacter*. Biopsies taken soon after successful treatment showed almost complete disappearance of any 'active' change in the mucosa, with loss of the bacteria. Other changes improved more slowly, but after 12 months most of these patients appeared near normal. Structural changes such as atrophy, metaplasia and fibrosis were relatively unaffected.

I was able to arrange a reliable quantification of the pathology, staging each of the main features on a 0–9 scale. Bacteria, polymorphonuclear leukocyte infiltration, 'active' distortion of the epithelium, mucus secretion and lymphocyte infiltration were the most useful features. Using this method, the pattern of the pathology remained remarkably similar in repeat biopsies for each patient while the bacteria were present. It remained the same in a follow-up study after seven years.[15]

I was also partly able to solve the problem of why duodenal ulcer, more so than gastric ulcer, is so closely related to a gastric infection. Barry included biopsies from the proximal end and the side of the ulcers. The tissue from the proximal biopsies usually resembled gastric mucosa, although often very scarred and almost unrecognizable. No Brunner's glands or other features of duodenal mucosa were present. Further investigation of partial gastrectomy specimens and animal stomachs showed that the very mobile gastric mucosa normally extends through the pylorus. When *Helicobacter* gastritis is present, it also extends through the pylorus. It seems reasonable that a point of maximum mucosal stress, such as the mucosa in the pyloric sphincter, should tend to ulcerate if inflamed. Gastric metaplasia, with *Helicobacter* and inflammation, is common beside the ulcers, although it is usually mild and superficial, and the significance is less certain.

After our studies, interest in *Helicobacter* spread widely. Many new species have been found in different animals, and *Helicobacter* now has its own dedicated journal and its own world congress. It has been one of the most widely published subjects of the past 15 years and no longer involves just pathologists, clinicians and microbiologists. There now is a spread of sophisticated expertise through most branches of medical study. It took about 10 years after our publications before treatment of *Helicobacter* infection became official; since the Sydney conference in fact.[16] But even now, it only applies to peptic ulcer. I find it very disappointing that chronic active gastritis is not considered worthy of more notice, but this is partly because of the rather weak relationship between the gastric pathology and the patients' symptoms, as we reported in 1984.[9]

In recent years, the pharmaceutical industry has been more helpful. Most firms were making money from the acid suppressant drugs, but now many firms are trying to be the first to produce a reliable, safe cure for *Helicobacter* infection. Results are variable, but promising.

During the past decade, Barry and I have received worldwide recognition for our pioneering work on the subject. Many organizations and countries have honored us, and although I have now retired, I still receive many requests to give lectures, or write articles (such as this). In conclusion, I will discuss a question I have been asked at several meetings. 'Dr Warren, do you think your findings result from brilliant research, luck, stealing other people's ideas or serendipity?' Well, in my opinion it is the latter. Serendipity includes luck, but is much more. I think I was the right person in the right place at the right time. My interests included gastric histology, gastritis and bacterial stains. When I first saw the organisms, I preferred to believe my eyes, not the medical textbooks or the medical fraternity. Our department had recently obtained an electron microscope. I enjoy solving logical puzzles; I did mathematics and statistics after medical studies just for the pleasure of seeing how they reduce complex masses of data to simple formulae. In addition, I am stubborn enough to keep going when everyone tells me I am wrong. All of these things came together in June 1979 and so my work was away. Brilliant research? I am a consultant pathologist, not a 'research worker', although research was involved. Stealing? I had no knowledge of anyone else's work, but of course 'No man is an island', to quote John Donne.[17]

References

1 Whitehead R, Truelove SC, Gear WML. The histological diagnosis of chronic gastritis in fibreoptic gastroscope biopsy specimens. *J Clin Pathol* 1972; **25**: 1–11.

2 Warren JR. Gastric pathology associated with *Helicobacter pylori*. In: Marshall BJ (ed.) *Gastroenterology Clinics of North America*, Vol. 29. Philadelphia: WB Saunders, 2000; 705–51.

3 Warren JR. Unidentified curved bacilli on gastric epithelium in active chronic gastritis. *Lancet* 1983; **1**: 1273.

4 Marshall BJ, Goodwin CS, Warren JR *et al*. Prospective randomized trial of duodenal ulcer relapse after eradication of *Campylobacter pylori*. *Lancet* 1988; **2**: 1437–42.

5 Salomon H. Ueber das Spirillum des Saugetiermagens und sein Verhalten zu den Belegzellen. *Zentralbl Bakteriol* 1896; **19**: 433.

6 Freedberg AS, Barron LE. The presence of spirochetes in human gastric mucosa. *Am J Dig Dis* 1940; **7**: 443–5.

7 Palmer ED. Investigation of the gastric mucosa spirochetes of the human. *Gastroenterology* 1954; **27**: 218–20.

8 Ito S. Anatomic structure of the gastric mucosa. In: Heidel US, Code CF (eds). *Handbook of Physiology*. Section 6: *Alimentary Canal*, Vol. 2: *Secretion*. Washington DC: American Physiological Society, 1967; 705–41.

9 Marshall BJ, Warren JR. Unidentified curved bacilli in the stomach of patients with gastritis and peptic ulceration. *Lancet* 1984; **1**: 1311–15.

10 Fung WP, Papadimitriou JM, Matz LR. Endoscopic, histological and ultrastructural correlations in chronic gastritis. *Am J Gastroenterol* 1979; **71**: 269–79.

11 Goodwin CS. *H. pylori*: 10th anniversary of its culture in April, 1982 (Editorial). *Gut* 1993; **34**: 293–4.

12 Marshall B. Unidentified curved bacilli on gastric epithelium in active chronic gastritis. *Lancet* 1983; **1**: 1273–4.

13 Morris A, Nicholson G. Ingestion of *Campylobacter pyloridis* causes gastritis and raised fasting gastric pH. *Am J Gastroenterol* 1987; **82**: 192–9.

14 Goodwin CS, Blincow ED, Warren JR, Waters TE, Sanderson CR, Easton L. Evaluation of cultural techniques for isolating *Campylobacter pyloridis* from endoscopic biopsies of gastric mucosa. *J Clin Pathol* 1985; **38**: 1127–31.

15 Forbes GM, Warren JR, Glaser ME, Cullen DJE, Marshall BJ, Collins BJ. Long-term follow-up of gastric histology after *Helicobacter pylori* eradication. *J Gastroenterol Hepatol* 1996; **11**: 670–3.

16 Tytgat GNJ, Axon ATR, Dixon MF, Graham DY, Lee A, Marshall BJ. *Helicobacter pylori*: Causal agent in peptic ulcer disease? Working party reports, World Congresses of Gastroenterology 26–31 August, 1990, Sydney, Australia; 36–45.

17 Donne, John (1572–1631). *Devotions Upon Emergent Occasions*. 1624.

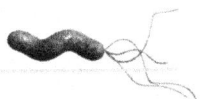

CHAPTER 15

The discovery that *Helicobacter pylori*, a spiral bacterium, caused peptic ulcer disease

Barry J. Marshall

Early days

I was born in 1951 in Kalgoorlie, Australia's largest gold mining town, located about 370 miles east of Perth. My father was a mechanical fitter and my mother a nurse, so I was exposed to both medical and engineering texts from a very early age. I think we were reasonably well off, even in those days, because my father's father was a publican, and hotels in mining towns such as Kalgoorlie were always very successful businesses. My first memory of a hospital may have been when my brother was born in 1954, or a few months later when he was admitted and nearly died from gastroenteritis. Our house did not have electricity, but we did have a kerosene refrigerator and a Model A Ford. I do recall that our toilet was a 'thunderbox' down the end of the backyard and that it was always necessary to check under the seat for red-back spiders before sitting down. For this reason, and also to 'kill the germs', I often took pleasure in pouring excessive amounts of creosote down the toilet. Thus, by four years of age I understood the basic principles of engineering, gastroenterology, and even treatment of infectious disease!

A few other memorable events in my early years might have directed me towards a career in medicine. At age five I was attacked by a dog and required numerous tetanus and penicillin shots in the same day. Two years later I suddenly developed an allergy to shellfish, which, with hindsight, must have been caused by dermal inoculation by lobster spines when my father was a fisherman in 1955. Finally, I clearly recall walking past a very attractive house in Kalgoorlie one day in 1956 and asking my mother why that family had two cars. The answer, of course, was that it was a doctor's house!

In high school, although interested in science and mathematics, I felt that my math skills were not strong enough to do electronic engineering, so I chose medical school as an alternative, which was at least as interesting, and should not require daily exposure to calculus! In the back of my mind I might also have had the idea that, if my medical career was successful, I would have enough resources to still do electronics as a hobby. As it happens, this seems to have turned out nicely because the computer and Internet continue to support much of the work I do.

I was first labeled as 'brash' by the journalist Suzanne Chazin in the Reader's Digest,[1] but, in retrospect, probably cultivated that attribute during medical school. The best example arose from an incident in 1972 after the pathology written examination. All the medical students were asked to complete an anonymous questionnaire regarding the teaching ability of the professors. Much to their dismay, one of the replies was rather abusive. One week later at the end of my successful pathology oral examination Professor Len Matz confronted me with my questionnaire sheet. Not one to stand on protocol he had traced my handwriting. I stood by my derogatory opinions and, luckily, my comments on Matz's lectures were even slightly favorable. If he had failed me Len Matz might have delayed the discovery of *Helicobacter pylori* by several years, resulting in suffering and misery to millions! It was no coincidence I suppose that Len Matz kept an eye on Robin and me 10 years later, helping us settle some very thorny issues on authorship (see Robin Warren's chapter[2]).

In that year also, I married Adrienne Feldman, a psychology student who, unlike myself, was nicely spoken, very well mannered, and never brash. In 1973 the first of our four children, Luke, was born soon after the 5th year medicine exam.

In spite of my brash exploits, I graduated with an MB BS (Bachelor of Medicine, Bachelor of Surgery) in 1975 and followed this with an internship and residencies in internal medicine at the Queen Elizabeth II Medical Centre (Sir Charles Gairdner Hospital). In those days I had no particular goals in medicine, but if I had to choose, was most interested in all aspects of clinical medicine including geriatrics, oncology and rheumatology. After failing the oral examination for the Australian College of Physicians in 1978, I moved to Royal Perth Hospital (RPH) in 1979, mainly because I would be exposed to more cardiology there as RPH was the only hospital performing open-heart surgery at that time. This plan was successful and I passed the first part of my physicians exam in 1979, and for the following three years took various internal medicine training posts at that hospital.

Early attempts at research

As part of the physician training at RPH, registrars were encouraged to submit a researched case report or clinical study for presentation at the yearly internal medicine trainee conference. This was my first attempt at research, with my 1980 presentation being the case of a 30-year-old man who apparently caught poliomyelitis from a Vietnamese refugee boat in Darwin Harbour, moored near to where he was swimming. The following year (1981) I had become interested in heat stroke and presented my investigation of Perth's hottest ever day (46°C on 12 December 1978), during which I had noticed double the mortality rate for elderly people, and quite a few cases of heat stroke that were mismanaged as 'cerebral-vascular accidents' by the emergency room teams around the city.

Investigation into heatstroke seemed to offer the right mix of clinical and basic research for me because the etiology of the changes was poorly understood and the popularity of short marathons ('fun runs') was increasing around the world. In addition, there was clearly a need for new technology that could monitor core body temperature during a marathon race. After some thought I devised a small mercury thermometer that could be inserted into the rectum and provide a maximum reading of the runner's core body temperature. To allow recovery of the device, a piece of fishing line was attached at the constriction near the bulb. My unfortunate resident, Graham Hankey (now a neurologist), was a keen marathon runner and together we spent several lunch breaks running up and down the RPH stair well, thermometers securely inside, in an attempt to raise our core body temperature above 40°C. Although the heatstroke interest was gradually replaced by *H. pylori* work, it did serve a useful purpose. I attended the Perth 'City to Surf' fun-run in April 1982 and predicted that it would be a disaster because the temperature that day was going to be about 30°C. As I expected, dozens of runners collapsed with hyperthermia and I attended one who developed status epilepticus. Whipping out a trusty mini rectal thermometer, I documented a core body temperature of 42.5°C, enough to cause brain damage. With the help of some of the bystanders we carried the runner to a nearby backyard swimming pool and floated him there until he cooled enough to recover consciousness. He made a full recovery but, sadly, that was the last time I ever used my invention. Later that day I collected blood samples for that patient and others in the race, but the hospital laboratory was closed by the time I completed the task. As the clotted blood needed to be spun, my solution was to tape the tubes to our overhead bedroom fan for the night, much to the dismay of my long-suffering wife. Actually, the technique worked quite well, but has never been patented!

Robin Warren and CLO, 1981

In July 1981, my medicine rotation took me to the gastroenterology division as the 'service' internal medicine trainee. The idea was to give me experience in gastrointestinal medicine, following which I would move on to my preferred area of rheumatology, never to see the inside of a stomach again. The first month there I spoke to my boss Dr Tom Waters about a research project. Tom was aware of two possible projects, the first of which was an analysis of approximately 20 000 endoscopy reports to ascertain the prevalence of various endoscopic findings in the RPH patients. I asked Tom what the second project was! He presented me with a list of 25 names, which he said had been given to him by one of the pathologists, Dr Robin Warren, who had been looking for the past 12 months for a clinical collaborator who would be interested in following up on some bacteria he had seen on stomach biopsies.

I looked down the list and was intrigued to see a patient whom I had referred for endoscopy during my previous internal medicine term. This 60-year-old woman with a past history of gastric ulcer had presented with nausea, abdominal pain, headache and mild splenomegaly. Endoscopy showed 'nodular gastritis of the antrum', but there was no ulcer. In desperation, and with no other diagnosis, her senior physician arranged a psychiatric consult, somehow extracted a diagnosis of depression, and then discharged the lady on amitriptyline. I saw her one week later, but she was no better, and still seemed perfectly sane to me, with a mental condition quite appropriate for a person with a chronic illness. This woman, and many like her, later fueled my interest in *Helicobacter* as a cause of nonulcer dyspepsia. (I telephoned that seminal patient while writing this chapter. At 82 years of age, she is well except for mild Parkinson's disease. Although she has never been treated for *H. pylori*, she no longer suffers from gastric symptoms other than being 'careful what she eats'. It is interesting to note that her original biopsy contained intestinal metaplasia. Perhaps this was an early atrophic gastritis that had led to burnout of her gastric ulcer disease. Her GP plans a urea breath test.)

That afternoon, I took the list down into the basement of RPH, where Dr Warren worked in the Pathology Department (Figure i). In those days, Robin used to drink strong black coffee and smoke small cigars. My previous encounters with him had only been at gastroenterology biopsy sessions, or when discussing the histopathology of one of my own patients, so I barely knew him. Robin spent the rest of the afternoon showing me slides of the curved bacteria he had seen, and explaining the histopathology of the gastric mucosa to me. Apparently, about two years earlier, he had seen what may have been bacteria on an H&E section of gastric mucosa, and had performed a

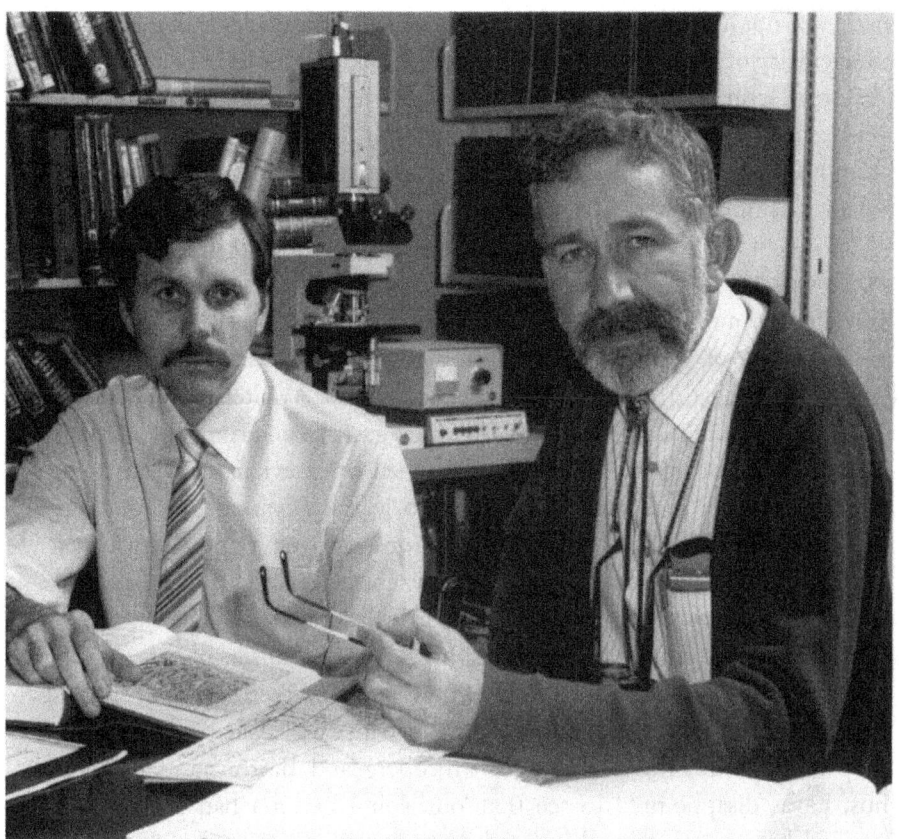

FIGURE 1 Barry Marshall and Robin Warren in July 1984.

silver stain, which then showed a striking appearance of apparently heavy colonization of the gastric mucosa by these curved bacteria.

I was interested in Robin's bacteria because, as he and I both knew, the stomach was supposed to be sterile. I did not know it then, but he had tried to recruit others into the work for some time, without success. Actually, as I soon discovered, Robin is one of those people who can never finish a conversation, always thinking of one more relevant point to make. Of course he did know an awful lot about gastric histology, but after a few hours in his office I felt my brain was full. I suppose he thought that I would need some convincing, but he presented such a good case for the bacteria as pathogens that I accepted the concept rather naturally after that. Apart from the obvious conflict between my attention deficit disorder and his obsessional perfectionism, we got on well. As I saw it, a new species of bacteria would make a nice publication, regardless of whether or not it actually caused a disease. I had no particular opinion as to the pathogenicity of the gastric organisms, but I was aware of publications in the literature describing *Campylobacter jejuni* as a newly discovered common cause of food-borne gastroenteritis and colitis. Thus both Robin and I had seen pictures of campylobacters and could appreciate that these gastric organisms did indeed have a very similar shape.

By the end of that afternoon I had a reasonable idea of what histological gastritis was, but had very little understanding of whether or not gastritis of itself was related to any clinical syndrome. In those days, our 'bible', if we had one, was the description of gastric mucosal histology and classification of gastritis by Richard Whitehead.[3] Robin loaned me his copy of Whitehead's book and I headed off to the medical library to read up on gastritis and campylobacters.

In the medical library at RPH, I searched for previous references to the curved bacteria. In a chapter by Susumu Ito in the *Handbook of Physiology*,[4] I found what appeared to be an excellent electron micrograph of a campylobacter-like organism happily attached to a gastric epithelial cell. Ito's chapter contained references of other observations, particularly that of Vial and Orrego,[5] who had described similar bacteria as 'spirilla' in the stomachs of cats and dogs. Vial's paper included references to Salomon[6] and Bizzozero[7] as cited by Eddie Palmer in *Gastroenterology* in 1954.[8] Palmer's paper was available to me and, in that paper, I found the citations for Freedberg and Barron[9] and Doenges.[10] Thus, I was disappointed to see that 'our' spiral bacteria had probably been described before. On the other hand, linkage with gastritis was not a major feature of the previous literature, because most of the studies were animal, post-mortem or gastrectomy material.

By 1981 RPH had online access to MEDLINE and I was able to search the current literature on campylobacters. New campylobacters were being discovered almost daily and a new category called 'campylobacter-like organisms' (CLO) was being added to the taxonomy to allow for new and poorly characterized campylobacter species. In humans, the main campylobacter was *C. jejuni*, but *C. fetus* was another known pathogen (although uncommon except in immunosuppressed individuals) and *C. sputorum* was a commensal that had been isolated from dental plaque. Thus, our organism could have been a commensal 'CLO' residing in the upper gastrointestinal tract.

My literature research also resurrected the series of papers from Siurala and others in which a cohort of normal Estonians had undergone repeated gastric biopsy studies.[11] Our interest by then was in the spiral bacteria and their prevalence in the normal population because Robin's biopsy series had been chosen for him by the gastroenterologists investigating abnormal endoscopy findings, and therefore did not tell us the prevalence of the bacterium in apparently healthy stomachs. Thus, at that time, it seemed likely that the new bacteria were commensals. In the days before PCR, there was no easy way for us to actually identify or classify these organisms except based on morphology or, if we could culture them, with biochemical tests.

In the following weeks I retrieved the case records of Robin's 25 patients, and coded them for clinical and pathological findings that could possibly be related to the presence of the spiral bacteria. Where possible, I called the patients by telephone and asked about diet, travel and past history. This was a highly selected group, with no control group (since all had the CLO on biopsy). The endoscopic diagnoses were duodenal ulcer (2), gastric ulcer (7), gastritis (12), and scars and erosions (4), and there was no apparent pattern in these 25 patients. Most had presented with abdominal pain, or were being managed for known peptic ulcer disease (PUD), or had presented with anemia.

In my sessions with Robin, he emphasized that these bacteria appeared to be associated with histologic gastritis, by which he meant infiltration of the lamina propria with various lymphocytic-type cells, as well as small collections of neutrophils, particularly around the necks of the superficial mucus glands. Robin also showed me oil immersion preparations of the histology of gastritis, revealing details of 'microerosions' and epithelial cell damage. He showed me some drawings he had made to describe these changes, which he felt were specific to the bacteria. In addition, in PAS sections, we could see that the intracellular mucus of affected cells was greatly diminished, such that these cells either had released their mucus or were no longer producing any and were stunted (for a detailed account see Warren[12]).

As mentioned earlier, the benchmark Scandinavian studies of gastritis had sampled a large group of Estonian volunteers, and had followed these persons longitudinally for more than a decade.[13] Although the bacteria were never described, most of the 'healthy volunteers' in that study were found to have various degrees of gastritis. In addition, the gastritis had apparently worsened with time, and progressed towards atrophic gastritis. Thus, the Scandinavian papers too, if read objectively, seemed to suggest that any organism associated with gastritis was likely to be a commensal. However, to me, all the literature on gastritis was extremely confusing because of the variations in terminology.

Whitehead's was the most precise description, whereby no etiology was attributed to the lesions, merely each component of the mucosa was quantitated. For example, the type of epithelium (mucus-secreting, acid-secreting or metaplastic) was described, followed by the degree of infiltration with various cells. The Scandinavian papers often discussed 'atrophic gastritis', but this was a difficult diagnosis to make in 1981, because biopsies were 2 mm specimens taken through the fiberoptic endoscope, whereas the original classifications of gastric histology were from gastrectomy specimens, such as those described by Magnus.[14] Thus, with fiberoptic endoscopy biopsies it was more appropriate to talk of intestinal metaplasia than extrapolating to the diagnosis of atrophic gastritis, although this might have been the endpoint for severe intestinal metaplasia.

From my reading it did appear that much of the population, at least in Scandinavia, had chronic gastritis that started in early adulthood and progressed throughout life until most of the population had intestinal metaplasia and, if much of the gastric mucosa was actually replaced by this process, also had gastric atrophy. A disappointing feature with many of these publications was that journal editors avoided publishing photographs of the histology. Instead, a few representative samples would be given, often at rather low power, followed by numerous data tables and statistical analyses of the results. Thus, it was not possible for me to be certain whether or not bacteria were present.

After discussing the negative preliminary findings from the 25 cases with my two bosses, Tom Waters and Chris Sanderson, I decided that we should try to culture these bacteria from fresh biopsies. I was still in the process of completing my training in internal medicine so I relied on my trainee status for help with my projects. Any collaboration from other staff was given on a goodwill basis and I was in no position to control any hospital resources. I approached John Pearman at the RPH Department of Microbiology. A few weeks later, a technologist there recalled an abstract from the Australian Society for Microbiology meeting authored by Michael Phillips and Adrian Lee describing the culture of a mucosa-associated spiral organism. The basic technique was to use nutritious media, such as brain–heart infusion blood agar, in a microaerophilic environment. By then, the RPH laboratory was routinely culturing stool for *C. jejuni* and had Skirrow's plates available, an inhibitory medium suitable for isolating campylobacters. We decided, however, that culture at 42°C, as is done for *Campylobacter*, was more of a selection criterion used for that bacterial species, and should not be used for isolation of this new organism. When simple blood agar culture failed, we tried Skirrow's plates and brain–heart infusion horse blood agar as suggested by Lee's group.

In the subsequent weeks, I obtained fresh gastric biopsies from about 20 consecutive patients attending for gastroscopy, in whom gastritis might have been suspected. Unlike the series of patients we had studied retrospectively, these biopsies were extra samples, taken at a distance from any endoscopic lesion. As soon as the biopsies were removed, I moistened them with a drop of saline and hand-delivered them to the Microbiology Department. There the specimens were smeared onto a slide and Gram stained. Within just a few cases we soon had quite good Gram stain preparations, showing sheets of

Gram-negative spiral organisms. This fired the enthusiasm of the microbiology team, who continued to process our specimens and attempted to culture them. All manner of media and atmospheres were used, but in the subsequent 6 months (August 1981–March 1982) all attempts to culture the spiral bacteria were unsuccessful, even though they could easily be seen on Gram stains and, of course, on Robin Warren's silver stained histology.

Our first treated case

In October 1981, although unable to culture the bacteria, we treated our first patient. During the endoscopy sessions I met an elderly Russian man with intractable abdominal pain. Because he did have some vascular disease, abdominal angina was a provisional diagnosis. At endoscopy, the stomach was red and our usual antral biopsies were taken. The Gram-stained biopsy showed numerous Gram-negative spiral organisms. By then, Robin and I had studied most of the literature related to campylobacters and we knew that CLO were sensitive to tetracycline. I approached the physician in charge of the patient, who agreed that a 14-day course with oral tetracycline was worth a therapeutic trial. In addition, both he and the patient agreed to return after that time (on day 14) to repeat the endoscopy and biopsy.

This was the first time I realized that our clinical research project was probably overstepping the bounds of what would normally occur in the management of a patient, and therefore might reasonably be the subject of ethics committee consideration. Taking an unnecessary biopsy was one thing, but using obscure findings from that specimen to justify antibiotic therapy was another. Nevertheless, we pressed on and I reviewed the patient two weeks after he was started on tetracycline. Robin and I were acutely aware that this was merely an anecdotal observation and so we were biased against observing any clinical response in this patient. The patient himself, however, was ecstatic in his discovery that an antibiotic treatment was able to completely eliminate his extremely severe and chronic gastric symptoms. As far as he was concerned, his stomach pain had been cured. Endoscopically, the stomach looked red as usual, but the histology had improved, with far fewer neutrophils in the mucosa and no bacteria.

I discussed the results of our experiment with the other gastroenterologists. What had we learned? Not really very much because on the basis of this one case we could not really show that the curved bacteria were pathogens or commensals. In addition, we still did not know the origin of this bug, or its prevalence in the community in Perth. Chris Sanderson's comment was succint, 'Barry, you should stop buggerizing around and do a proper study.'

A prospective study, 1982

By November 1981 I was extremely enthusiastic about the CLO project and determined to take it to the next step, but my gastroenterology term had almost finished and allocations for 1982 had already been decided. In the first six months, I was to be a hematology registrar looking after the bone marrow transplant patients, and in the second half of the year I was to be the physician at Port Hedland Hospital, a rotation 2000 km north of Perth. However, because the Hematology Department was quite close to Gastroenterology, it did seem possible that I could continue to run a research project in the first few months of the year. By then also, Robin and I had developed a degree of confidence in our methodology; that is, location of biopsies, transport methods and staining, and we believed that we could easily carry out a study on 100 or so patients.

In the evenings during 1981, I had continued with my hobby of computing and electronics, and by the end of the year I had built a computer capable of word processing and was able to type up a consent form and protocol for a proposed study of 100 patients to be performed by the gastroenterologists at RPH in the first half of 1982.

In 1982, Kentucky Fried Chicken was the most popular fast food in Perth, and my father was an engineer at the largest chicken processing plant in the city. My reading had revealed that many campylobacter species were present in birds and that *C. jejuni* was particularly common in chickens. So as well as our human studies I was carrying out parallel studies trying to culture and find campylobacters in chickens. This was one of the many early theories we had as to the origin of these organisms. If they had not been properly described before, then it was possible that some new event in Western society was causing humans to be infected with these bacteria. It was also possible that our bacteria were Australian, and thus could have come from any one of the many unique marsupial animals. Additionally, the recent introduction of acid-reducing drugs such as Tagamet (cimetidine, a histamine-receptor blocker) could have reduced the gastric acidity of our patients to such an extent that they were susceptible to colonization from these bacteria. Additionally, the organism could have come from crevasses between the teeth, or been present in dairy products and milk, or been contracted during holiday travel to Asia, which was a common destination from Perth.

Thus, our protocol consisted of a pre-endoscopy questionnaire for all patients, giving details of symptoms, medication use, diet, pets and travel. Then, at endoscopy the following morning, patients would have two antral mucosal biopsies taken, the first for Robin Warren (silver-stained histology), and the second for microbiology (Gram stain and an attempt to culture).

Because John Pearman was not the chief of RPH Microbiology in those days, he suggested that I gain approval of this protocol from his boss, Professor Stuart Goodwin. Although I met with Professor Stuart Goodwin in his office at the end of 1981, and obtained permission to carry out the study with RPH Microbiology laboratory staff attempting to culture the gastric bacteria, as far as I recall, I never saw Stuart again until 1983. Tom Waters, Chris Sanderson and John Pearman were the only other collaborators named on the protocol. (Eighteen months later, Stuart Goodwin pressed me to write up the microbiological side of the discovery so that the West Australian team could claim naming rights to the new organism. I was advised against it by David McGechie at Fremantle hospital, but eventually I agreed, no doubt encouraged by Stuart's offer to put me first on that paper, and himself fourth. I was later to regret this, as it gave Stuart a claim to the original work and his paper[15] almost beat ours to press!)

As stated in the protocol, our 100-patient study aimed to answer the following questions.

> Is the observed bacterium present in normal stomachs?
> Can the presence of the bacterium be correlated with the type and severity of the gastric pathology?
> Can the organism be cultured?
> In those patients who undergo a further gastroscopy and biopsy for whatever reason, does persistence or disappearance of the organism correlate with the patient's symptoms?

The study was to be a pilot one after which we proposed to use it as the baseline for a more elaborate trial with a control group and incorporating follow-up endoscopy and biopsy after treatment of affected patients with the appropriate antibiotic. If at this stage the organism still had not been cultured, immunological methods would also be undertaken for its identification. FIGURE 2 is the simple consent form I used to recruit patients into the study and from my recollection, only one patient declined to take part.

The study commenced early in 1982, when I was working as a hematology registrar. I would look at the endoscopy list for the coming day and, at the end of my working day, would interview and recruit the next day's endoscopy patients into the study. In the morning, before work and later at the morning tea break, I would accost elective day-cases and ask them to take part in the study before their endoscopy. At the endoscopy itself, my senior colleagues would be ordered by the study nurse, Dorothy Hayes, to collect the two biopsies and keep them chilled until I was able to deliver them to the laboratory in my tea break.

```
                    APPENDIX B PROTOCOL

INVITATION TO PARTICIPATE IN A RESEARCH PROJECT AT ROYAL PERTH HOSPITAL

      During 1982 a study is being conducted at Royal Perth Hospital on
patients undergoing stomach examinations.

      We are doing this study to see if bacteria (germs) in the stomach are
responsible for indigestion and other complaints.  These bacteria are
sometimes seen when we take a biopsy (a small sample of tissue from the
stomach) and look at it under the microscope.  We need to know whether
normal people have these germs as well as sick people.

      For this reason we would like to take a stomach biopsy on everyone
undergoing gastroscopy.

What will it entail?    Apart from signing this form you will not be aware
that anything was done.  The biopsies are two or three pieces of tissue
2 mm in diameter (this size →O← 2ᵐᵐ) removed from the stomach through
the gastroscope.  They are often taken in any case if an abnormality is
found, but if you agree to take part in this research project these biopsies
will definitely be taken.

Is it painful?    No it is totally painless.

Is it risky?    The risk is very small.  It is possible that bleeding or
puncturing of the stomach could occur, but no one at Royal Perth Hospital
has ever come to harm from this complication and it is very very rare.
Your doctor will take special care when performing the biopsy.

Will it help me?    Probably not, however, if a severe infection of your
stomach is found your doctor may wish to give you a course of antibiotics
to clear it.

How will I find out the results?    Your doctor will inform you or you may
contact Dr. Marshall at the Hospital (on page during working hours).  If you
have any other questions ring Dr. Marshall or ask the sister on your ward to
get him to see you.

      I understand and agree that gastric biopsies may be taken from me
during gastroscopy for research purposes.




     _____  Signed    ......................

                                       Date      ......................

                                       Witness   ......................
```

FIGURE 2 The consent form used for the 1982 CLO study. Regrettably, patients these days have to read many more pages of 'legalese' in order to take part in research studies.

I also collaborated with a statistician so that data collected by Robin (histology and bacteria scores) remained blind, as did microbiology results. I was not able to spend a lot of time looking at the histology or microbiology during that period, because it might have affected the blindness of the prospective study. Nevertheless, I continued to be disappointed in the first two months when, in spite of being told that quite a few patients did have the bacteria, on no occasion was the organism able to be cultured.

Culture success, 8 April 1982

The first culture of *H. pylori* was partly luck. In 1982, the Easter holiday occurred from the 9th (Good Friday) to the 12th (Easter Monday) of April. On Thursday 8 April, we had biopsied a middle-aged man with a history of duodenal ulcer. At that time, my recollection is that the Microbiology Department was in the midst of a manpower crisis, with a methicillin-resistant *Staphylococcus aureus* (MRSA) epidemic in one of the wards, requiring hundreds of potentially infected staff to be screened as possible carriers of the organism. Unbeknown to us, junior microbiology staff in the 'feces lab' where our biopsies had been relegated, were treating them much as they did feces cultures or throat swabs. Thus, expecting to see complete overgrowth of the agar plate after 48 hours, the plates were routinely examined at 48 hours and, if no unusual organisms were present, they were discarded. However, because of the workload over Easter 1982, an oversight occurred and the busy weekend microbiology technician did not examine the research plates on Saturday morning. Thus, the plates remained in the incubator until the next working day, Tuesday 13 April. On that day, the small transparent colonies of *H. pylori* were evident. The organisms were subcultured, and it was not until the following week that John Pearman telephoned me in an excited voice to say that the new bacteria had been cultured. I recall he showed me some unimpressive blood agar plates and a Gram stain in which the organism certainly did not resemble the curved and spiral forms present in the histology. By then, however, they had already cultured the bacterium from another patient and were moderately confident that it was the CLO we were seeking. In the following weeks, 11 more of these new organisms were isolated from our patients but, as I was blinded to the data, I was not to know who actually had the bacteria until about six months later.

That study was completed in May 1982. The various laboratories coded their results and mailed them to the statistician. I was busy winding up my hematology term and, in addition, Adrienne and I were organizing ourselves for the 2000 km plane trip and temporary accommodation in Port Hedland with our four children. On the last two days before we left Perth, while Adrienne was packing up our belongings and driving our car onto a road transport truck, I spent the weekend at RPH. Although our study had been mainly to determine the prevalence of the bacteria in the endoscopy population, and its clinical correlation with gastritis, I decided that it would be important to include the clinical details of our patients in the report. Thus, I retrieved and photocopied the 100 endoscopy reports so that, before the microbiology and histology results were known to me, I could encode the clinical findings and include this in the 'prospective blinded database'.

I took all my references and textbooks up to Port Hedland, and was lucky enough in that location to have both a good supply of microbiology books in the local state health laboratories and, for the first time, some spare time in the evenings to study the endoscopy reports and encode these into meaningful numeric data. I tried to separate patients into various types of ulcer (i.e. duodenal, gastric or both) or esophageal disease (hiatus hernia and oesophagitis) or just red stomach (gastritis) or apparently normal cases. The resulting clinical scores were then mailed back to the statistician and were returned to me around September 1982. In addition, I continued my literature searching by correspondence and was greatly assisted by the librarians at RPH library.

Winter in Port Hedland was beautiful, every day sunny with a temperature in the 80s (°F). My remaining spare time was mostly taken camping around the remote north-west of Western Australia and seeing the sights. By September, however, the place was starting to warm up with most days over 100°F and many of the nights unpleasantly hot. Thus, more time was spent in our air-conditioned house, with me able to work both on the data and the results of the literature searches.

When the data analysis arrived it was very obvious that there was an extreme correlation with the presence of these bacteria and the presence of inflammation in the gastric mucosa. Our statistician used the SPSS program, which only produced results significant to five figures, and for this reason, most of our correlations between bacteria and gastritis came out with a *P*-value of zero. However, with a new Hewlett-Packard calculator he purchased especially for this job, Robin Warren was able to calculate that the *P*-value on a Fisher's exact test was more like 10^{-12}.

Most of the other data (e.g. symptoms, diet, travel, pets, drug use) bore no relationship to the presence of the bacteria, except that abdominal pain and 'burping' (eructation) were significantly more common in individuals with the bacteria than in those without. Overall, at least 65 of the patients had the bacteria, and in nearly all of these histologic gastritis was present.

Bacteria and ulcers, October 1982

The correlation between the bacterium and endoscopic appearance was interesting. Of 13 patients in the study who were found to have duodenal ulcer, all 13 had the bacteria. This association was therefore highly significant ($P < 0.001$). Because the overall infection rate had been 65%, it was like tossing a coin and seeing 'heads' 12 times in a row ($0.5^{-12} = 0.00024$). If all ulcers were taken into account (gastric and duodenal), then 26 of 30 patients had the bacteria, a finding that was also significant ($P < 0.01$). If the association was compared against CLO presence in normal endoscopy cases, the P-value was very low indeed.

After double-checking my original endoscopy report codes and considering the implications of these data for several days, I realized that the converse of this association appeared to be true; that is, people without the new bacterium could not develop peptic ulcer. The four exceptions, according to my notes, were persons who had been taking nonsteroidal antiinflammatory drugs.

While I was in Port Hedland things were not idle at RPH. Our electron microscopist, John Armstrong, had previous experience with identification of bacteria. By telephone and letter I arranged to supply him with bacterial cultures for negative stains, as well as glutaraldehyde-fixed mucosal biopsy specimens. With his technologist, Willy Wee, he was able to demonstrate the morphology of the new organism, particularly the flagella detail and the nearby bacterial morphology. With this information at hand, I spent several weeks poring through my old copy of *Bergey's Manual of Determinative Bacteriology*.[16] Our characterization of these bacteria showed they were microaerophilic and spiralled like campylobacters, but (from John Armstrong's pictures) with sheathed flagella, similar to vibrios. Thus, morphologically, they did seem to be a new species.

In November 1982 I wrote to Michael Phillips and Adrian Lee to receive their input on the new organisms because it did appear that they were related in some way to the mucosal flora of the mouse colon. He and Michael Phillips had already cultured a spiral organism from this site, which in retrospect, was the first known isolation of a helicobacter, probably *H. muridarum* (see chapter by Lee *et al.*[17]).

My literature search focused on gastritis, pulling out various articles written in the 1970s where the histology of the gastric mucosa had been studied by various means, particularly by the 'Swiss roll' technique. In this technique, gastrectomy specimens are opened along the greater curve and strips of mucosa are taken vertically from the pylorus up to the corpus. These are then rolled and fixed, so that when cut they give a 'Swiss roll' appearance, with visible histology from the duodenum up to the gastric corpus. These studies had shown that in most peptic ulcer patients, gastritis was most severe in the antrum, fading out as it travelled up towards the corpus. I again reviewed the paper written in the *American Journal of Gastroenterology* by colleagues at RPH, Wye Poh Fung, John Papadimitriou and Len Matz.[18] They had been interested in the correlation between endoscopy and gastric mucosal histology, and had done quite a number of biopsies. In their article, they had even pointed out a couple of these organisms, but had not followed up the observation. Like many others, they had found a rather poor correlation between endoscopic findings (gastritis, red stomach, erosions etc.) and mucosal inflammation on histology. The converse of their conclusions did seem to be useful, however; that is, when the stomach appeared totally normal, gastritis was unlikely to be present. As Robin and I became more interested in the electron microscopic appearance of the mucosa and these bacteria, we were able to confirm our findings by looking at some of the old electron micrographs taken from the Fung study, which were in the collection at the Electron Microscopy Department.

One major problem with the new bacterium was that John Pearman's enteric laboratory had a clinical emphasis and the only 'PhD scientist' associated with it was Dr Doug Annear, a MRSA specialist. Before Doug became peripherally involved, I sent the RPH microbiology laboratory identification tables for spirillaceae from Bergey's Manual so that progress could be made with taxonomic identification of the organism. After some weeks Helen Royce returned a preliminary report to me, which I believe gave a negative result for urease (although I have misplaced the original data sheet).

Synthesis, October 1982

In October 1982, I presented the preliminary findings from our study to the local College of Physicians meeting, where it received a patronizing and mostly negative response. The main objection from the gastroenterologists was that our study had found a strong correlation between gastritis in the stomach and ulcer in the duodenum. This seemed out of place and incorrect, because 'everyone knew' that gastritis was associated with gastric ulcers, but not especially with duodenal ulcers. I had no answer for this criticism, as I was not formally trained in gastroenterology and my reading (apparently selective) had taught me that gastritis was more likely to be associated with duodenal ulcers than with gastric ulcers.

Clearly, I needed to recheck my facts. I traced this information back to its source, which was a paper by Magnus at the Mayo Clinic in the early 1950s.[14] In that study of stomachs from motor vehicle accident fatalities and partial gastrectomy specimens, Magnus had found quite a high prevalence of antral gastritis. In addition, he had observed that 100% of 256 patients with duodenal ulcer had chronic gastritis of the antrum versus 93% of 284 with gastric ulcer. Thus, the ulcer research community appeared to have skipped over the paradox that ulcers in the duodenum were more likely to be associated with gastritis than ulcers in the stomach. This fact did not mesh well with the current understanding of peptic ulcer etiology, and had therefore been ignored. Was gastroenterology a science or a religion? I decided it was the latter.

At the end of 1982 I was at a turning point in my career. I had not arranged an internal medicine position at RPH and the gastroenterology post had already been allocated. Whereas Adrienne would have been happy to go back to work and support me I was less keen on taking over her role while also trying to somehow follow the research line. Alternatively, private practice would have meant severely restricting the time I could spend on the research. I was rescued by senior colleagues from Fremantle Hospital who had been at my presentation in October. A senior registrar post in general medicine and gastroenterology was available.

Publish or perish, October 1982

It was also time to publish. By the final months of 1982, Robin had been looking at his data for three years, but had become too busy to actually finish writing up his pre-1981 data. From my preliminary look at the literature I could see that it was only a matter of time before someone else made the same connections; in fact, I was amazed that it hadn't already been done. In October 1981 I attempted to construct a letter to *The Lancet* concerning our data and mailed a first draft of this to Robin Warren, but received no reply for several weeks. Eventually, Robin and I discussed the letter by phone, and had further correspondence about it. He was concerned that a joint author letter made it appear that I was also involved with his original observations of spiral bacteria and gastritis that he had made in the 18 months prior to our collaboration. In reply, I felt that the endoscopic, microbiologic and clinical work, which I had supervised, was really responsible for our present understanding of the importance of the organism (i.e. that it could be etiologically related to peptic ulcer and gastric cancer). My literature search had also allowed us to gain considerable confidence that our observations were correct, thereby allowing us to be more forceful and place our observations in a top medical journal, rather than a more specialized pathology journal. I believed that my exhaustive literature review proved that the new bacterium was almost certainly the cause of ulcers. Feeling rather paranoid and very isolated in the remote town of Port Hedland, I reviewed the protocol for our study, which noted that Robin planned to publish his current findings in a pathology journal. I was rather disappointed that Robin apparently planned to 'go it alone' with a letter to *The Lancet*. I called him and discussed this, then wrote to him agreeing that it was his decision to make, but suggesting that a single letter from him would have to be sanitized so as not to steal the thunder of the collaborative work. Robin apparently discussed the whole situation with Len Matz and, eventually, we reached a compromise; we would write two letters, which I mailed at the end of January 1983.

Several weeks later we received an air-mail letter from David Fox, who was subeditor at *The Lancet*, stating he was having trouble with our letters and could not understand why there were two. After that, I believe we each called Fox to discuss the issue of authorship of the work and he finally agreed to publish separate letters, with Robin's original observations being described in the first letter, followed by my letter, which included our collaborative work and discussion of the available literature. My decision not to have co-authors on my letter was, like Robin's, somewhat selfish I agree, but I felt that most of the effort up to that point had been mine. In addition, I was still annoyed about the fact that the microbiology staff had been discarding the cultures for six months before the CLO was 'accidentally' grown over the Easter break. When I finally needed expert input in order to determine the taxonomy of the bacterium, it had been more or less left up to me. (Later I also discovered the error of the negative urease test, the story of the defective incubator (see Robin's chapter[2]), and that all my serum samples had been discarded because the microbiology refrigerator was defrosted.) To reinforce my decision, I received a letter from John Armstrong, our electron microscopist, who had really contributed a lot to understanding the taxonomy of the new organism and now provided excellent electron micrographs. John's statement was 'I have no wish or claim to be involved in authorship of articles on this subject – just in case you might have thought otherwise!!' Finally, in October 1982 Burman published a discussion of authorship, which appeared to justify my stance.[19]

In early 1983, while *The Lancet* stewed over our letters, I commenced my new post at Fremantle Hospital and was able to confirm very quickly that our observations of the bacteria at RPH also applied to other parts of the city, the majority of peptic ulcer patients there also having the organism. This gave us more confidence in the importance of the observations. Eventually, *The Lancet* agreed to publish the letters, which were first seen in print in June 1983[20] and were quite spectacular, because they included the silver stain illustrations of Robin's first case, plus negative stains showing two helicobacters with dramatic sheathed flagella. The journal also agreed not to delete my claim that these organisms were important in the etiology of peptic ulceration and gastric cancer. In retrospect, David Fox may have had the last laugh because, at least on the front cover of *The Lancet*, the letters were cited as a single entry with two authors. In addition, to confuse readers further, Robin was cited as Dr J Warren, and I was cited with my full name as Dr Barry Marshall.

Fremantle Hospital, 1983

It was an exciting time in 1983 for those on the trail of *Helicobacter* and peptic ulcer. My job as senior medical registrar at Fremantle Hospital was under the tutelage of Ian Hislop in Gastroenterology. Although Ian agreed that the possible connection between gastritis and peptic ulcer was likely to be important, we differed on the role of gastritis in nonulcer dyspepsia (this controversy still rages). I had approval for a protocol allowing us to biopsy patients undergoing endoscopy, and within a few weeks, had confirmed all the observations from RPH. My second colleague there was microbiologist Dr David McGechie, who had attended a previous Campylobacter workshop and who was a 'campylobacteriologist' with a new research laboratory and excellent microaerophilic culture techniques in CO_2 incubators. He was enthusiastic about supporting the project, so within a few weeks, we had dozens of helicobacters growing and were preparing to preserve samples.

My third colleague, because Robin Warren did not have an appointment at Fremantle Hospital, was the pathologist Ross Glancy. Between the four of us, we soon had a system for collecting gastric mucosal biopsies from patients attending for endoscopy, and were able to culture the spiral bacteria in about 90% of cases in which bacteria were visible on histology. Initially, we were happy to culture the organisms to confirm that they were associated with duodenal ulcer, but within a few months I collaborated with chief technologist Peter Rogers who helped me to further characterize the bacterium, including antibiotic susceptibility studies.

When on night shift at Fremantle, I often had hours to spare during which I could visit the medical library and thumb through years and years of gastroenterology journals. I knew that if these bacteria were common in Australia, they were probably quite common elsewhere, and therefore should appear in at least a few publications describing gastritis. In my literature searching, I came across two articles that showed very clear illustrations of active gastritis. The first of these was by Wiersinga and Tytgat describing a case of acute gastritis in a man who had Zollinger–Ellison syndrome.[21] The acute gastritis had resulted in achlorhydria. The other publication, also in *Gastroenterology*, was by Ramsey *et al.* in which they described an epidemic of gastritis that occurred in Texas in 1977.[22] Neither of the articles included electron microscopy, so we could not be certain that the bacteria were present;

however, the observations prompted me to write to both Tytgat and Ramsey (answered by Walter Peterson), asking for a section of their histology. A month or so later I was pleased to receive a histological section from Guido Tytgat and although he was by no means a convert, I was reassured to find that at least one of the senior gastroenterologists in Europe was interested in the spiral organism. My letter to the Texas group was less successful, in that Walter 'Pete' Peterson was in the midst of moving the gastroenterology laboratory and pathology department to new premises, and was therefore unable to resurrect the histologic sections and study them for the spiral organism. Some six months later, however, he and colleagues were able to perform silver stains on the sections and confirm that patients did have the spiral organism. Several publications, including a chapter in this book, have resulted from those data.

Meanwhile, in February 1983, Robin Warren and I wrote an abstract for submission to the Gastroenterological Society of Australia meeting, which was to be held in Perth (Figure 3). We were sure the abstract would be accepted and, because the meeting was local, it would cost us very little to attend the conference and present it. Regrettably, however, as shown in Figure 4, our abstract was not accepted, with the condolence letter from the secretary stating that, 'of 67 abstracts submitted we could only accept 56', thus our material must have been rated in the bottom 10%!

David McGechie suggested that the microbiologists may now be more interested in the organism and he gave me the telephone number of Martin Skirrow in England. Martin was at that time publishing numerous papers describing new spiral organisms, usually campylobacters, isolated from various animals. That evening, I called Martin Skirrow and told him about the new organism. He was interested, and agreed that I should send him some of our cultures for characterization studies. He also suggested that I submit an abstract to the Campylobacter Workshop that was to be held that year in Brussels and, as he was on the abstract committee, he agreed that it would almost certainly be accepted. Robin and I rewrote the earlier, rejected abstract and submitted it with subsequent success.

In 1983 there was still no collaborative evidence that the spiral bacteria were causing either gastritis or peptic ulceration, except the association we had seen. Clearly, there were two pieces of experimental data we needed to obtain. The first of these was to produce the infection in an animal (i.e. fulfil Koch's postulate that bacteria could cause gastritis and peptic ulcer) and secondly, we needed to show that eradication of the organism in the individual led to healing of the gastritis and the associated PUD. It was already apparent that we were not going to get an objective audience. Everything we claimed flew in the face of accepted dogma. It was undercutting the basis of gastroenterology,

SPIRAL BACTERIA IN GASTRITIS AND ASSOCIATED DISEASE.

BARRY J. MARSHALL J. ROBIN WARREN

Spiral gastric bacteria have been noted on antral mucosal biopsies by J.R.W. since 1979, usually in association with active chronic gastritis. To determine whether they were commensals or truly associated with this pathological entity, a clinical trial was set up. 100 patients undergoing elective gastroscopy gave informed consent to have antral biopsies taken, each also filled in a detailed questionnaire and the endoscopists' reports were added and correlated with the other data at completion of the trial. The relevant results were as follows:-

1. The bacteria were present in patients with active chronic gastritis. (P = .001).

2. The bacteria were present in patients with duodenal ulcer, (P = .01), and gastric ulcer. (P = .05).

3. The bacteria were cultured in 12 patients and both microbiological and electron microscopic evidence is at hand to support the thesis that these bacteria are a new genus with characteristics of campylobacters, spirillae, and vibrios.

It is likely that the gastric spiral bacteria are aetiologically related to gastritis and therefore to gastritis associated diseases; i.e. duodenal ulcer and gastric ulcer. They may be responsible for the high relapse rate in ulcers treated with Cimetidine.

FIGURE 3 Abstract submitted to the Gastroenterology Society of Australia, February 1983.

which had experienced a funding boom with the advent of the H2 receptor blockers, the world's most widely used drugs. It didn't help that I was a 31-year-old, living in the most isolated city in the world, who did not have a university job even in my home town. I realized that I was going to have to do this on my own.

Early in 1983, I wrote to several of the large manufacturers of ulcer drugs (i.e. Smith Kline and French, Glaxo, and Gist-Brocades, the makers of a bismuth tablet called DeNol) asking if they were interested in the new bacterium as a cause of ulcers. I was also applying for government grants with the National Health and Medical Research Council (NHMRC), and even approaching the directors of my father's chicken processing factory. All of them wrote encouraging letters back, but were unable to support my research. No-one was interested in revolutionizing the world of gastroenterology, partly because the concept was so outlandish and partly also because there was very little pharmaceutical research being undertaken in Australia at the time, with nearly all drug companies acting as subsidiaries of American- or European-controlled entities. Therefore, funding for new projects required substantial applications from substantial individuals with long lead times. However, the

GASTROENTEROLOGICAL SOCIETY OF AUSTRALIA

145 Macquarie Street,
SYDNEY.   2000

Telephone 27 3288

17th March, 1983

Dear Dr. Marshall,

I regret that your research paper was not accepted for presentation on the programme of the Annual Scientific Meeting of the Gastroenterological Society of Australia to be held in Perth in May, 1983.

The number of abstracts we receive continues to increase and for this Meeting 67 were submitted and we were able to accept 56.

There were a large number of high quality abstracts which made it extremely difficult to choose those which should be accepted for presentation, and as you know, this is now done by a National Abstract Selection Committee which reviews the abstracts without knowledge of the Authors concerned.

The National Programme Committee would like to thank you for submitting your work, and would hope that this might be re-submitted in the future, perhaps following critical review from your colleagues.

My kindest regards,

Yours sincerely,

for Terry D. Bolin,
Honorary Secretary.

FIGURE 4 Rejection letter from the Gastroenterology Society of Australia, 1983. On the returned abstract, the score '59' had been written in pencil. Some members of the society later spread the rumor that the abstract had been submitted late; however, the delivery receipt (kept by the author) shows that it was received on time.

Gist-Brocades Pharmaceutical Company in Australia sent me several references about their product 'DeNol', which was also known at the time as tripotassium di-citrato bismuthate. According to the literature, and in contrast to the findings of ulcers treated with H2 blockers (i.e. cimetidine and ranitidine), duodenal ulcers could be shown to heal more perfectly, with histological healing, when they were treated with bismuth. In addition, two recent papers had shown that after treatment with bismuth, up to 40% of patients appeared to be cured of their PUD,[23] whereas there were few cures with H2-receptor blockers, almost all patients relapsing in the subsequent year or so.

I was intrigued by these publications, because I recalled seeing incidental bacteria in the electron micrographs in the paper by Fung, Papadimitriou and Matz at RPH.[18] In one of the more recent papers,[24] quite good electron microscopic descriptions of duodenal ulcer borders were included with several round bacteria present on the surface that was cut in section. In addition, these bacteria did not appear to be present on the post-treatment images. This suggested to me that the treatment that caused less relapse (i.e. cure) in a proportion of ulcer patients could actually be eradicating the bacteria. I then searched the literature on bismuth, and found that it had been used as an antibacterial agent for hundreds of years. In the pre-penicillin era, contaminated wounds were often packed with bismuth-soaked dressings, and bismuth was also used as an antimicrobial in culture plates designed to prevent *Proteus mirabilis* from swarming. Additionally, prior to 1935, bismuth injections were used to treat syphilis, much in the way that arsenicals were used. Thus, bismuth had a good track record as an antimicrobial, particularly for slow-growing, spiral, mucosa-associated organisms, such as spirochetes.

The following week, I obtained some liquid DeNol and asked Neil Stingemore, who was assisting that week, to make antibiotic sensitivity disks. After dipping the disks in the DeNol and applying them to heavily inoculated blood agar plates, we placed the experiment in the incubator over the weekend. On Monday we were excited to find there was a large zone of inhibition around the bismuth disk, showing that it had inhibited the spiral organism with an effect almost equivalent to an antibiotic. Subsequent experiments over the next week or so showed that there was very little inhibition seen with the H2-receptor blockers. Thus, our experimental data seemed to fit with the observations of several investigators; that is, ulcer relapse was diminished and some patients were cured when the inhibitory bismuth salts were used.

In about April 1983, Ian Hislop and I received permission to carry out a prospective study in which ulcer patients would be treated with either DeNol (bismuth) or cimetidine, and followed up endoscopically to see if their ulcers healed or relapsed. In this study, we would also study the gastroduodenal mucosa, in order to see if healing of gastritis occurred, or if the bacteria were eradicated. During the remainder of 1983, we asked patients, about 20 in each group, to take part in this prospective study. Unfortunately at that time DeNol was only available as a liquid, which meant that patients were required to take a 4-times daily dose of pink liquid with a pH of approximately 10 and a strong ammoniacal odor. The treatment continued for 2 months, so patients needed to be extremely motivated to complete it. The study was supposed to be investigator-blind, but because I was managing the patients and fielding the telephone calls, there was no way we could keep it totally blinded. Nevertheless, we did recruit approximately 15 patients into each group before terminating the study at the end of the year because we could see that the numbers were too small to achieve significance (unless something dramatic occurred) and there were approximately equal numbers of ulcer relapses present in each group. Thus my colleagues were a little disappointed at the results of this study, but I took the time to blindly score the biopsies taken during and post-treatment for gastritis and CLO. Once I did this, I could show that in some patients the histology dramatically improved while they were on the bismuth, whereas there was virtually no change in patients treated with the H2-receptor blockers. Thus, I could see that although the treatment had no effect on ulcer relapse, it appeared that only 1 of 10 patients in the bismuth group had achieved eradication of the bacterium. Failure could have been the result of poor compliance, or just that the antibacterial effect of this bismuth drug was somewhat overrated in other studies (later studies confirmed it was probably the latter).

In 1983 it was important to use DeNol in our antibiotic treatment protocol because it was a proven ulcer-healing drug, and we believed that it would have been unethical to compare a proven therapy, such as H2-receptor blockers with antibacterial treatments not containing DeNol. Antibiotics would have been unproven as ulcer-healing agents and it is unlikely that we would have been able to have such a study approved by the Ethics Committee because patients might have been at risk of relapsing with bleeding or perforation from their peptic ulcer. Thus it was convenient and ethical to do studies in which the antibiotic treatment arm always included bismuth.

As mentioned earlier, patients taking the liquid DeNol for our study must have been extremely motivated because of the horrible taste of the medication. We had intended to randomize patients on the basis of their hospital numbers (odd *vs* even), but when patients told us they could not possibly take DeNol they were allocated instead to the H2-receptor blocker treatment group. At the end of the study it appeared to me that most of our private patients had been allocated to H2-receptor blocker, whereas most of the hospital patients had been allocated to DeNol! This was a lesson that made me take care in future to ensure that I did not compromise the blindedness of the treatment arms in my prospective randomized studies.

A lucky event occurred during the prospective study. One of the patients who relapsed in the study attended my clinic, where I treated him again with DeNol. By this time, DeNol chewing tablets were available, which were much more convenient. While chewing the tablets he developed a sore mouth, which I thought may have been caused by periodontal disease, and so I added metronidazole to his bismuth for the last five days of his ulcer treatment. We had not studied susceptibility to metronidazole prior to this, because it was used primarily for anaerobic infections (the spiral organism was micro-acrophilic). Subsequently, when the patient's ulcer completely healed and I was able to take a further biopsy at follow-up endoscopy, he was one of the first in whom the spiral bacteria had been eradicated. Thus, it seemed to me that there was some synergism between metronidazole and bismuth.

In susceptibility studies on approximately 10 strains, nine were found to be susceptible to metronidazole, and thereafter we added metronidazole when treating peptic ulcer patients for their spiral bacteria. In that year I treated approximately 10 patients with severe relapsing PUD, and was able to eradicate the infection in eight using this combination. In all eight patients there were no further episodes of peptic ulcer in approximately six months of observation, whereas in the two patients who still had the bacteria, peptic ulcer and peptic ulcer symptoms, including ulcer bleeds, continued. Because I knew the history of these patients in the previous six months when they had quickly relapsed in our prospective study, I was impressed that the eradication of the spiral bacteria certainly seemed to have had a beneficial effect.

By mid-1983, Martin Skirrow had written to report that he had cultured the organism and was interested in it as a possible new type of *Campylobacter* species; at least it grew in the same conditions as *Campylobacter* and was spiral and flagellated etc. By then also we had studied numerous cultures of the organism by electron microscopy with our colleagues at RPH (Robin Warren and John Armstrong) and could show that they had a different morphology to the previously described campylobacters. In our two letters that were published in *The Lancet* (FIGURE 5) we had included excellent photographs of the histology and electron microscopic appearance of the organisms, which Robin and I had both felt was important because, without the illustrations, the letters would probably have gone unnoticed or been far less convincing. Subsequent to this, I successfully applied to Fremantle Hospital for a grant that enabled me to travel to the UK and Belgium later that year to present our findings at the Campylobacter Workshop in Brussels in September. Guido Tytgat, who had earlier sent me one of his histological sections, was also well connected with the

THE LANCET

No 8336   BOSTON, MASS. AND LONDON · SATURDAY 4 JUNE 1983   VOL.1 FOR 1983

LETTERS TO THE EDITOR

FIGURE 5 Citation of the letters on the front page of *The Lancet*, June 4 1983.

Gist-Brocades company that manufactured DeNol and, perhaps because of his interest, they also agreed to partly sponsor my trip to Europe.

In September 1983 on the way to the European Campylobacter Workshop meeting, I visited Martin Skirrow in Worcester, UK, and attended an endoscopy session at the Worcester Infirmary. The first patient that afternoon was an 80-year-old woman with a gastric ulcer. I remember that the biopsy accidentally flicked out of the forceps and landed on the floor before being put into the transport medium for culture. Nevertheless, Martin's registrar, Cliodna McNulty, was able to successfully isolate the organism three days later, which showed that the spiral bug was not merely an Australian phenomenon, but was present in ulcer patients in the UK as well. From there I travelled to Brussels, where Martin Skirrow allowed me to use some of his poster space for a hastily assembled poster on the new spiral bacterium. I was also able to present the data from our 100-patient study with the additional finding that the G + C content of the new bacterium was very similar to that present in campylobacters. The reaction was mixed.

As a result of our letters to *The Lancet* in 1983 and my presentation in Brussels in September that year, several groups around the world started work on the new spiral organism. Most notably, Martin Skirrow's group in Worcester continued to biopsy patients undergoing endoscopy, and were able to culture the bacteria from many patients. George Buck cultured it in Galveston, Texas and subsequently wrote several papers. Martin Blaser became interested, and with colleagues in Denver, produced the early serologic papers. Adrian Lee recruited a PhD student and subsequently Stuart Hazell took the organism to David Graham's laboratory in Texas.

In between my medical duties of 1983, I continued to revamp the computer and word processor in my garage. Finances were tight, so this computer ultimately only had 48K of RAM, but ran the main word processor available at that time, 'Wordstar', and saved documents to floppy disk. Because I did not have secretarial support, the word processor at least enabled me to send out letters to all and sundry asking about their experiences with gastritis and possibly with the spiral bacteria. As well, I started to write the description of our 100-patient study from 1982. Without proper organization of the data, it was rather difficult, because Robin and I were trying to mesh the histology, microbiology and clinical data from 100 patients. We partially achieved it with the statistical analysis we had available, but much of it had to be done manually. It took us several drafts of the paper before we finally agreed on the final format of the data. In addition, my enthusiasm caused some difficulty in my relationship with Robin. Typically, I would do a draft of the paper one weekend and deliver it to Robin sometime during the following week. Robin would then very carefully go through the manuscript at length, correcting and rewriting it. Meantime, by the following weekend, I would have created another totally different draft of the paper, and as he submitted to me his corrections, I would submit him the further draft, much to his dismay! Luckily, we were both helped by our spouses. We would sometimes get together for joint sessions with our wives to arbitrate. Adrienne would edit most of my version, cutting it down by at least 50%. Robin's wife, Win, was a psychiatrist and some of the thoughtful discussion in the paper was put down by her. Thus, much further analysis ensued and many drafts of the paper were passed back and forth before we were reasonably happy with its final format, towards the end of 1983. We probably never would have sent it off if our wives had not insisted it was complete and vetoed any further revisions. Finally, in about January 1984, we had a version of the paper that was suitable for submission to *The Lancet*.

By the end of 1983, my experiments with metronidazole combinations had led me to a paper by Satoh *et al.* describing how metronidazole prevented peptic ulceration in a rat model.[25] The surprising finding was that stress-induced ulcers in rats (usually produced by tying rats in strait jackets and dipping them in ice water) did not form when the rats were pretreated with metronidazole or were germ-free. Thus, that team had some suggestive data to support an infectious cause for peptic ulcer, or at least some role for bacteria. In their references they mentioned that *Pseudomonas* had been seen in peptic ulcers by Steer and colleagues, which led me to the paper by Steer and Colin-Jones. I was horrified to find that they had described the bacteria in association with gastric ulcer in a large number of patients.[26] Unfortunately for them, those investigators had decided that the organisms were *Pseudomonas*, an error that may have been because it was not possible to reliably culture *Campylobacter* in the 1970s, and *Pseudomonas* was a common contaminant of the biopsy channels in endoscopes. I showed this publication to Robin, who agreed that, even though we were almost ready to mail our paper, we should refer to Steer's paper as previous evidence for the presence of the bacteria. Thus, in a final re-write, we added it to our Discussion and References. John Armstrong commented that the electron microscopic appearance of the organisms in Steer's paper was enough to tell him that they were not *Pseudomonas*.

Koch's postulates, 1984

In January 1984, my 12-month appointment as gastroenterology registrar at Fremantle Hospital came to an end, but David McGechie was able to organize a similar trainee post in the Microbiology Department, which meant I would be able to work full time on the bacteria for another year while I continued to apply in vain for research funding. In 1984, there were several groups around the world obtaining results that paralleled those of our group in Perth. Because of our letters to *The Lancet*, our research had become at least partially respectable and in 1984, the abstracts we submitted to the Gastroenterological Society of Australia were accepted. Also in 1984, I began a collaboration with Stuart Goodwin at RPH in an attempt to infect pigs with the organism. We chose the pig because it also suffers from PUD and was large enough to easily take an endoscope. Our experiment merely consisted of biopsying and culturing gastric mucosa at baseline and at periods after inoculation with helicobacter isolates from humans.

In order to make the experiment parallel the human situation as far as possible, our piglets were allowed to eat RPH food, and they were always fasted for 12 hours after Thursday evening so that we could perform endoscopy on them on Friday morning. This experiment continued during the first few months of 1984 and was generally a failure, in that we could not isolate the bacteria from the pigs and no gastritis developed during the experiment. By that time also, I had treated several patients for their infections and was starting to treat patients who merely had gastritis, but no peptic ulcer, which increased the number of subjects available for our studies, and gave us quite a bit of experience with various antibiotic regimens, usually given in combination with bismuth. Thus, we were able to eradicate the infection with amoxicillin and bismuth, erythromycin and bismuth and, our favorite combination, metronidazole and bismuth. Typically, this treatment was given as a 14-day course, followed 2–4 weeks later by endoscopy and biopsy.

In April or May 1984, at a time when our pig experiments were failing, I presented Grand Rounds on the bacterium, and subsequently presented some of our findings to the local hospital scientific meeting. In particular, I showed data from a blinded histologic study where healing of gastritis occurred in conjunction with bismuth treatment. Perhaps because of my enthusiasm, I could not get the audience to look objectively at my data. One expert grudgingly admitted to seeing 'subtle' changes when as far as I was concerned, the changes were dramatic! Robin Warren could certainly back me up on this, and by then Ross Glancy at Fremantle Hospital was also convinced. Once again I realized that beliefs on gastritis were more akin to a religion than having any basis in scientific fact. I knew I would need to obtain more data to convince the skeptics.

As our pig experiments progressed, the pigs became larger and more aggressive, such that it was more and more difficult to catch the animals each Friday after they had been fasting for 12 hours, and it was quite difficult to keep them sedated during the procedure. One pig even had a cardiac arrest and required a resuscitation effort. In addition they were, at 40 kilograms, almost too large for the endoscope to reach the duodenum, so new equipment would have been required if the experiment continued. Stuart Goodwin had cultured all manner of campylobacters from the animals, but could not detect any colonization with the new organism.

At this time also, I had been rather frustrated by the Editors of *The Lancet*. Once again, they had procrastinated with our publication. They had been unable to find reviewers who could agree that our paper was important, general enough and interesting enough to be published. We suggested other reviewers, but it was not until May 1984 that the paper was accepted and eventually published in June. In spite of the opinions of the first reviewers, it was accompanied by a prominent editorial. What I think happened was that Cliodna McNulty in Martin Skirrow's laboratory repeated our study with similar findings and submitted a letter in April. With this letter being readied for publication in May 1984,[27] *The Lancet* was finally able to find a reviewer, Dr Mair Thomas, in London who advised them to accept our paper. In the same issue, a letter from Weiss Langenberg in Amsterdam marked an important milestone in the *H. pylori* story, the discovery of the bacterium's urease.[28] Apparently, Zanan had asked her to perform an API test on the new gastric bacteria, which had been isolated from one of Tytgat's patients, and in the panel of tests normally available on the API was a urease well. Langenberg presented her data and was told to re-check it, because it was not then known that *H. pylori* was urease positive. Of course, the organism continued to be positive on every test and its remarkable urease production was then noted by the investigators in their letter to *The Lancet*. The third letter accompanying our paper was the polyacrylamide gel electrophoresis of the new organism performed by Pearson in Southampton, who was able to show that it did not resemble the known campylobacters.

As already mentioned, I was becoming increasingly frustrated in my efforts to get appropriate peer review of the work. I had only six months to go in my current job with no idea whether I would finally get funding for the full-time double-blind trial I planned for 1985. On top of this, the animal work was becoming a nightmare. That year was the centenary of Koch's postulates. It seemed like a good enough omen. I discussed the idea of swallowing the bacteria with my colleagues David McGechie and Ian Hislop, who were both rather noncommittal about the experiment, so I did not press them further on it. I also decided not to publicize the idea either at the hospital by going through the Ethics Committee or at home. I didn't like my chances of getting either official approvals!

By then I had eradicated the organism in quite a few patients, and Peter Rogers and I were becoming confident that our antimicrobial susceptibility studies could predict treatment outcome. In early June, I arrived 30 minutes before the endoscopy clinic began and asked to be endoscoped by Ian Hislop. He complied and, rather diplomatically, did not ask why this was necessary. The biopsies showed that my gastric mucosa was normal without any signs of infection. That same day, we were able to culture *H. pylori* from a middle-aged man with heartburn, dyspepsia and associated mild gastric erythema. Histology showed active gastritis. Sensitivities were performed and the organism was found to be susceptible to metronidazole, so I treated that patient with a

2-week course of bismuth and metronidazole. One month later, the patient was re-endoscoped and found to be cured of the infection. By then we had subcultured a large amount of his spiral organism, and a solution of a heavily inoculated 4-day culture on blood agar was prepared for me by technician Neal Noakes. I premedicated myself with cimetidine 400 mg, and swallowed about 30 mL of the solution in peptone broth just before midday on 12 June 1984.

The week of the experiment was rather busy for me because we had developed a passive hemagglutination serologic test for *H. pylori* and were having some success with it, but had been beaten to publication by Eldridge and colleagues who described the use of a complement fixation test to detect antibody to spiral organisms in a letter to *The Lancet* on June 2.[29] Thus, during my self-administration experiment, I was testing large numbers of blood donors trying to estimate the prevalence of the infection in our population and also trying to determine the accuracy of the test in our patients, both of which involved a lot of preparation and the testing of hundreds of samples in the evenings and over the weekend.

On about the 7th day after ingestion of the bug broth, I woke up before dawn and vomited. The nausea and vomiting in the morning continued for 3 days and surprised me, in that the vomitus consisted mainly of clear secretion without any acid. On the 10th day, Ian Hislop performed another endoscopy on me and I remember that this was a very difficult day for me because I felt very tired and generally unwell, and had fasted from midnight the day before. However, we had such a busy endoscopy list that it was necessary for me to work all morning and not place myself on the list until all the cases were finished. In addition, it was usually normal for me to spend the lunch break performing Gram stains on the specimens of all the patients who had taken part in the endoscopy list, then returning to write up the reports for their antibiotic treatment if the Gram stains were positive. Thus, my morning work did not finish until approximately 2 pm and Ian Hislop was not available until the end of his clinic, approximately 4 pm. My second endoscopy was very uncomfortable and I remember I gagged excessively during the procedure. The Gram stain of the biopsy a few minutes later was positive and the organism was cultured during the next three days. The histology report from Ross Glancy was as follows: 'Sections show gastric mucosa of antral type. There is a moderate predominantly active inflammatory cellular exudate with polymorphs present within the superficial lining epithelium and glandular epithelium. A minor increase in chronic inflammatory cells is seen within the lamina propria. A moderate degree of mucin depletion is seen and there are inflammatory/reactive nuclear changes. Moderate numbers of spiral bacteria are seen in the H&E preparation' (FIGURE 6). As expected, the silver stain revealed masses of CLO

(FIGURE 7). On that day, pleased with the heavily infected biopsy results, I first told my wife about the experiment. With hindsight I probably chose a bad time. All mothers have those odd weeks when they cope rather less well than usual and Adrienne was having one of those. She had been in a motor car accident two weeks before and had a couple of cracked ribs and whiplash, so she was struggling a bit to keep up with a 2-year-old and three other children. When she found that my flu-like illness of the past few days was self inflicted, she was rather upset. She was quite convinced that the new bug was a very nasty pathogen and she wasn't interested in either herself or the kids becoming part of the experiment. I tried to reassure her, claiming that 99.9% of the scientific community believed it was a harmless commensal and that it was still possible that they were correct. I may have weakened that argument when I had to depart in mid sentence to go and throw up yet again. In the last few days of the illness, although never awake enough to save any liquid from my morning vomits, I did notice a very strange thing. There was no acid in the vomit. The liquid I produced was clear and completely bland. After putting up with me vomiting for a few more nights, moaning and groaning all night and having breath like a sewer, Adrienne finally demanded that I immediately commence antibiotics or be evicted from the household to sleep under a bridge. So it was

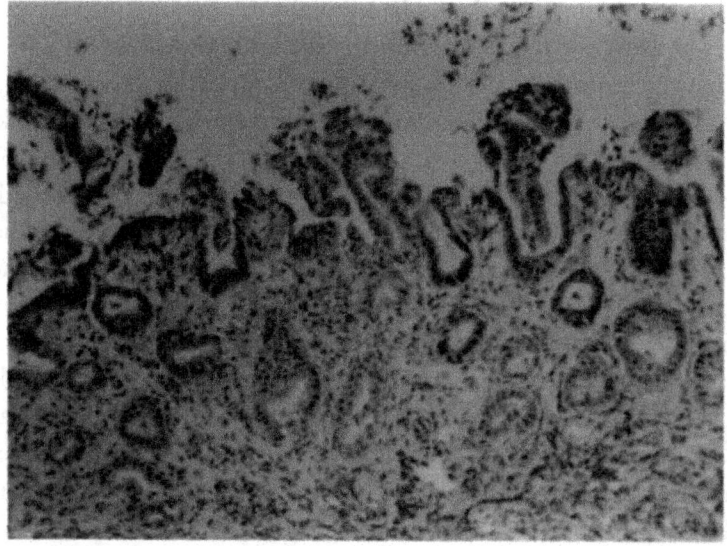

FIGURE 6 Section of the gastric biopsy taken on day 10 of the Koch's postulates experiment. The epithelial cells are abnormal, polymorphonuclear and mononuclear cells are present in the lamina propria, and edema is present (H&E, ×250).

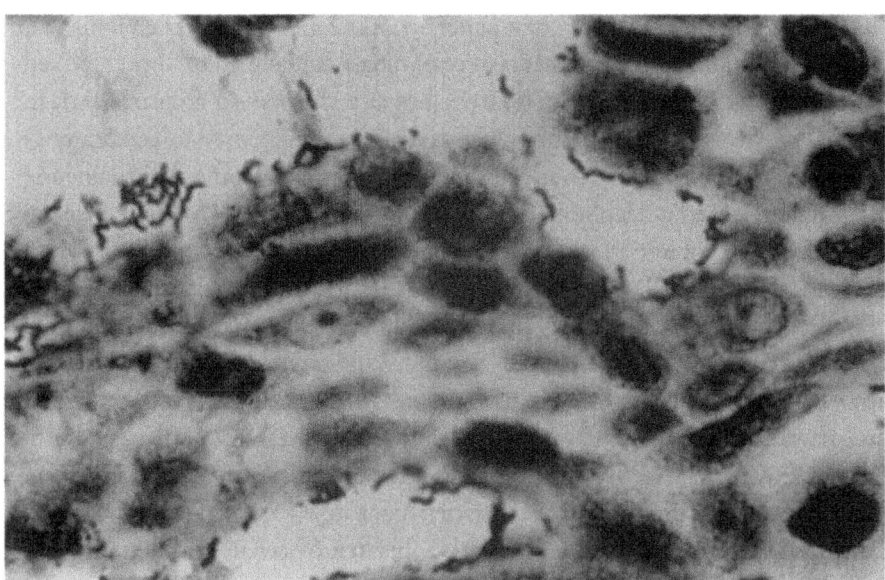

FIGURE 7 Silver stain of the author's biopsy taken on day 10 of the experiment. Epithelial cells have rounded up in shape without intracellular mucin, and have many closely adherent black *H. pylori* organisms.

that 14 days after taking the spiral bacterium, pockets readied with 3 g of tinidazole, I underwent further endoscopy. Numerous samples were taken in order to accurately document the histology, but, regrettably, the spiral bacterium had by then totally disappeared and most of the mucosal biopsies had returned to normal.

After writing up that experiment some months later and having it reviewed by my colleagues, the comment was made that I had left a lot out of the manuscript. Several other people had noted halitosis during the week of the experiment, but had not told me. At the same time I was browsing through a 1919 edition of Osler's *Principles and Practice of Medicine*, which had been given to me as a present by my father-in-law. In the chapter on gastritis I came upon a beautiful description of my illness, the well-known syndrome (in 1919) of 'gastritis with hypochlorhydria'. I re-read the paper of Ramsey *et al.* and realized that the acute illness I had experienced had already been described. I therefore rewrote a more complete version of the paper, which was subsequently published in the *Medical Journal of Australia* in 1985.[30]

Actually, the first publication of the Koch's postulates experiment was six months earlier, but in a less reputable journal, the 'Star' (a tabloid newspaper in the USA). A few weeks after our paper in *The Lancet* had been published, Robin and I had taken our wives out to celebrate. Adrienne and I always looked forward to nights out with Win Warren because she was so amusing and, in addition, as we were now ex-smokers, it was an opportunity to celebrate by stealing a few cigarettes from her. Anyway, after returning home slightly inebriated, Robin received a telephone call from a journalist in the USA who insisted on asking very probing questions about whether or not the spiral bug was a pathogen. The reply was 'yes', and Dr Marshall had proved it by drinking a brew of the bug, thus infecting himself. The article that followed prompted many ulcer sufferers in the United States to approach their GPs asking for Pepto-Bismol and antibiotics. Naturally, they usually received a cool reception and so were forced to write to us, typically addressed to 'Dr Warren, Perth Hospital, Australia'. Actually, the story was thoughtfully written and based on fact, and the experiment was also written up a few years later by Laurence Altman in his book 'Who Goes First', a history of self-experimentation in medicine (FIGURE 8).

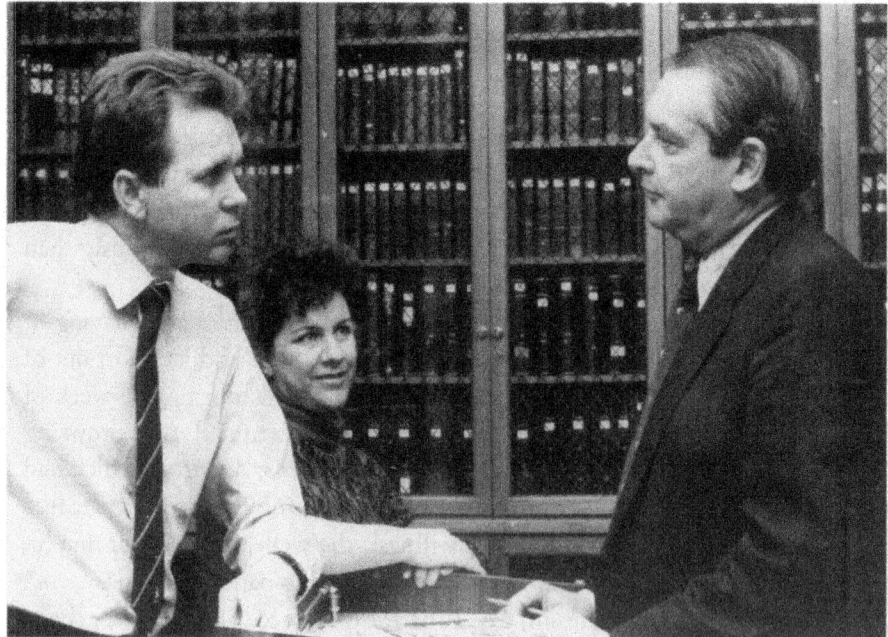

FIGURE 8 The author with wife Adrienne and Laurence Altman at the signing of Altman's book 'Who Goes First'. (Taken at the University of Virginia in 1987. The University of Virginia has a historical collection of Walter Reed's archives. In Reed's experiment, one of the assistants died from yellow fever.)

Conspiracy theories

Was there a conspiracy to keep the *H. pylori* story under wraps? In some ways yes, but this was fired more by inertia and bad advice than by malice. I give the example of the Smith Kline and French company. At the time (1984) SK&F was the most profitable drug company in the world, selling Tagamet, the first H2-receptor blocker (for ulcers). After presenting my data in April that year, I was approached by Peter Seville, their Australian research director, who proposed that I educate him about the bacteria so that he could have the head office review the whole concept, and perhaps fund some research. Regardless of the outcome, Peter offered to buy me an IBM-compatible PC and a database program to manage all my biopsy data.

After two days at Fremantle watching and learning, Peter wrote letters to his research directors and traveled to Philadelphia. Some of the ideas in those letters were very provocative, and likely threatening, to the Tagamet company. For example, the three key concepts proposed by Seville were (i) an antibiotic–Tagamet combination treatment, (ii) a serological test to see who might need the new therapy even before they developed ulcers, and (iii) a vaccine to prevent ulcers altogether. In his preamble, Seville stated 'This places me in an extraordinary position, in that I be asked [by Marshall] to fund a project that may well see the demise of cimetidine as an agent for the prevention of relapse of peptic ulceration, cimetidine being replaced by long-term antibiotics.' In response, perhaps after consulting with the company's gastroenterology advisors, memos were circulated to the effect that Seville should not be encouraged further on his weird crusade. Undeterred, Seville still paid for my computer, and was indirectly responsible for accurate data tables being presented in several of my subsequent papers.

Other H2-receptor blocker companies ignored the CLO, and effectively drowned out much of the related research by funding hundreds of acid reduction trials, which probably delayed the acceptance of *H. pylori* for a few years. Finally, around 1994, patents on the H2-receptor blocker, ranitidine, expired and after that no-one really had a personal stake in its success. In its place, the proton-pump inhibitor/antibiotic combinations were developed, which now dominate *H. pylori* therapy, as discussed in the final chapter of this book by Peter Unge.[31]

At the end of 1984 I found that our application for performing a prospective double-blind study of bacterial eradication in duodenal ulcer patients had been funded by the Australian government. The NHMRC was not totally convinced of the worth of the project, so it only funded the first year with a necessary review after the project had been going for 6–8 months. For the first time I would be funded to work full time on the organism. It also meant a bit of a pay rise because NHMRC researchers are better paid than registrars.

In late 1984 I was contacted by the Proctor & Gamble company in Cincinnati, which had been in touch with Martin Skirrow in the UK, and were preparing a trial there of Pepto-Bismol. This medication (bismuth sub-salicylate) had been acquired by P&G as part of their portfolio when they purchased the Norwich company. Pepto-Bismol was regarded as 'snake oil' by many, but it had recently shown promise in studies in which it prevented traveler's diarrhea. The possibility that bismuth compounds could be used to treat a bacterium that possibly caused peptic ulcer was naturally very interesting to P&G, so they wanted to talk with me and further develop the idea. Thus, as I mailed off the Koch's postulates experiment and the susceptibility data we had collected at Fremantle Hospital to the *Medical Journal of Australia*, I boarded a plane for a pre-Christmas visit to the USA. That was an interesting excursion, because I initially spent three days in San Francisco and visited Stanford University to present a seminar to the Gastroenterology Division at the Veteran's Affairs Hospital there, and subsequently traveled to Cincinnati where we commenced development of a patenting program, ultimately securing the idea of treating the new spiral bacterium with bismuth and antibiotic combinations. Towards the end of that trip, I traveled to Dallas where the epidemic of achlorhydria had occurred. By then 'Pete' Peterson had resurrected the biopsies and performed a study comparing the prevalence of the spiral bacterium in persons involved in the epidemic with a control group. Unfortunately, most of the control group also had the spiral bacterium! Thus, it could still have been a commensal, or almost everyone in Dallas in 1980 was already infected with the bug. I suspect that the control group were nurses or gastroenterologists and therefore were infected because of their workplace (see chapter by Peterson *et al.* for more detail[32]).

Before finalizing the protocol of our prospective double-blind study in 1984, I discussed it with Pete Peterson and also the clinical pharmacology group at SK&F research. Both these groups told me that the study was too complicated, and that the numbers were too small to be statistically significant. I continued with the planned protocol, however, because it was essential that at least one of our groups had eradication of the spiral organism. Thus, there were four treatment groups: bismuth alone; cimetidine alone; bismuth with antibiotic; and cimetidine with antibiotic. This should have allowed us to have a dose-ranging effect, whereby benefits were most marked when complete eradication of the bacterium occurred compared with suppression only or lesser degrees of eradication (i.e. H2-receptor blocker alone). As it turned out, our second metronidazole combination (Tagamet with metronidazole) was useless in so far that only one patient in that group had eradication of the organism. Unfortunately for us, metronidazole alone merely caused a change in the organism, which became totally resistant to that antibiotic and was not eradicated. Nevertheless, at the end of the study we did see some 'dose effect'. The relapse rate was highest in patients given cimetidine.

I was able to complete that study 15 months early and left Australia to take a position at the University of Virginia in August 1986, expecting to find a receptive audience in the USA. I was disappointed. It was to be another eight years before the bacteria was finally accepted there, following the consensus conference held by the National Institutes of Health in February 1994.

References

1   Chazin S. The doctor who wouldn't accept no. Readers Digest, 1993.
2   Warren JR. The discovery of *Helicobacter pylori* in Perth, Western Australia. In: Marshall BJ (ed.) Helicobacter *Pioneers: Firsthand Accounts from the Scientists who Discovered Helicobacters, 1892–1982*. Melbourne: Blackwell Science Asia, 2002; 151–64.
3   Whitehead R (ed.) *Gastrointestinal and Oesophageal Pathology*. Edinburgh: Churchill Livingstone, 1989.
4   Ito S. Anatomic structure of the gastric mucosa. In: Heidel US, Code CF (eds). *Handbook of Physiology*. Section 6: *Alimentary Canal*, Vol. 2: *Secretion*. Washington DC: American Physiological Society, 1967; 705–41.
5   Vial JD, Orrego H. Electron microscope observations on the fine structure of parietal cells. *J Biophys Biochem Cytol* 1960; **7**: 367–72.
6   Salomon H. Ueber das Sprillum des Saugetiermagens und sein Verhalten zu den Belegzellen. *Zentralbl Bakteriol* 1896; **19**: 433–42.
7   Bizzozero G. Ueber die Schlauchformigen Drusen des Magendarmakanals und die Bezienhungen ihres Epithels zu dem Oberflachenepithel der Schleimhaut. *Arch Mikr Anat* 1983; **42**: 82–152.
8   Palmer ED. Investigation of the gastric mucosa spirochetes of the human. *Gastroenterology* 1954; **27**: 218–20.
9   Freedberg AS, Baron LE. The presence of spirochetes in human gastric mucosa. *Am J Dig Dis* 1940; **7**: 443–5.
10 Doenges JL. Spirochetes in the gastric glands of *Macacus rhesus* and of man without related diseases. *Arch Pathol* 1939; **27**: 469–77.
11 Siurala M, Isokoski M, Varis K, Kekki M. Prevalence of gastritis in a rural population. *Scand J Gastroenterol* 1968; **3**: 211–23.
12 Warren JR. Gastric pathology associated with *Helicobacter pylori*. In: Marshall BJ (ed.) *Gastroenterology Clinics of North America*, Vol. 29. Philadelphia: WB Saunders, 2000; 705–51.
13 Kekki M, Villako K, Tamm A, Siurala M. Dynamics of antral and fundal gastritis in an Estonian rural population sample. *Scand J Gastroenterol* 1977; **12**: 321–4.
14 Magnus HA. Gastritis. In: Jones FA (ed.) *Modern Trends in Gastroenterology*. London: Butterworth, 1952; 323–51.
15 Marshall BJ, Royce H, Annear DI *et al.* Original isolation of *Campylobacter pyloridis* from human gastric mucosa. *Microbiol Lett* 1984; **25**: 83–8.
16 Buchanan RE, Gibbons NE (eds). *Bergey's Manual of Determinative Bacteriology*, 8th edn. Baltimore: Williams & Wilkins, 1974.

17 Lee A, Phillips M, O'Rourke J. We grew the first *Helicobacter* and didn't even know it! In: Marshall BJ (ed.) Helicobacter *Pioneers: Firsthand Accounts from the Scientists who Discovered Helicobacters, 1892–1982*. Melbourne: Blackwell Science Asia, 2002; 131–42.

18 Fung WP, Papadimitriou JM, Matz LR. Endoscopic, histological and ultrastructural correlations in chronic gastritis. *Am J Gastroenterol* 1979; **71**: 269–79.

19 Burman KD. 'Hanging from the masthead': reflections on authorship. *Ann Intern Med* 1982; **97**: 602–5.

20 Warren JR, Marshall B. Unidentified curved bacilli on gastric epithelium in active chronic gastritis. *Lancet* 1983; **1**: 1273–5.

21 Wiersinga SM, Tytgat GN. Clinical recovery owing to parietal cell failure in a patient with Zollinger–Ellison syndrome. *Gastroenterology* 1977; **73**: 1413–17.

22 Ramsey EJ, Carey KV, Peterson WL *et al.* Epidemic gastritis with hypochlorhydria. *Gastroenterology* 1979; **76**: 1449–57.

23 Martin DF, Hollanders D, May SJ, Ravenscroft MM, Tweedle DE, Miller JP. Difference in relapse rates of duodenal ulcer after healing with cimetidine or tripotassium dicitrato bismuthate. *Lancet* 1981; **1**: 7–10.

24 Gregory MA, Moshal MG, Spitaels JM. The effect of tri-potassium di-citrato bismuthate on the duodenal mucosa during ulceration: An ultrastructural study. *S Afr Med J* 1982; **62**: 52–5.

25 Satoh H, Guth PH, Grossman MI. Role of bacteria in gastric ulceration produced by indomethacin in the rat: cytoprotective action of antibiotics. *Gastroenterology* 1983; **84**: 483–9.

26 Steer HW, Colin-Jones DG. Mucosal changes in gastric ulceration and their response to carbenoxolone sodium. *Gut* 1975; **16**: 590–7.

27 McNulty CA, Watson DM. Spiral bacteria of the gastric antrum. *Lancet* 1984: **1**: 1068–9.

28 Langenberg W, Tytgat GN, Schipper ME, Rietra PJ, Zanen HJ. Campylobacter-like organisms in the stomach of patients and healthy individuals. *Lancet* 1984; **1**: 1348–9.

29 Eldridge J, Lessells AM, Jones DM. Antibody to spiral organisms on gastric mucosa. *Lancet* 1984; **1**: 1237.

30 Marshall BJ, Armstrong JA, McGechie DB, Glancy RJ. Attempt to fulfill Koch's postulates for pyloric Campylobacter. *Med J Aust* 1985; **142**: 436–9.

31 Unge P. *Helicobacter pylori* treatment in the past and in the 21st century. In: Marshall BJ (ed.) Helicobacter *Pioneers: Firsthand Accounts from the Scientists who Discovered Helicobacters, 1892–1982*. Melbourne: Blackwell Science Asia, 2002; 203–15.

32 Peterson WL, Harford W, Marshall BJ. The Dallas experience with acute *Helicobacter pylori* infection. In: Marshall BJ (ed.) Helicobacter *Pioneers: Firsthand Accounts from the Scientists who Discovered Helicobacters, 1892–1982*. Melbourne: Blackwell Science Asia, 2002; 143–50.

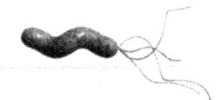

CHAPTER 16

Helicobacter pylori treatment in the past and in the 21st century

Peter Unge

Introduction

Today's knowledge about *Helicobacter pylori* infection was not easily achieved. There was a delay from the very first day the bacterium was cultured by Marshall and Warren until the association between *H. pylori* and peptic ulcer disease (PUD) was widely accepted, mainly because of a lack of therapies suitable for use in blind studies. In this review I would like to give a short summary of the history of PUD, its association with *H. pylori* and the development of today's recommended eradication regimens.

The early history of peptic ulcer disease

In 1586, Marcellus Donatus of Mantua made an autopsy-based description of a gastric ulcer and about 100 years later, in 1688, Johannes von Murault made a record of a duodenal ulcer. A further 100 years later, in 1799, Matthew Baillie published detailed descriptions of ulcers and their clinical histories. However, PUD is most likely not a disease of the post medieval period only; mummies from Egypt have been found with signs of peptic ulcer as the possible cause of death. Modern gastroenterology, though, was born on the morning of 6 June 1822, when Dr William Beaumont treated a severe wound of Alexis St Martin, whose stomach was left permanently exposed through his abdominal wall as a result. The experiments done by Beaumont in this human model of the stomach proved the presence of hydrochloric acid in the gastric juice, the relationship between emotional state and gastric secretion and digestion, and delineated the details of gastric motor activity. Ulcer of the stomach was a

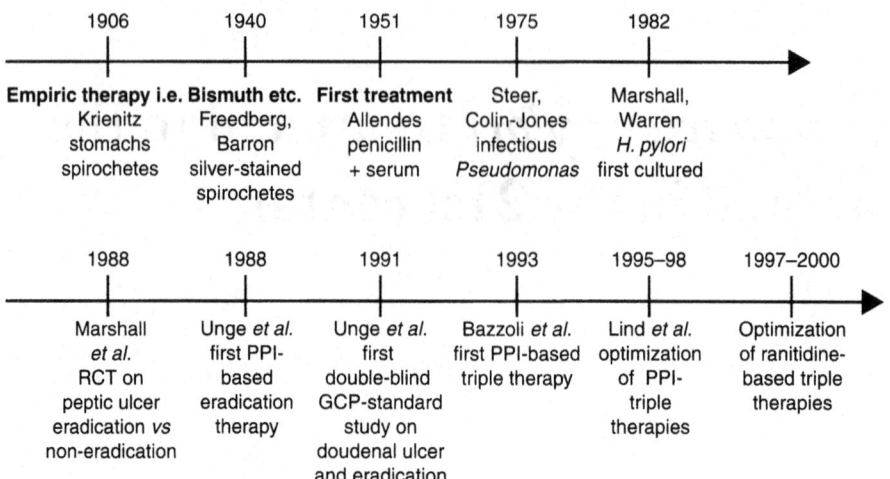

FIGURE I Time-line for the discovery of *Helicobacter pylori* as an ulcerogenic bacterium and the development of effective therapy for the cure of peptic ulcer disease.

common autopsy finding in the second half of the 19th century and its diagnosis based on clinical findings was described by Brinton.[1] For severe pain he recommended opium alone or in combination with bismuth, and cure of the ulcer could, according to Brinton, be achieved by proper diet. The dictum 'no acid–no ulcer' was published in 1910 by K. Schwartz, who assumed that it was an imbalance between gastric acid and gastric defence mechanisms that caused the development of ulcers.[2] Peptic ulcer disease was clearly caused by gastric juice corrosion and neutralization of gastric acid became a popular therapeutic option, as recommended by Bertram Sippy.[3]

The history of the gastric microflora

Spiral organisms had been observed in the stomachs of dogs by Giulio Bizzozero in 1893, and in 1906 Dr W. Krienitz found spirochetes in the stomachs of patients with gastric carcinoma[5] (FIGURE I). The Danish scientist Johannes Fibiger claimed he could induce gastric cancer in mice by feeding them with a nematode and was awarded the Nobel prize for his work.[6] Intermittent reports of spirochetes in the stomach appeared over the next 36 years and one of the most important publications was by James Doenges in 1938, who described 'spirochetes' in the stomach from victims undergoing routine autopsy.[7] Two years later, Stone Freedberg and Louis Barron observed spirochetes in stomachs resected from living patients (FIGURE 1) and the spirochetes were easily visualized by silver impregnation.[8]

A major step was taken by J. Allende in 1951 when he published a book on treatment of gastric ulcer with penicillin and convalescent serum,[9] but unfortunately, the spirochetes were not regarded as part of the gastric microflora until 1975, when Steer and Colin-Jones observed bacteria in gastric biopsy specimens with gastric ulcer (FIGURE 1), but not from normal stomachs.[10] They classified the bacteria as *Pseudomonas aeruginosa*, but stated that they were not contaminants. In the search for an infectious cause of chronic gastritis and PUD, Robin Warren and Barry Marshall observed a small, curved bacterium that could only be visualized with silver staining[11,12] (FIGURE 1). Today, it is unequivocal that gastric infection by *H. pylori* is the major etiological factor in chronic active (type B) gastritis and PUD, and that eradication of *H. pylori* reduces the relapse rate of peptic ulceration. Several studies have also shown an association between infection with *H. pylori* in early life and subsequent development of gastric carcinoma,[3] which has led to the International Agency for Research on Cancer of the World Health Organization classifying *H. pylori* as a Group I carcinogen.

The organism as a target for therapy

Helicobacter pylori infection is one of the most common in the world, but the organism is very tenacious and cannot be successfully treated with normal antimicrobial monotherapy. Animal models have so far not been reliable screening models for evaluating the efficacy of treatment regimens and trials in infected humans are still the gold standard. The bacterium has found a niche in the neutral environment of the gastric mucosa, but is also present in the gastric lumen in an acidic environment. There is significant inflammation in infected stomachs, histologically classified as chronic active gastritis, and the immune reaction causes an increased and easily detected level of IgG antibodies against *H. pylori*. The bacterium is fragile in the *in vitro* environment and sensitive to a large number of antibiotics, but when it comes to *in vivo* therapy *H. pylori* is not an easy target. Most antimicrobials are either not effective or only partly effective and the gold standard in the evaluation of therapeutic efficacy *in vivo* has been controversial. Differences exist in assessment methods and their sensitivity, specificity and predictive value. Authorities have changed the approved combination of tests necessary for regulatory purposes and recommendations on assessment of *H. pylori* and the designs of clinical trials have been published by the European *Helicobacter pylori* Study Group.[13]

Antimicrobial therapy of *Helicobacter pylori*

General aspects of antimicrobial therapy

Helicobacter pylori is sensitive to a number of antimicrobials *in vitro*, but only a few have a clinical effect[14–16] and the acidic gastric environment has been blamed for deficiencies in drug delivery. Oral formulations of antibiotics or antimicrobials with medium- or low-acid stability might be expected to be less effective, but a pronounced alteration in the secretion of gastric acid might open an opportunity for acid-labile drugs. Intravenous administration of antimicrobials is, at least theoretically, a suitable method to improve drug delivery to the bacterium, but has not been confirmed in large controlled trials.

Bismuth-containing compounds are usually only partially absorbed and have a local inhibitory effect on the organism. Intraluminal concentrations of antibiotics have been claimed to be a key factor and local therapy is effective,[17] but it may be that the local effect of antibiotics, such as amoxicillin, is not so important, as it has been found that amoxicillin in a formulation that stayed in the gastric lumen for more than 8 hours did not have a beneficial advantage over the immediate release formulation.[18] Frequent and irregular gastric emptying may affect local antibacterial potential.

Gastric secretion of the antimicrobial has been suggested as a favorable property facilitating the transportation of the drug to the target, *H. pylori*. Macrolides, such as clarithromycin and azithromycin, are concentrated in the gastric mucosa and secreted into the gastric lumen and they have a detectable effect on the organism. Amoxicillin is concentrated in the gastric mucosa, but without significant secretion into the gastric lumen. Development of resistance towards nitroimidazoles and/or macrolides varies in grade and frequency and the clinical impact has been poorly elucidated. No plasmid-transferred resistance has been reported for *H. pylori*.

Initial antibacterial therapies for *H. pylori* infection

Old Swedish recommendations for treatment of ulcer disease such as 'Rapp-Antes droppar' include a significant amount of bismuth in the specified mixture, and 'Pepto-Bismol' has been, and still is, a frequently used over-the-counter drug in the USA for symptom relief of dyspeptic symptoms. Skornetsky and Gavrilenko reported from Russia that metronidazole therapy had a modest ulcer healing effect and possibly a relapse-prevention property also.[19] There has been extensive use of bismuth in various formulations and salts for at least 150 years,[20] and recently lower relapse rates after treatment with bismuth compounds were reported by McNulty *et al.*[21] and Coghlan *et al.*[22] In 1986, Goodwin, Armstrong and Marshall treated one patient with bismuth plus amoxicillin, which eradicated the bacterium, and the gastritis returned to normal mucosa;[23] later reports confirmed the efficacy of the bismuth–amoxicillin combination.[24] Monotherapy with amoxicillin was studied by Yeung *et al.* and a 15% success rate was achieved.[25] Blind, randomized, controlled studies, designed according to Good Clinical Practice (GCP), of eradication of *H. pylori* and cure of PUD with a double-blind design were not reported before 1990.

Acid-inhibitory drugs for peptic ulcer disease

During the second half of the 20th century there was a strong focus on acid as the most important and possibly the only factor, other than NSAID and aspirin, in the development of PUD. Anticholinergic drugs with a moderate acid-inhibitory property were standard therapy in combination with antacids. The discovery of the H2-receptor and the development of an antagonist are milestones in the successful race to develop acid-inhibitory drugs. About 10 years later the proton pump was identified and the proton-pump inhibitor (PPI), omeprazole, was tested and approved in many countries. Uncomplicated ulcers, as well as refractory ulcer and NSAID- or aspirin-induced ulcers, could now be healed. However, the healing process did not last very long and the majority of ulcer patients had at least one relapse within six months. Maintenance therapy was invented, documented and recommended. It was possible to keep almost all patients in remission for a long time only by pronounced acid inhibition. In 1986, the focus of PUD research had reached an impasse.

The discovery of *H. pylori* and its role in PUD caused a major paradigm shift and the use of acid-inhibitory drugs was all but eliminated because almost all patients suffering from ulcer disease seemed to be cured. Barry Marshall, one of the most active 'inventors' of the bacterium, combined tinidazole and bismuth in the very first large randomized study, the results of which were published during Christmas 1988.[26] One year later, the very first report on omeprazole plus amoxicillin as eradication therapy was published.[27] Acid inhibition again became an essential part of the eradication strategies that were developed during the last decade of the 20th century.

Bismuth

One of the most quoted studies on bismuth in the treatment of peptic ulcer was published by Coghlan *et al.* in 1987.[22] Triple therapies including bismuth, tetracycline and nitroimidazole were shown in 1988 by Borody to eradicate

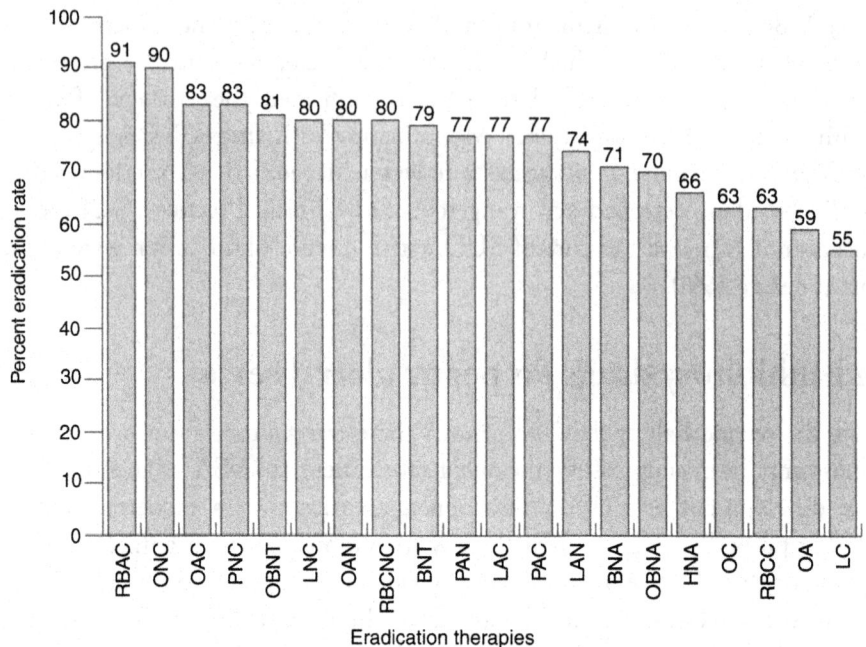

FIGURE 2 Eradication therapies ranked by efficacy based on all available studies. Eradication rates (%) are given above the bars.

RBAC, ranitidine bismuth/amoxicillin/clarithromycin; ONC, omeprazole/nitroimidazole/clarithromycin; OAC, omeprazole/amoxicillin/clarithromycin; PNC, pantoprazole/nitroimidazole/clarithromycin; OBNT, omeprazole/bismuthdicitrate or bismuthsubsalicylate/nitroimidazole/tetracycline; LNC, lansoprazole/nitroimidazole/clarithromycin; OAN, omeprazole/amoxiciellin/nitroimidazole; RBCNC, ranitidine bismuth/nitroimidazole/clarithromycin; BNT, bismuthdicitrate, subsalicylate or nitrate/nitroimidazole/tetracycline; PAN, pantoprazole/amoxicillin/nitroimidazole; LAC, lansoprazole/amoxiciIlin/clarithromycin; PAC, pantoprazole/amoxicilin/clarithromycin; LAN, lansoprazole/amoxicillin/nitroimidazole; BNA, bismuthdicitrate; subsalicylate or nitrate/nitroimidazole/amoxicillin; OBNA, omeprazole/bismuthdicitrate-bismuthsubsalicylate/nitroimidazole/amoxicillin; HNA, H2-antagonist/nitroimidazole/amoxicillin; OC, omeprazole/clarithromycin; RBCC, ranitidine bismuth/clarithromycin; OA, omeprazole/amoxicillin; LC, lansoprazole/clarithromycin.

the infection in nearly 90% of patients,[28] and in the Amsterdam study of the same year, published in *The Lancet*, authors were permitted for the first time to use the word 'cure' in the title of a paper on peptic ulcer. All this prompted the World Congress of Gastroenterology to recommend treatment of severe duodenal ulcers with eradication regimens.[29] Over the following years there were many reports on bismuth as part of triple or quadruple therapies and bismuth-based triple therapy was one of the recommended therapeutic options advised by Consensus Meetings until today.[30] The efficacy of the most common therapies is evaluated in a systematic review[31] and summarized in FIGURE 2.

Proton-pump inhibitor-based therapies

Helicobacter pylori cannot survive in an acidic environment without its urease activity, which creates and maintains a neutral pH status close to the bacterium. Consequently, acid was regarded as a negative factor for *H. pylori* and one of the important downregulators of the infection. Paradoxically, inhibition of gastric acid secretion was subsequently also found to be inhibitory, thus assisting in the eradication of the infection. On the other hand, most antibiotics were acid labile and their antibacterial activity was much lower in a more acidic environment.

Dual therapies

The hypothesis that acid is more harmful to the antibiotics than to the bacterium was studied in the first trial on the interaction between omeprazole and amoxicillin performed between April and June 1988 and published in 1989.[27] This double-blind, randomized study clearly showed that omeprazole alone and amoxicillin alone had a limited effect on the infection in contrast to the combination, which cured more than 60% of the infected patients. Four years later, the first double-blind study performed according to GCP was published.[32] The new dual therapy was used in a large number of trials and also recommended as the treatment of choice by the Swedish Consensus Meeting in 1993 and was one of the therapies of choice by the NIH Consensus Meeting in February 1994.[30] Clarithromycin, the most effective antibiotic as monotherapy, was later studied in combination with PPI such as omeprazole and lansoprazole (FIGURE 2). The overall efficacy was less than ideal (70–80%), but better than the amoxicillin/PPI combination (50–70%).

Triple therapies

Highly effective PPI-based triple therapies have been carefully studied since F. Bazzoli presented the first report at the 'Digestive Diseases Week' meeting in 1993 and published in 1994.[33] Data on a slightly less effective PPI-based triple therapy were published in 1993 by Bell *et al*,[34] but PPI-based triple therapies have been most aggressively documented since 1996, after the first double-blind pilot study, MACH 1, that compared the three available PPI-based triples.[35] Results from this large international multicentre study, involving almost 800 patients, demonstrated that it was possible to achieve *H. pylori* eradication rates of up to 96% and elicited the comment in *The Financial Times* that 'The race is on'.

The role of the acid-inhibitory compound as part of the triple therapy had to be defined. From the results of the MACH 2 study, it is clear that the addition of omeprazole is mandatory to achieve high success rates.[36] A significant reduction in the eradication rate was found in the omeprazole-free treatment groups (i.e. clarithromycin/amoxicillin: 26%; clarithromycin/metronidazole: 69%) as compared with the omeprazole-containing groups (omeprazole/clarithromycin/amoxicillin: 94%; omeprazole/clarithromycin/metronidazole: 87%).

PPI/amoxicillin/nitroimidazole

The triple combinations of omeprazole plus amoxicillin and metronidazole or tinidazole, the Bell therapy, and lansoprazole plus amoxicillin and metronidazole or tinidazole, have been frequently studied[31] (FIGURE 2) and are effective in about 80% (omeprazole) and 74% (lansoprazole) of cases; data on the pantoprazole/amoxicillin/nitroimidazole combination are probably comparable to the omeprazole combination. The lansoprazole dose is comparable to less than 40 mg omeprazole, which may explain the lower efficacy in the lansoprazole studies. Resistance to metronidazole seemed to be a weak, but negative predictive factor, and significant side-effects were in the range of 5–20%.

PPI/amoxicillin/clarithromycin

There are four important combinations that have been studied: omeprazole/amoxicillin/clarithromycin, named the Bordeaux regimen because it was first studied in France,[37] lansoprazole/amoxicillin/clarithromycin and pantoprazole or rabeprazole[38] with amoxicillin/clarithromycin. Omeprazole was the most frequently used PPI and the overall mean efficacy was 83%. Study quality was a major positive predictor probably because of the high drug compliance and the low number of patients lost to follow-up in the blind studies. Resistance to clarithromycin was a negative predictive factor for success. The lansoprazole combination was effective in 77% and study quality did not change the mean cure rate substantially. The pantoprazole and rabeprazole combinations were equally effective in the overall evaluation. Significant side-effects were in the range 5–20%. Data on efficacy (excluding the rabeprazole data) are shown in FIGURE 2.[31]

PPI/nitroimidazole/macrolide

Data from Bazzoli and coworkers in Italy in 1994 showed 100% efficacy in the very first study of the combination of omeprazole/nitroimidazole/clarithromycin.[33] The overall pooled result of that combination today is 90% efficacy and again there is a higher mean cure rate, 92–94%, in controlled studies.[31] Resistance to clarithromycin was a negative predictive factor for success. Metronidazole was the most commonly used nitroimidazole and twice daily dosing for seven days was preferred. Roxithromycin was less effective (65% cure rate) than clarithromycin when combined with omeprazole, and data on the use of azithromycin instead of clarithromycin indicates an efficacy of 76%.[31] The combination of lansoprazole/nitroimidazole/clarithromycin was effective in 80% and pantoprazole/nitroimidazole/clarithromycin in 83% of cases. Again, side-effects were in the range of 5–20% and the data on efficacy are shown in FIGURE 2.[31]

Mucosal protective agent-based triple therapies

Mucosal protective agents, such as sucralfate and sofalcone, have an inhibitory effect on *H. pylori*, clearing, but not eradicating the bacteria, with a mean over-all cure rate of 72%. Sofalcone in combination with ranitidine and clar-ithromycin has been less effective and the overall success rate was 36%.[31]

H2-antagonist/nitroimidazole/amoxicillin combination

The most commonly used H2-antagonist has been ranitidine, but there are a few studies on cimetidine and a few on famotidine and roxatidine triple thera-pies. Overall success rates have been 65%, but in the original first study by E. Hentschel the efficacy was 88%.[39] Variations in study design and size have not significantly affected the result; treatment for less than 10 days was slightly inferior in result compared with longer treatment periods. Side-effects were in the range of 10–20%.

Quadruple therapies

PPI/bismuth-based combinations

The PPI/bismuth-based quadruple therapies have been reported to be very effec-tive, but pooled data show only 81% efficacy for the omeprazole/bismuthdicitrate or bismuthsubsalicylate/nitroimidazole/tetracycline combinations and 70% efficacy for the omeprazole/bismuthdicitrate or bismuthsubsalicylate/nitroimida-zole/amoxicillin combinations.[31] These combinations might be more likely to overcome metronidazole resistance and are recommended as the second-line therapy in the Maastricht 2, 2000 Consensus report.[40]

Bismuth–ranitidine/plus two antimicrobials

Bismuth–ranitidine is a salt and in this review I have regarded it as two drugs. The earlier efficacy and safety data on the bismuth–ranitidine/clarithromycin combination came from studies that were designed to show the ulcer preventive effect of the eradication regimen, not primarily assess the eradication rate (FIGURE 2). The use of ITT-analysis may be too conservative, but any other approach could also be criticized.[31] A large number of patients were not followed up and consequently were regarded as treatment failures. Eradication rates when bismuth–ranitidine is combined with clarithromycin plus amoxicillin or with clarithromycin plus nitroimidazole are 91% and 80%, respectively (FIGURE 2).[31]

Development of resistance

Resistance is usually defined as 'reduced sensitivity of the bacterium to a given concentration of the antimicrobial', but whether this definition allows resistance data to predict the clinical outcome is controversial. *Helicobacter pylori* develops resistance to nitroimidazoles, macrolides and tetracycline. Metronidazole resistance is probably of less importance when using PPI-based triple regimens, but bismuth-based triple therapies appear more vulnerable. Clarithromycin resistance is regarded as more likely to predict treatment failure, although recent data show a minor clinical impact of *in vitro* resistance to clarithromycin,[41] but the data are far too limited to draw any conclusions. A cut-off level for potential amoxicillin resistance has yet to be defined.

In China, considerable experience has been reported with furazolidone-based PPI triple regimens, which appear to be an alternative in patients who are penicillin allergic or who have failed previous therapy, and are well described by Xiao *et al.* in their chapter.[42]

Current research on new therapeutic options

Combination therapy is efficacious, but extended use of antimicrobials is probably increasing the risk for resistance development and also the risk for severe adverse events. New chemical entities are under development, as are vaccines, but until today there have not been any reports of successful vaccines or effective monotherapies. Probiotics (competitive harmless bacterial flora such as lactobacilli in yoghurt) are attractive alternatives, reflecting the long-held impression that various dietary factors can affect a person's propensity to develop ulcers.[43] Nevertheless, this concept requires much basic and clinical research before it can take on the dominant role of the triple therapies.

Summary of antimicrobial therapies

The ideal therapy for *H. pylori* eradication is still lacking, but of those available, the PPI- and ranitidine/bismuth-based triple therapies seem effective and tolerable enough to be used in the clinical setting.

Conclusions

The effort in finding *Helicobacter pylori* and reporting it to a very reluctant scientific society has been one of the big steps in medical history and maybe even more importantly so in the lives of patients with PUD. This disease will be eradicated through the use of effective therapy, but the memory of the explorers will remain.

References

1 Brinton W. *On the Pathology, Symptoms and Treatment of Ulcer of the Stomach* (Facsimile of the Original 1857 edition). Oxford: Oxford Historical Books, 1990.

2 Schwartz K. Ueber penetrierende Magen und Jejunalgeschwure. *Beitr Klin Chir* 1910; **67**: 96–128.

3 Sippy BW. Gastric and duodenal ulcer: medical cure by efficient removal of gastric juice. *JAMA* 1915; **64**: 30.

4 Bizzozero G. Ueber die Schlauchformigen Drusen des Magendarmkanals und die Bezienhungen ihres Epithels zu dem Oberflachenepithel der Schleimhaut. *Arch Mikr Anat* 1893; **42**: 82–152.

5 Krienitz W. Ueber das Auftreten von Spirochaeten verschiedener Form im Mageninhalt bei Carcinoma Ventriculi. *Dtsch Med Wochenschr* 1906; **28**: 872.

6 Fibiger J. Investigations on Spiroptea Carcinoma and the Experimental Induction of Cancer. Nobel Lecture, December 12, 1927.

7 Doenges JL. Spirochaetes in the gastric glands of *Macacus rhesus* and humans without definite history of related disease. *Arch Pathol* 1939; **27**: 469–77.

8 Freedberg AS, Barron LE. The presence of spirochaetes in human gastric mucosa. *Am J Dig Dis* 1940; **7**: 443–5.

9 Allende JAS. *La ulcera de estemago y su tratamiento por la asosiacion de suero de convaleciente y penicilina.* Gutenberg: Hijo de Ramirez-Guadelajar, 1951.

10 Steer HW, Colin-Jones DG. Mucosal changes in gastric ulceration and their response to carbenoxolone sodium. *Gut* 1975; **16**: 590–7.

11 Warren JR. Unidentified curved bacilli on the gastric epithelium in active chronic gastritis. *Lancet* 1983; **1**: 1273.

12 Marshall B. Unidentified curved bacilli on the gastric epithelium in active chronic gastritis. *Lancet* 1983; **1**: 1273–5.

13 Working Party of the European Helicobacter pylori Study Group. Guidelines for clinical trials in *Helicobacter pylori* infection. *Gut* Suppl. 1997; **2**.

14 Loo VG, Sherman P, Matlow AG. *Helicobacter pylori* infection in a pediatric population: in vitro susceptibilities to omeprazole and eight antimicrobial agents. *Antimicrob Agents Chemother* 1992; **36**: 1133–5.

15 Millar MR, Pike J. Bactericidal activity of antimicrobial agents against slowly growing *Helicobacter pylori*. *Antimicrob Agents Chemother* 1992; **36**: 185–7.

16 Rubinstein G, Dunkin K, Howard AJ. The susceptibility of *Helicobacter pylori* to 12 antimicrobial agents, omeprazole and bismuth salts. *J Antimicrob Chemother* 1994; **34**: 409–13.

17 Kimura K, Kenichi I, Saifuko K *et al.* One-hour topical therapy for the eradication of *H. pylori*. *Am J Gastroenterol* 1994; **90**: 205–14.

[18] Unge P, Gad A, Back S *et al.* Local treatment for *H. pylori* eradication in duodenal ulcer patients comparing modified and immediate release amoxicillin tablets. *Gastroenterology* 1994; **106**: AI269.

[19] Skornetsky BD, Gavrilenko Ya V. The ulcerative disease of the duodenum treatment by metronidazole. *Military Med J* 1977; **8**: 37–40.

[20] Collins R, Coghlan JG, O'Morain C. *Helicobacter pylori* and ulcer treatment. In: Rathbone BJ, Heatley RV (eds). Helicobacter pylori *and Gastroduodenal Disease.* Oxford: Blackwell Scientific Publications, 1992; 244–58.

[21] McNulty CAM, Gearty JC, Crump B *et al. Campylobacter pyloridis* and associated gastritis: investigator blind, placebo controlled trial of bismuth salicylate and erythromycin ethylsuccinate. *BMJ* 1986; **293**: 645–9.

[22] Coghlan JG, Gilligan D, Humphries H *et al. Campylobacter pylori* and recurrence of duodenal ulcers: a 12-month follow-up study. *Lancet* 1987; **ii**: 1109–11.

[23] Goodwin CS, Armstrong JA, Marshall BJ. *Campylobacter pyloridis,* gastritis and peptic ulceration. *J Clin Pathol* 1986; **39**: 353–65.

[24] Unge P, Gad A, Gnarpe H, Nilsson B. Bismuth compound, Cavedess, in combination with amoxycillin in patients with *Campylobacter pylori* infection. *Deutsch Klin Wochenschr* 1989; **67**(Suppl. XVIII): PI75.

[25] Yeung CK, Fu KH, Yuen KY *et al. Helicobacter pylori* and associated duodenal ulcer. *Arch Dis Child* 1990; **65**: 1212–16.

[26] Marshall BJ, Goodwin CS, Warren JR *et al.* Prospective randomized trial of duodenal ulcer relapse after eradication of *Campylobacter pylori. Lancet* 1988; **ii**: 1437–42.

[27] Unge P, Gad A, Gnarpe H, Ohlsson J. Does omeprazole improve antimicrobial therapy directed towards gastric *Campylobacter pylori* in patients with antral gastritis? A pilot study. *Scand J Gastroenterol* 1989; **24**(Suppl. 167): 49–54.

[28] Borody T, Cole P, Noonan S *et al.* Long-term *Campylobacter pylori* recurrence post-eradication. *Gastroenterology* 1988; **94**: A43.

[29] Rauws EAJ, Tytgat GNJ. Cure of duodenal ulcer associated with eradication of *Helicobacter pylori. Lancet* 1990; **335**: 1233–5.

[30] NIH Consensus Conference. *Helicobacter pylori* in peptic ulcer disease: NIH Consensus Development Panel on *Helicobacter pylori* in Peptic Ulcer Disease. *JAMA* 1994; **272**: 65–9.

[31] Unge P. Antibiotic treatment of *Helicobacter pylori* infection. In *Current Topics in Microbiology and Immunology: Gastroduodenal Disease and Helicobacter pylori: Pathophysiology, Diagnosis, and Treatment.* Heidelberg: Springer Verlag, 1999; 261–300.

[32] Unge P, Gad A, Eriksson K *et al.* Amoxicillin added to omeprazole prevents relapse in the treatment of duodenal ulcer patients. *Eur J Gastroenterol Hepatol* 1993; **5**: 325–31.

[33] Bazzoli F, Zagari RM, Fossi S *et al.* Short-term low dose triple therapy for the eradication of *Helicobacter pylori. Eur J Gastroenterol Hepatol* 1994; **6**: 773–7.

[34] Bell GD, Powell KU, Burridge SM *et al. Helicobacter pylori* eradication: efficacy and side-effect profile of a combination of omeprazole, amoxicillin and metronidazole compared with four alternative regimens. *Q J Med* 1993; **86**: 743–50.

[35] Lind T, Veldhuyzen van Zanten S, Unge P *et al.* Eradication of *Helicobacter pylori* using one-week triple therapies combining omeprazole with two antimicrobials: The MACH I Study. *Helicobacter* 1996; **1**: 138–44.

[36] Lind T, Megraud F, Unge P *et al.* The MACH 2 Study: Role of omeprazole in eradication of *Helicobacter pylori* with 1-week triple therapies. *Gastroenterology* 1999; **116**: 248–53.

[37] Lamouliatte H, Dorval ED, Picon L *et al.* Fourteen days triple therapy using lansoprazole amoxicillin and tinidazole achieves a high eradication rate in *H. pylori* positive patients. *Acta Gastroenterol Belg* 1993; **56**(Suppl.): 139.

[38] Nguyen HN. Proton pump inhibitors in comparison. *Dtsch Med Wochenschr* 2000; **125**(Suppl. 12): S20–1.

[39] Hentschel E, Brandstatter G, Dragosics B *et al*. Effect of ranitidine and amoxicillin plus metronidazole on the eradication of *Helicobacter pylori* and the recurrence of duodenal ulcer. *N Engl J Med* 1993; **328**: 308–12.

[40] Malfertheiner P. Current concepts in the management of *Helicobacter pylori* infection: The Maastricht Consensus Report 2, 2000. *Aliment Pharmacol Ther* 2001 (in press).

[41] Megraud F, Lehn N, Lind T *et al*. Antimicrobial susceptibility testing of *Helicobacter pylori* in a large multicenter trial: the MACH 2 Study. *Antimicrob Agents Chemother* 1999; **43**: 2747–52.

[42] Xiao S-D, Shi Y, Liu W-Z. How we discovered in China in 1972 that antibiotics cure peptic ulcer In: Marshall BJ (ed.) Helicobacter *Pioneers: Firsthand Accounts from the Scientists who Discovered Helicobacters, 1892–1982*. Melbourne: Blackwell Science Asia, 2002; 99–104

[43] Sakamoto I, Igarashi M, Kimura K, Takagi A, Miwa T, Koga Y. Suppressive effect of *Lactobacillus gasseri* OLL 2716 (LG21) on *Helicobacter pylori* infection in humans. *J Antimicrob Chemother* 2001; **47**: 709–10.

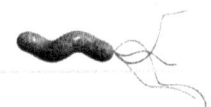

Index

217